# Vegetarian Nutrition in Health Improvement

Guest Editors

**Luciana Baroni**
**Gianluca Rizzo**

MDPI

Basel • Beijing • Wuhan • Barcelona • Belgrade • Novi Sad • Cluj • Manchester

*Guest Editors*
Luciana Baroni
Scientific Committee
Scientific Society for
Vegetarian Nutrition
Venice
Italy

Gianluca Rizzo
Independent Researcher
Messina
Italy

*Editorial Office*
MDPI AG
Grosspeteranlage 5
4052 Basel, Switzerland

This is a reprint of the Special Issue, published open access by the journal *Nutrients* (ISSN 2072-6643), freely accessible at: https://www.mdpi.com/journal/nutrients/special_issues/691PV8Y018.

For citation purposes, cite each article independently as indicated on the article page online and as indicated below:

| Lastname, A.A.; Lastname, B.B. Article Title. *Journal Name* **Year**, *Volume Number*, Page Range. |
|---|

**ISBN 978-3-7258-6292-4 (Hbk)**
**ISBN 978-3-7258-6293-1 (PDF)**
**https://doi.org/10.3390/books978-3-7258-6293-1**

# Contents

# About the Editors

**Luciana Baroni**

Luciana Baroni is a medical doctor, specialist in Neurology, Geriatrics, Gerontology, with an International Master's Degree in Nutrition and Dietetics. She is the President of the Scientific Society of Vegetarian Nutrition (SSNV), a non-profit organization, which she founded in 2000. In her clinical practice, she is engaged in the diagnosis and treatment of neurodegenerative diseases, and has been the author and editor of numerous articles and publications on health, nutrition, and lifestyle. In addition to this, she has delivered numerous lectures and courses on vegetarian nutrition, as well as having been a guest on various radio and television programs. In 2015, she conceived and published the VegPlate method, an updated food guide for vegetarian nutrition. She currently serves as the co-author and coordinator of the Master's Degree in Vegetarian Nutrition and Dietetics at the Polytechnic University of Marche, Italy.

**Gianluca Rizzo**

Gianluca Rizzo is a freelance nutritionist and independent researcher. He holds a Bachelor of Science in Biology, a PhD in Biotechnology, a 2nd Level Master's Degree in Food Supplements, and a Master's in Advanced Study in Nutraceuticals from the University of Messina. During his PhD and postdoctoral studies for the Telethon Foundation, he deepened research into the role played by oxidative stress related to iron metabolism in neurodegenerative diseases. As an author, reviewer, Section Board Member, as well as a Topic, Guest and Associate Editor for peer-reviewed journals, he is an expert in the field of human nutrition and is currently employed by the University of Messina (Italy). In addition to this, he has been an invited speaker and scientific manager for current medical education courses. His research interests primarily focus on the vegetarian diet, vegan diet, plant-based diet, soy, soy foods, phytoestrogens, isoflavones, vitamin B12, cobalamins, homocysteine, B vitamins, polyunsaturated fatty acids, vitamin D, dietary supplements, oxidative stress, and antioxidants.

# Preface

This Reprint, Vegetarian Nutrition in Health Improvement, brings together current scientific contributions exploring how lacto-ovo vegetarian and vegan dietary patterns influence human health across a lifespan. Its scope includes mechanistic, clinical, and public health perspectives, offering a multidisciplinary overview that connects metabolic pathways with epidemiological evidence and translational outcomes. The aim is to clarify the physiological effects, nutritional adequacy, and potential of plant-based diets in preventing and managing chronic diseases such as cardiovascular disorders, diabetes, obesity, and age-related decline.

The motivation for assembling this Reprint stems from the increasing global interest in plant-based eating as a strategy not only for individual well-being but also for sustainability and equity within food systems. Despite the popularity of vegetarian diets, misconceptions and knowledge gaps persist, particularly regarding micronutrient balance, protein quality, and long-term health effects. The Editors therefore sought to provide a rigorous scientific resource that integrates diverse research findings into a coherent narrative.

This Reprint is aimed at clinicians, nutritionists, researchers, educators, and policymakers who require evidence-based guidance on vegetarian nutrition. It also serves readers interested in the evolving interface between diet, health promotion, and environmental responsibility, fostering a shared understanding of how plant-based nutrition can contribute to a healthier and more sustainable future.

**Luciana Baroni and Gianluca Rizzo**
*Guest Editors*

nutrients

MDPI

*Editorial*

# Vegetarian Nutrition in Health Improvement

**Gianluca Rizzo [1,*] and Luciana Baroni [2,*]**

1 Independent Researcher, 98121 Messina, Italy
2 Scientific Society for Vegetarian Nutrition—SSNV, 30171 Venice, Italy
* Correspondence: drgianlucarizzo@gmail.com (G.R.); luciana.baroni@scienzavegetariana.it (L.B.)

There is a growing interest in vegetarian diets among the world population, and this has implications for public health. The current literature offers numerous sources for understanding the possible beneficial effects of plant-based foods on human health [1–4]. However, the wide variability of vegetarian diets, from the vegan diet that excludes any food of animal origin to the lacto-ovo-vegetarian one that includes dairy products and eggs, suggests the need to further expand knowledge on the subject. The Special Issue entitled "Vegetarian Nutrition in Health Improvement" aimed to collect experimental studies and literature reviews that could enrich the current state of the art on vegetarian nutrition and its effectiveness in improving health, to stimulate more effective policies for health and environmental sustainability, as well as prevention of chronic–degenerative diseases.

We know that the consumption of red meat, in particular processed meat, is associated with negative effects on health. For this reason, Niedermaier and colleagues conducted a 30-year simulation study on the impact of reducing or eliminating red meat and processed red meat on colorectal cancer (CRC) risk in Germany (Contribution 1). Currently, the mean consumption of red meat and processed meat among German men is 329 g and 427 g per week, respectively. Women have a lower consumption than men, with an age-standardized mean amount of 203 g and 224 g per week for red meat and processed meat, respectively. Reducing the mean consumption of both red meat and processed meat by 75 g or 150 g per week could reduce the burden of CRC by 1.1% and 6.5%, respectively. However, eliminating red meat and processed meat could reduce the incidence of CRC by 2.9% and 9.6%, respectively. This effect seems to be more pronounced among men compared to women.

The transition to a vegetarian diet also involves replacing animal-based foods with plant-based alternatives. For example, soymilk can be consumed as a substitute for cow's milk. However, a lack of knowledge about the benefits of plant-based options, as well as concerns regarding taste, may pose obstacles to this transition. To identify potential predictors of soymilk consumption among the American population, Storz and colleagues conducted a cross-sectional study on participants from two different datasets of the National Health and Nutrition Examination Surveys (NHANES) (2015–2016 and 2017–2020, respectively) (Contribution 2). The total NHANES 2015–2016 sample for analysis comprised 5264 participants with a full dataset, of which 132 reported soymilk consumption. This may be extrapolated to represent 4,427,078 U.S. Americans. The NHANES 2017–2020 pre-pandemic cycle included 8511 participants with a full dataset, of which 187 reported soymilk consumption. This may be extrapolated to represent 3,460,784 U.S. Americans. In the multivariate logistic regression analysis, the authors found a direct association between soymilk consumption and moderate physical activity (OR: 2.36, 95% CI: 1.40–3.99, $p$: 0.003), as well as a high level of education (OR: 1.84, 95% CI: 1.01–3.33, $p$: 0.045). However, no association was observed between sex and soymilk consumption. Since individuals who consumed soy milk made up only 1.5 to 2% of the population sample, identifying strategies to promote soymilk consumption as a healthy choice for both personal health and the environment is essential.

Plant foods are not only a source of nutrients, but they also provide raw materials for the biotechnological extraction of health-beneficial molecules. This is the case of *Rhaponticum carthamoides* (Willd.) Iljin, a perennial plant belonging to the Asteraceae family, endemic to Eastern Europe, whose root extract (RCE) has been studied for its alleged benefits on lipid metabolism. In a comparative analysis conducted by Todorova and colleagues, RCE was tested in vitro on human preadipocytes (Contribution 3). The authors observed an anti-adipogenic and lipolytic effect by measuring the lipid accumulation and concentrations of free fatty acids and glycerol in the culture medium, respectively. The effect was due to both RCE and some secondary metabolites derived from it, whose presence was confirmed through the development and validation of a method based on high-performance thin-layer chromatography (HPTLC).

Although a plant-based diet has shown several health benefits, especially for chronic conditions, it must be well-planned. Among the at-risk nutrients often discussed, adequate protein intake is one of the most debated aspects. Plant proteins may have a reduced biological value compared to proteins of animal origin due to the presence of limiting amino acids and also due to the presence of fiber, protease inhibitors, and other plant matrix molecules, which reduce digestibility. To investigate this aspect, Bartholomae and Johnston conducted an intervention study on 17 minimally active vegan men who received a 5-day eucaloric diet containing 0.8 g/kg/d protein (Contribution 4). Protein sufficiency was assessed by nitrogen balance with 24 h urine collection on the fifth day of intervention. The authors observed a significant absolute and relative negative nitrogen balance (−1.38 g/d, 95% CI: −2.00 to −0.75, $p < 0.001$ and −18.60 mg/kg/d, 95% CI: −27.32 to −9.88, $p < 0.001$, respectively) that did not correlate with age, free-fat mass, or years being vegan. The results of this study confirm that a vegetarian diet, and in particular a vegan one, should ensure a higher protein intake than the U.S. recommended dietary allowance (RDA) for protein of 0.80 g/kg/d for adults, as also stated by experts and organizations in the field of vegetarian nutrition.

A vegetarian diet may be useful not only for the prevention and support of metabolic diseases but also for the management of disorders common in developed countries. Although the link between gastroesophageal reflux disease (GERD) and dietary choices remains unclear and understudied, some evidence suggests that nutrition may play a role in managing the disease both in the short and long term. Rizzo and colleagues explored this relationship through a cross-sectional study on 1077 adult participants of the INVITA study (Investigation on Italians' Habits and Health) through a survey based on an online questionnaire (Contribution 5). In total, 37.3% of participants followed a vegan diet, with a prevalence of women, while the prevalence of GERD in the reference sample was 9%. As expected, the quality of life was statistically lower in individuals with GERD, based on the SF-36 questionnaire. Furthermore, the logistic multivariate analysis, adjusted for confounders such as BMI and smoking habits, showed that adopting a vegan diet compared to other animal-based dietary patterns significantly reduced the risk of GERD (OR: 0.47, 95% CI: 0.28–0.81, $p$: 0.006). This evidence suggests that a vegetarian diet can help improve the quality of life and manage disorders associated with GERD through simple lifestyle interventions.

Another aspect that affects the quality of life and long-term prognosis is frailty in senescence. This is relevant considering the increase in the aging population and the resulting health burden. Qi and colleagues conducted a prospective study including 2883 participants aged 65 years and above from the Chinese Longitudinal Healthy Longevity Survey (CLHLS) from 2008 to 2018 to explore the association between diet and frailty (through the frailty index) (Contribution 6). The authors assessed the participants' eating habits through a food frequency questionnaire, defining the score for the overall plant-based diet index (PDI), healthful plant-based diet index (hPDI), and unhealthful plant-based diet index (uPDI). Using the Cox proportional hazard model corrected for covariates, a lower frailty risk was associated with adherence to a plant-based diet (HR: 0.86, 95% CI: 0.77–0.95, $p < 0.01$) and a healthful plant-based diet (HR: 0.83, 95% CI: 0.75–0.93, $p < 0.001$), when the highest tertile score was compared with the lowest. In contrast, adherence to an unhealthful plant-based diet was associated with a higher risk of frailty (HR: 1.21, 98% CI: 1.08–1.36, $p < 0.01$). While at baseline, only individuals without predisposition to frailty were included, at the end of the follow-up 1987 individuals suffered from pre-frailty or frailty, and the association between the frailty index and the plant-based diet indices was linear, with a more marked effect among men than women in the subgroup analysis (in women, statistical significance persisted only in the association with uPDI). This underlines how important it could be to plan a well-balanced vegetarian diet.

In a cross-sectional web-based survey with 2180 adult participants, Stenico and coworkers investigated the eating habits of an Italian sample living in Italy and abroad, following a vegan diet for at least one year (Contribution 7). Based on the results of structured and semi-structured questionnaires on food frequency, sociodemographics, and difficulties in daily management and relationships with health professionals, the participants were predominantly women and were motivated by ethical principles in their food choices. While ethical and environmental motivations were associated with the level of education, the duration of adherence to the diet was negatively associated with the environmental motivations and positively associated with the ethical ones. The length of time following the vegan diet was also positively associated with the consumption of plant-based cheeses and vegetable burgers and negatively associated with the consumption of cereals, legumes, and soy foods. Additionally, there was a strong awareness of the need for vitamin B12 supplements and a focus on following food guides for health. However, a skeptical approach from the medical community and health professionals emerged, raising concerns about the limited support for those who choose this dietary pattern.

Although the prevalence of plant-based foods in the diet has been reported to be associated with metabolic benefits, such as reduced cardiovascular risk, which food groups and macronutrients are specifically related to these benefits remains to be explored in depth. Jakše and colleagues conducted a secondary analysis from a Slovenian cross-sectional study (Whole-Food Plant-Based Diet Lifestyle Program) involving 151 individuals who had followed a well-structured plant-based diet for a long period (4.1 ± 2.5 years, on average) and maintained an active lifestyle (5541 ± 4677 total METs) (Contribution 8). From the multivariate analysis adjusted for confounders, the authors highlighted associations between foods such as fruits and whole grains and improved cholesterol levels, including total cholesterol (TC), high-density lipoprotein cholesterol (HDL-C), and low-density lipoprotein cholesterol (LDL-C). At the same time, an association between HDL-C levels and the consumption of legumes, nuts, and seeds was found. The study also pointed out associations between cholesterol levels and fiber, carbohydrates, and different types of fatty acids, even if the effects were weak ($0.16 < r < 0.32$). Moreover, some unexpected findings emerged, such as the negative association between HDL-C levels and higher consumption of legumes or nuts and seeds, as well as the lack of a significant association between food groups and blood pressure and the absence of a beneficial relationship between fiber intake and LDL-C levels. However, it must be noted that the study population had a homogeneous concentration of cardiovascular markers, which were within the normal range.

A narrative review and a systematic review were also included in this thematic collection.

Hernández-Lougedo and colleagues conducted a systematic review of the literature on the relationship between athletic performance and vegetarian nutrition (Contribution 9). After applying inclusion criteria, they selected six studies: three cross-sectional studies and three clinical trials. Two studies did not differentiate between types of vegetarian diets, one study focused on lacto-ovo-vegetarians, and the other three specifically involved participants following a vegan diet. Only one of the clinical trials was randomized and included a blinded omnivorous or vegetarian dietary intervention. Although overall differences in performance and health between diets were not evident, specific differences did emerge. The best performers in endurance activities (races under 21 km and half marathons) were individuals following a vegetarian diet, except for marathon or ultra-marathon events, where omnivores performed better. Omnivores showed better adaptation to environmental conditions, with significant differences observed between omnivorous and vegetarian women. Muscle mass in vegetarians was significantly lower than in omnivores. However, in cycle ergometer endurance tests, vegetarians showed a performance advantage over omnivores. No significant differences were observed regarding strength parameters. Given the still fragmentary nature of the data, further studies are needed to fully understand the influence of diet on physical performance, particularly in relation to specific parameters and sports disciplines.

A vegetarian diet has often been proposed as a beneficial dietary approach for chronic kidney disease (CKD), due to the greater tolerance of plant proteins compared to animal proteins and better compliance compared to the canonical low-protein diets commonly used in these cases. Narasaki and colleagues conducted a narrative review of the literature to investigate the available information on the potential influence of vegetarian nutrition on CKD (Contribution 10). A vegetarian diet has shown benefits for various conditions that exacerbate CKD, such as hypertension and diabetes. Additionally, it can be beneficial for reducing oxidative stress, inflammation, metabolic acidosis, and the accumulation of uremic toxins. Many of the benefits of plant-based foods come from the presence of phytochemicals and fiber. The adoption of a vegetarian diet in CKD patients has been debated due to the high phosphorus and potassium content in plant foods, which could worsen the renal burden associated with mineral metabolism disorders. However, the literature data suggest that phosphorus in plant foods is much less absorbable and bioavailable than that found in animal products. Phosphorus in vegetables is complexed with macromolecules that reduce the risk of hyperphosphatemia, as demonstrated in comparative studies with similar intake levels between plant and animal foods. Similarly, the risk of hyperkalemia does not seem relevant enough to justify the avoidance of plant foods, except for some processed items such as fruit juices, dried fruits, and sauces. The relationship between diet and end-stage kidney disease remains to be clarified.

Overall, plant-based diets appear to have positive implications for health, if appropriate adjustments are made compared with guidelines for the general population. Health professionals can play a crucial role in managing vegetarian diets, avoiding misinformation, and promoting sustainability for individuals, society, and the environment. Consumers' knowledge about plant-based foods needs to be enhanced.

**Author Contributions:** Writing—original draft preparation, G.R.; writing—review and editing, L.B. All authors have read and agreed to the published version of the manuscript.

**Funding:** This research received no external funding.

**Conflicts of Interest:** The authors declare no conflicts of interest.

**List of Contributions:**

1. Niedermaier, T.; Gredner, T.; Hoffmeister, M.; Mons, U.; Brenner, H. Impact of Reducing Intake of Red and Processed Meat on Colorectal Cancer Incidence in Germany 2020 to 2050—A Simulation Study. *Nutrients* **2023**, *15*, 1020. https://doi.org/10.3390/nu15041020.
2. Storz, M.A.; Brommer, M.; Lombardo, M.; Rizzo, G. Soy Milk Consumption in the United States of America: An NHANES Data Report. *Nutrients* **2023**, *15*, 2532. https://doi.org/10.3390/nu15112532.
3. Todorova, V.; Savova, M.S.; Ivanova, S.; Ivanov, K.; Georgiev, M.I. Anti-Adipogenic Activity of Rhaponticum Carthamoides and Its Secondary Metabolites. *Nutrients* **2023**, *15*, 3061. https://doi.org/10.3390/nu15133061.
4. Bartholomae, E.; Johnston, C.S. Nitrogen Balance at the Recommended Dietary Allowance for Protein in Minimally Active Male Vegans. *Nutrients* **2023**, *15*, 3159. https://doi.org/10.3390/nu15143159.
5. Rizzo, G.; Baroni, L.; Bonetto, C.; Visaggi, P.; Orazzini, M.; Solinas, I.; Guidi, G.; Pugliese, J.; Scaramuzza, G.; Ovidi, F.; et al. The Role of a Plant-Only (Vegan) Diet in Gastroesophageal Reflux Disease: Online Survey of the Italian General Population. *Nutrients* **2023**, *15*, 4725. https://doi.org/10.3390/nu15224725.

6. Qi, R.; Yang, Y.; Sheng, B.; Li, H.; Zhang, X. Plant-Based Diet Indices and Their Association with Frailty in Older Adults: A CLHLS-Based Cohort Study. *Nutrients* **2023**, *15*, 5120. https://doi.org/10.3390/nu15245120.
7. Stenico, A.; Zarantonello, D.; Vittadello, F.; Kob, M. A Comprehensive Examination of Vegan Lifestyle in Italy. *Nutrients* **2024**, *16*, 86. https://doi.org/10.3390/nu16010086.
8. Jakše, B.; Godnov, U.; Fras, Z.; Fidler Mis, N. Associations of Dietary Intake with Cardiovascular Risk in Long-Term "Plant-Based Eaters": A Secondary Analysis of a Cross-Sectional Study. *Nutrients* **2024**, *16*, 796. https://doi.org/10.3390/nu16060796.
9. Hernández-Lougedo, J.; Maté-Muñoz, J.L.; García-Fernández, P.; Úbeda-D'Ocasar, E.; Hervás-Pérez, J.P.; Pedauyé-Rueda, B. The Relationship between Vegetarian Diet and Sports Performance: A Systematic Review. *Nutrients* **2023**, *15*, 4703. https://doi.org/10.3390/nu15214703.
10. Narasaki, Y.; Kalantar-Zadeh, K.; Rhee, C.M.; Brunori, G.; Zarantonello, D. Vegetarian Nutrition in Chronic Kidney Disease. *Nutrients* **2024**, *16*, 66. https://doi.org/10.3390/nu16010066.


## References


1. Dinu, M.; Abbate, R.; Gensini, G.F.; Casini, A.; Sofi, F. Vegetarian, Vegan Diets and Multiple Health Outcomes: A Systematic Review with Meta-Analysis of Observational Studies. *Crit. Rev. Food Sci. Nutr.* **2017**, *57*, 3640–3649. [CrossRef] [PubMed]
2. Oussalah, A.; Levy, J.; Berthezène, C.; Alpers, D.H.; Guéant, J.-L. Health Outcomes Associated with Vegetarian Diets: An Umbrella Review of Systematic Reviews and Meta-Analyses. *Clin. Nutr.* **2020**, *39*, 3283–3307. [CrossRef] [PubMed]
3. Storz, M.A. What Makes a Plant-Based Diet? A Review of Current Concepts and Proposal for a Standardized Plant-Based Dietary Intervention Checklist. *Eur. J. Clin. Nutr.* **2022**, *76*, 789–800. [CrossRef] [PubMed]
4. Selinger, E.; Neuenschwander, M.; Koller, A.; Gojda, J.; Kühn, T.; Schwingshackl, L.; Barbaresko, J.; Schlesinger, S. Evidence of a Vegan Diet for Health Benefits and Risks—An Umbrella Review of Meta-Analyses of Observational and Clinical Studies. *Crit. Rev. Food Sci. Nutr.* **2023**, *63*, 9926–9936. [CrossRef] [PubMed]

nutrients MDPI

*Systematic Review*

# The Relationship between Vegetarian Diet and Sports Performance: A Systematic Review

**Juan Hernández-Lougedo [1], José Luis Maté-Muñoz [2,*], Pablo García-Fernández [2], Edurne Úbeda-D'Ocasar [1], Juan Pablo Hervás-Pérez [1] and Blanca Pedauyé-Rueda [1]**

[1] Faculty of Health Sciences, Camilo José Cela University, 28692 Madrid, Spain; jlougedo@ucjc.edu (J.H.-L.); eubeda@ucjc.edu (E.Ú.-D.); jphervas@ucjc.edu (J.P.H.-P.); blanca.pedauye@ucjc.edu (B.P.-R.)
[2] Department of Radiology, Rehabilitation and Physiotherapy, Complutense University of Madrid, 28040 Madrid, Spain; pablga25@ucm.es
* Correspondence: jmate03@ucm.es

**Abstract:** Introduction: In recent years, the vegetarian diet has increased in popularity among athletes. The aim of this review is to ascertain the differences in variables related to performance, nutritional intake, and health in athletes according to whether they are omnivores or vegetarians. Methodology: A literature search was carried out in different databases: PubMed, Web of Science, Dialnet, and Cochrane. The keywords used were "vegetarian diet", "vegan diet", "exercise", "sport", and "performance". After applying different inclusion criteria, six studies were included in the review. Results: No significant differences were obtained in variables related to physical performance (adherence exercise, Vo2Máx, muscle power, and sprint test) or health (body composition, psychological well-being, and social relationships), but dietary intake was significantly higher in carbohydrates and lower in proteins in vegetarian athletes ($p < 0.05$). Conclusions: It cannot be affirmed that vegetarian subjects have a higher sports performance, for which more research should be carried out.

**Keywords:** vegetarian diet; vegan diet; performance; sport and exercise

## 1. Introduction

The population's diet has changed over the years, which has led to an increase in the consumption of plant-based foods in Western countries [1–4].

A vegetarian is defined as a person who does not consume any type of meat, including poultry, seafood, fish, or products containing them. However, within vegetarianism, there are different groups, some less restrictive than others. From less restrictive to more restrictive, we find the ovolactovegetarians who do include dairy products and eggs in their diet, the lactovegetarians who only include milk, and the vegans who do not include any type of food of animal origin [5–7] (Table 1).

The reason why people choose to consume such foods varies greatly depending on their age:

- Adolescents for reasons of animal or environmental concern.
- Adults who wish to improve their health.

Historically, this type of food is related to health, culture, and religious factors [8,9]. The origin of this diet is found in ethical–religious and medical movements, since it was used as a ritual of health and purity of the body. For example, in China, a large part of the population continues to maintain a vegetarian diet and it is also in traditional Russian medicine, in India meat is not consumed because it is considered an act of violence, and in the Buddhist religion, meat consumption was not introduced until the end of the Second World War [10].

**Table 1.** Types of diets.

| | 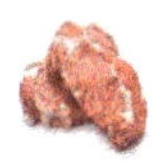 | 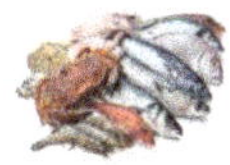 |  | 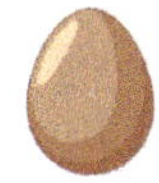 | 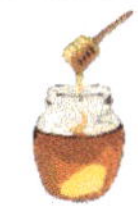 | 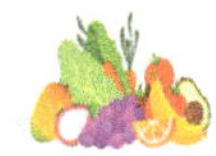 |
|---|---|---|---|---|---|---|
| | | | **Non-vegetarian** | | | |
| **Omnivorous** | + | + | + | + | + | + |
| | | | **Vegetarian-based** | | | |
| **Ovo-lacto-vegatarian** | − | − | + | + | + | + |
| **Ovo-vegetarian** | − | − | − | + | + | + |
| **Lacto-vegetarian** | − | − | + | − | + | + |
| **Vegan** | − | − | − | − | − | + |

However, in Europe, vegetarianism began in the Renaissance, and from that moment, began to expand. It was in 1847 when a group of vegetarians met and formed the first vegetarian society in Europe, which was named "Vegetarian Society" [10].

The benefits of this diet, as evidenced by the American Dietetic Association, are an improvement in health and in the prevention and treatment of pathologies. It has been shown that the chances of developing cardiovascular pathologies are lower, while some cancers have shown improvements in the biochemical parameters of the organism. It should be noted that vegetarians are not only characterized by their eating style, but also by generally engaging in more physical activity and consuming less harmful products [11].

However, this diet not only has the benefits outlined above, but it also has some negative aspects. The main disadvantage is the possibility of suffering from nutritional deficiencies, especially in vitamin B12, zinc, iron, calcium, omega-3 fatty acids, and protein [7,11].

To ascertain the effects that this diet may have on sports performance, we need to compare the nutritional contributions of the foods that make up the vegetarian diet with that of the omnivorous diet.

According to The Academy of Nutrition and Dietetics, a well-planned vegetarian diet can meet the macronutrient and energy needs of an athlete [12,13]. Vegetarian diets can vary widely in terms of calorie content and fiber, just like omnivorous diets. It is important for vegetarian athletes to focus on a balanced and nutrient-rich diet that supports their performance and overall health. As for the carbohydrate requirements of sportsmen and sportswomen, mainly in endurance sports, athletes need to replenish their glycogen stores, as the success of their sports performance will depend on this. This is why carbohydrate intake recommendations are between 3 and 12 g/kg/day depending on the volume, intensity, and type of exercise effort [11]. Vegetarian diets do not meet the daily protein recommendation, but it should be kept in mind that, in the case of athletes, the requirements are higher, and these depend on the sports: 1–1.6 g/kg in endurance sports and 1.4–2 g/kg for strength athletes [11,14]. It has been shown that people who follow a vegetarian diet can cover their protein requirements of high biological value if they consume eggs and dairy products, as well as legumes and nuts. With respect to fats, the requirement for athletes is like that of non-athletes (20–35% of total daily calories), and these should be healthy fats [11].

When planning a diet for an athlete, the total energy requirement must be taken into account, along with the basal metabolism, the energy expenditure generated by the physical exercise performed, and the thermogenic effect of food, which represents between 3% and 10% of the total energy expenditure [15]. Some of the methods used to calculate it are the equations, such as Harris–Benedict or Mifflin–St-Jeor, using electronic devices such as watches or cell phones, or direct and indirect calorimetry.

Hydration is a key factor in successful performance, as it optimizes thermoregulation during exercise [16]. Correct fluid levels should be monitored before, during, and after exercise. Ideally, fluid loss should not exceed 2%, as higher values decrease cognitive function and performance. Athletes can lose between 0.3 and 2.4 liters of body fluid per hour of exercise through sweat, depending on variables, such as environment, gender, body size, and exercise duration [15].

We must also take into account the intake of micronutrients, which, according to several studies, is deficient when a vegetarian diet is followed [17]. The main mineral that research should be focused on is iron. The type of iron suitable for vegetarians is non-heme iron, and the amount that is absorbed will depend on whether it is consumed with enhancers (vitamin C and citric acid) or inhibitors. Iron is important in an athlete's performance as it is involved in the delivery of oxygen to the muscle. According to Fuhrman and Ferreri (2010), it is not necessary to take supplements if an adequate amount of food containing this mineral is consumed, except in cases of anemia, low ferritin, or menorrhagia. Something similar happens with zinc, which is consumed in foods that contain a large amount of this micronutrient, although such foods also inhibit its absorption. Supplementation is recommended due to its importance in the functioning of the immune system function [18]. These studies have linked vegetarian diets with vitamin B12 deficiency, which is associated with cardiovascular pathologies [18]. These same authors mention the importance of an adequate supply of vitamin D in athletes, since it is directly related to the musculoskeletal system, and the best sources of vitamin D are sun exposure and/or the consumption of fortified foods.

Injured athletes should control caloric intake to lose as little muscle mass as possible during the period when there is the least amount of movement. During this period, athletes should increase protein intake by 1.2–1.5 g/kg to aid healing tissue formation while reducing muscle loss [15].

In terms of performance in strength and endurance sports, it can be stated that the vegetarian diet provides the necessary nutrients for good performance, provided that the diet is well planned. In strength sports, protein intake is especially relevant, although with the intake of plant proteins, such as legumes, seeds, nuts, and whole grains, the recommendations can be met [5]. In addition, there are now a large number of foods enriched with micro-nutrients, which can help vegetarian or vegan athletes reach the recommended intakes.

Some of the athletes, both strength and endurance, who eat a vegetarian or vegan diet are Derek Tresize and Carla Lewis, bodybuilder and velocity athlete [19], respectively, as well as in intermittent sports, such as soccer or tennis, as we find in the cases of Saul Ñiguez and Novak Djokovic.

This review aims to assess the effects of vegetarian and omnivorous diets on various aspects of athletic performance, health-related parameters, and nutritional intake.

## 2. Materials and Methods

### 2.1. Acquisition of Evidence

For this systematic review, we followed the protocol according to the standards and guidelines of the PRISMA statement for systematic reviews and meta-analyses, which aims to improve the reporting of future systematic reviews [20].

### *2.2. Eligibility Criteria*

We included articles that met the following inclusion criteria: (a) publications in the last ten years (from 2013 to 2023); (b) written in English or Spanish; (c) clinical trials and randomized controlled clinical trials using a placebo or control group; (d) relationship between diet and sports performance; (e) women of working age (intervention group performing a physiotherapeutic intervention; (f) cytokine analysis. Exclusion criteria were (i) animals were used for research. (ii) clinical trials without results or not completed. (iii) literature reviews.

### *2.3. Sources of Information*

The literature search was conducted between September 2022 and September 2023. The aim of the search was to find out whether athletic performance changed as a function of the diet the athlete would take. The databases used were Web Of Science (WOS), PubMed, Cochrane, and Dialnet.

### *2.4. Search Strategies*

The keywords we used for the document search were "vegetarian diet", "vegan diet", "performance", "sport", and "exercise". The search strategy was ("vegetarian diet" OR "vegan diet") AND (performance OR sport OR exercise). At the end of the search, we had 263 articles that met the search criteria, after reading the abstracts, methods, and objectives, exclusion criteria were applied:

- Articles with a publication date prior to 2013.
- Articles that were written in a language other than English or Spanish.
- Articles in which animals were used for research.
- Articles that were literature reviews.
- Articles that did not link diet to sports performance.

### *2.5. Data Extraction Process*

An exhaustive reading and evaluation of the six studies finally selected were carried out, to which the PEDro scale was applied to assess their methodological quality, evaluating the design of the study, the source of obtaining the subjects, whether the study was randomized, whether there was concealment, whether there was blinding, and what the outcome of the study was like. The PEDro scale of the synthesis results can be found in more detail in Section 3.5.

In addition, the PRISMA 2020 checklist [20] was used to collect the most relevant data for each of the studies, author and year, type of study, sample characteristics, objectives, type of intervention, intervention time, diet, ergogenic aids, program, healthy variables, and performance variables. Figure 1 shows the process followed in selecting the articles used for the literature review according to PRISMA declaration. The results of the data extraction will be presented in Supplementary Materials.

### *2.6. Risk of Bias Assessment of Individual Studies*

Risk of bias is a tool developed by the Cochrane Collaboration to assess the methodology of scientific evidence. It is useful in systematic reviews for the individual analysis of included CTs and RCTs. In this sense, the present systematic review has followed the Cochrane Handbook 5.1.0 [21] to assess the risk of bias.

The Cochrane Handbook 5.1.0 presents six levels of bias: selection bias, conduct bias, detection bias, attrition bias, reporting bias, and other bias. Each level has one or more specific items in a Risk of Bias table, and each item includes a description of what happened in the study and an assessment where the assignment of "low risk", "high risk", or "unclear risk" of bias is included [21].

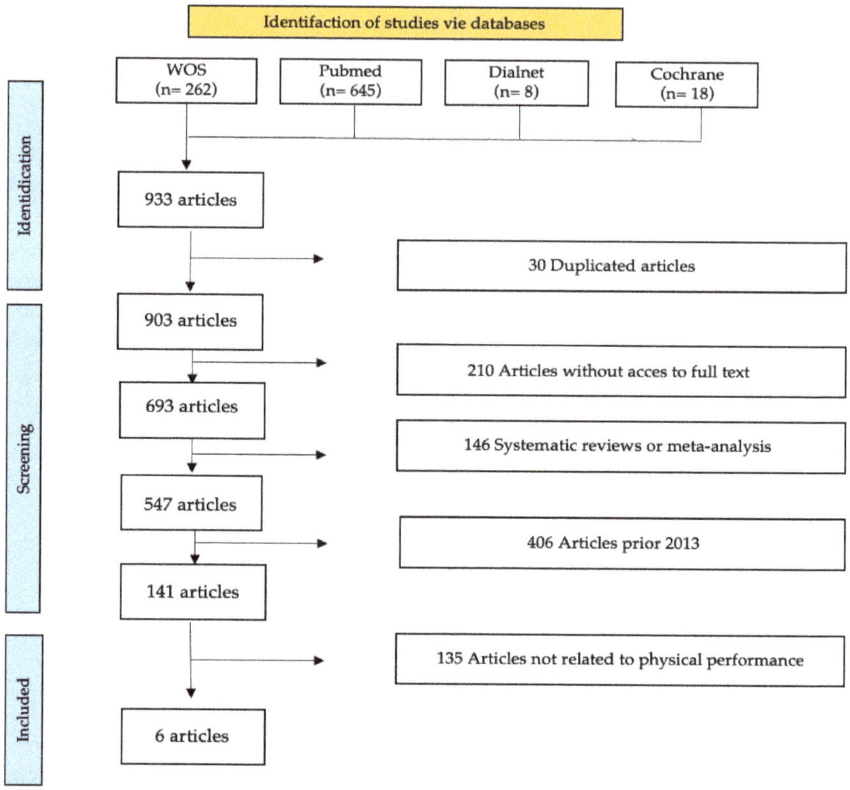


**Figure 1.** Flow diagram according to the PRISMA declaration.

*2.7. Synthesis Methods*

The synthesis methods used in the present review are the eligibility criteria that were determined in Section 2.2 of Material and Methods and the analysis of methodological quality using the PEDro scale, which is based on the Delphi checklist developed by Verhagen [22]. The checklist has a total of 11 items. The first item refers to external validity and is not considered for the final score, items 2–9 refer to internal validity, and items 10 and 11 indicate whether the statistical information provided by the authors allows for an adequate interpretation of the results.

Therefore, the maximum score is 10 points, and the minimum is 0. Only items that are answered affirmatively are scored. Studies with a score of 9–10 were of excellent methodological quality, 6–8 were of good quality, and 5 were of fair or acceptable quality. The PEDro scale can be found in more detail in Section 3.5.

Further to the synthesis measures, we assessed whether the studies included in the analysis met their objectives set at the start of the study.

*2.8. List of Variables*

Table 2 details the study variables found in the articles found for this systematic review.

Table 2. List of variables of the results.

| | |
|---|---|
| Physical health | Quality of life questionnaire (WHOQOL-BREF).<br>Psychological well-being and social relationships.<br>% of subjects performing one endurance modality or the other according to sex and diet. |
| Body composition | Body mass.<br>Lean mass.<br>Fat mass. |
| Performance | Relative, absolute, and maximum oxygen consumption.<br>Maximum number of extensions and push-ups.<br>Maximum performance.<br>Muscular strength.<br>Respiratory Coefficient.<br>Macronutrient oxidation.<br>International Physical Activity Questionnaire.<br>Fatigue index.<br>Average and peak power. |
| Energy, macronutrient, and micronutrient intake | Basal metabolic rate (BMR).<br>Dietary profile.<br>Dietary intake.<br>Energy, macronutrients, and Fe intake. |

## 3. Results

### 3.1. Selection of Studies

During the initial phase of the search, 933 studies were identified from different databases. After eliminating duplicates, 903 studies remained.

To refine the selection, we applied date filters (2013–2023) and chose to select only clinical trials and randomized clinical trials, which were available in English or Spanish, leaving us with 141 articles. After reviewing the titles and abstracts, 135 studies that did not fit the study topic were discarded. After a detailed reading, a total of six studies that met the inclusion criteria were selected and subjected to a qualitative analysis, using database filters for date and type of study. Mendeley was used to search for duplicates.

### 3.2. Characteristics of the Studies

Of the total articles included in this review, 33.33% were published in 2016 [23,24], 16.67% in 2018 [25], 16.67% in 2020 [26], and 33.33% in 2021 [27,28]. A total of 3363 individuals participated, with 1921 females, of whom 543 were vegetarians, 652 vegans, and 726 omnivores; and 1442 males, with 305 vegetarians, 352 vegans, and 785 omnivores.

The articles were cross-sectional studies, trial-control studies, or randomized clinical trials. Of the six studies included in this systematic review, five present a group of athletes eating a vegetarian or vegan diet and a control group composed of athletes eating an omnivorous diet. A single observational study compares subjects according to diet and sport modality, 10 km, half marathon, and marathon. More detailed information can be found in the descriptive table of each of the studies in Table 3.

**Table 3.** Table of results for each study.

| Ref. | Subjects | Program | Variables | Performance/Health |
|---|---|---|---|---|
| [25] | 281 subjects<br>123 omnivorous diet<br>158 vegetarian diet<br>Control group: 10 km<br>2 diet groups:<br>Omnivores and vegetarians * or vegans<br>3 distance groups:<br>10 km<br>Half marathon<br>Marathon/Ultra marathon | WHOQOL-BREF<br>Quality of Life Study | Physical health | Physical health:<br>84.6% omnivorous women<br>85.4 vegetarian women<br>87.4 male omnivores<br>87% male vegetarians<br>10 km fem: 84.3%<br>10 km men: 87.4%<br>$\frac{1}{2}$ Marathon fem: 87.8%<br>$\frac{1}{2}$ Marathon men: 86.5%<br>Women's marathon: 86.5%<br>Men's marathon: 86.4% |
| [23] | NCAA Division 1 Athletes<br>27 vegetarians *<br>43 omnivores | Their meals for the last 7 days were recorded.<br>Oxygen consumption → Bruce protocol<br>Fatigue → Borg RPE<br>Leg extensions and push-ups → dynamometer | Body composition | Body mass<br>Vegetarian *: −11%<br>Lean mass<br>Vegetarian *: −7%<br>Fat mass<br>Vegetarian: 25.5%<br>Omnivores: 26.9%<br>Vegetarians: 19.2%<br>Omnivores: 19.2% |
| | | | Relative/absolute maximal oxygen uptake | Relative maximal oxygen uptake<br>Vegetarian *: +13%<br>Absolute Maximum Oxygen Consumption<br>No significant differences |
| | | | Maximum number of extensions and push-ups. | Maximum number of extensions and push-ups<br>No significant differences |

**Table 3.** *Cont.*

| Ref. | Subjects | Program | Variables | Performance/Health |
| --- | --- | --- | --- | --- |
| | | | Energy, macronutrients, and Fe intake | Energy consumption per week<br>Vegetarian: 106.1 kcal/kg/week<br>Omnivores: 85.6 kcal/kg/week<br>Vegetarians: 108.8 kcal/kg/week<br>Omnivores: 91.7 kcal/kg/week<br>Carbohydrates *<br>Vegetarians: 53%<br>Omnivores: 48%<br>Protein *:<br>Vegetarians: 12%<br>Omnivores: 17%<br>Saturated fats:<br>Vegetarians: 8.3%<br>Omnivores: 11.6%<br>Iron (Fe) *<br>Vegetarians: 19.4 mg<br>Omnivores: 15.4 mg |
| [24] | 74 subjects with type 2 diabetes mellitus<br>Treatment → oral hypoglycemic agents.<br>2 groups:<br>Lactovegetarians (maximum 1 daily serving of skimmed dairy products)<br>Control (omnivorous diet) | Duration:<br>12 weeks<br>Diet:<br>Vegetarian: 60% HC, 15% protein, 25% fat<br>Omnivore: 50% HC, 20% protein, 30% fat<br>Exercise:<br>Frequency: 2 days/week<br>Intensity: 60% HR max<br>Duration: 1 h | Maximum performance<br>Maximum oxygen consumption<br>Respiratory Coefficient<br>Fasting fat and protein carbohydrate oxidation<br>Adherence to exercise | Performance:<br>Vegetarians: +23 W<br>Control: +4 W<br>Maximum oxygen consumption<br>Vegetarians: 3 mL/kg/min<br>Control: −1 mL/kg/mi<br>Respiratory quotient<br>Did not change significantly in any of the groups<br>Oxidation of fats and proteins<br>No significant change in either group<br>Fasting carbohydrate oxidation<br>Vegetarians: 0.3–0.3 mL/kg/min<br>Control: 0.4–0.1 mL/kg/min<br>Adherence to exercise<br>Vegetarians: 90.3%.<br>Control Group: 80.6% |

**Table 3.** *Cont.*

| Ref. | Subjects | Program | Variables | Performance/Health |
|---|---|---|---|---|
| | | | BMR | BMR<br>Vegetarians: 2050–2100 kcal<br>Control: 1950–1970 kcal |
| [27] | Subjects: 2864<br>Omnivores (OMV): 1272<br>Vegetarians * (VEGT): 598<br>Vegans (VEG): 994 | Standardized questionnaire of the NURMI study | % of subjects performing one endurance modality or the other according to sex and diet | Women<br>MVNO / VEGT / VEG<br><21 km: 23% / 29% / 30%<br>MM: 40% / 38% / 43%<br>M/UM: 37% / 33% / 27%<br>Men<br>MVNO / VEGT / VEG<br><21 km: 11% / 14% / 14%<br>MM: 29% / 32% / 31%<br>M/UM: 60% / 54% / 55%<br>MM: half marathon; M: marathon; UM: ultra marathon |
| [26] | 56 healthy young women<br>Vegan: 28<br>Omnivores: 28 | Cycloergometer endurance test:<br>Warm-up → 2 min at 50 W<br>Every 2 min →↑ 25 W<br>Frequency → 70–80 rpm<br>Test of strength:<br>1 RM test on leg and chest presses | $VO_2$ max.<br>Muscular strength<br>Dietary profile | $VO_2$ max: ↑ 3.5 mL/kg/min in vegans than in omnivores.<br>Submaximal endurance: ↑ 6.1 min in vegans than in omnivores.<br>No significant differences in strength.<br>Dietary profile:<br>Carbohydrates: ↑ 7.7% in vegans<br>Protein: ↑ 9.2% in omnivores<br>Total fat: no significant differences<br>Saturated fats: ↑ 7.1% in omnivores<br>Vitamin B12: ↑ 2.86 mcg in omnivores<br>Iron: ↑ 13.3 mg in omnivores |

**Table 3.** *Cont.*

| Ref. | Subjects | Program | Variables | Performance/Health |
|---|---|---|---|---|
| [28] | 18 subjects:<br>9 vegans<br>9 omnivores | Familiarization session<br>Fasting 10–12 h<br>Warm up: 5 min at 80 rpm + 4 s sprints at the end of minutes 2 and 4.<br>3 min break<br>Main part: 4 sprints of 30 s<br>5 min rest between sprints | International Physical Activity Questionnaire<br>Fatigue index<br>Average and peak power | No significant differences in any parameter of physical activity volume/intensity.<br>There was no significant difference in fatigue.<br>Peak power: ↑ in the 1st and 2nd sets compared to the 3rd and 4th sets. No significant differences between groups.<br>Average power: No significant differences between series or between groups. |
| | | | Dietary intake | Dietary intake:<br>Carbohydrates: ↑ 17.9% in vegans<br>Protein: no significant differences<br>Fat: ↑ 21.4% in omnivores<br>Saturated fats: ↑ 36.5% in omnivores |

* Vegetarians without specifying whether it is a lactovegetarian or ovolactovegetarian diet.

### 3.3. Results of Individual Studies

The results of the data extraction will be presented in Table 3.

### 3.4. Risk of Bias in Individual Studies

A risk of bias assessment of the individual studies was performed, allowing a more accurate picture of the quality of the available evidence and the reliability of the results obtained.

The risk of bias assessment figures for each study included in this systematic review are shown below. Each figure will show the result of the risk of bias assessment for each domain assessed, allowing us to identify the strengths and weaknesses of each study. In this way, we will gain a more detailed understanding of the quality of the included studies and their impact on the overall results of the systematic review.

In the risk of bias graph (Figure 2), it can be seen that the incomplete short- and long-term outcome data and selective reporting is 100% low risk; while blinding of participants, personal, and outcome assessment is 83.3% low risk; other source of bias is 50% low risk; and randomized sequence generation and allocation concealment is 83.3% high risk.

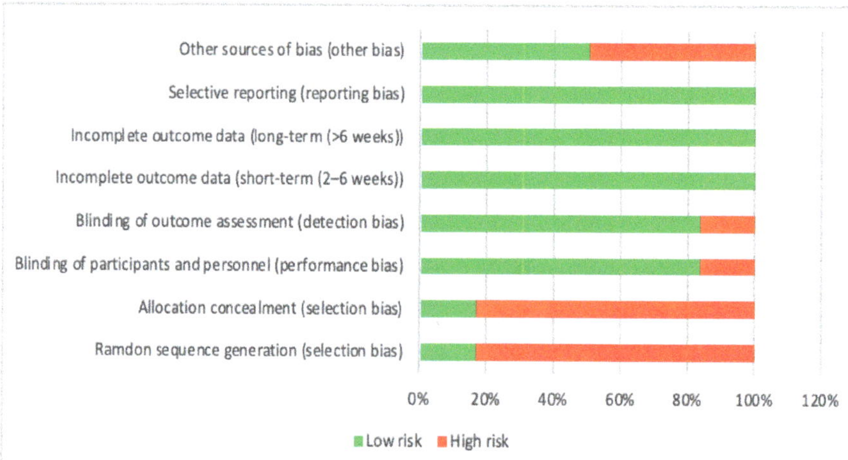


**Figure 2.** Risk of bias.

In the present review, the articles with the greatest bias are those that are not randomized and that do not blind the group assignment [23,25–28]. The article with the greatest bias is due to the lack of blinding of the subjects and the evaluators, as well as other biases such as only specifying the depurative modality [25]. In some articles there are other types of biases, such as not specifying exercise variables [27] or that the calculated dietary intake was based on a 3-day recall [25,26].

Furthermore, in the risk of bias summary (Figure 3), it can be seen which author and item has a low risk, unclear risk, and high risk.

### 3.5. Results of the Synthesis

The articles included in the review were assessed using the PEDro methodological quality scale, shown below in Table 4. The final score obtained ranged from 5 to 10. Five studies were classified as being of good quality and one of fair quality. The studies achieved a mean value of 6.16 ± 0.75.

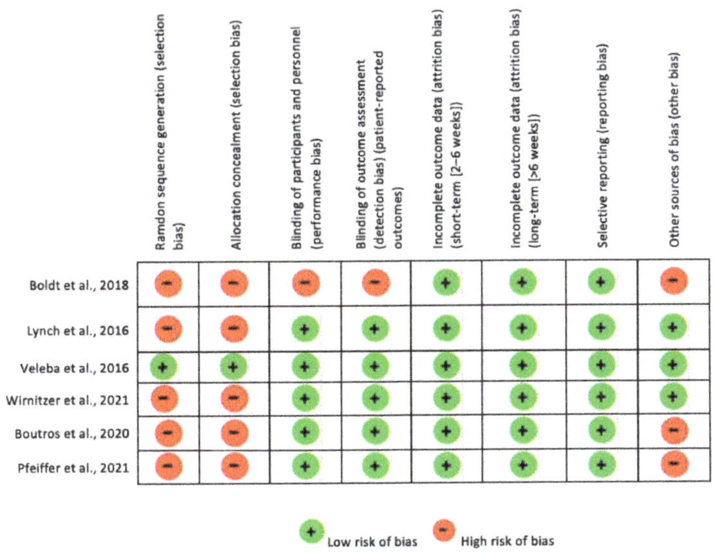


**Figure 3.** Risk of bias summary [23–28].

**Table 4.** Methodological assessment PEDro scale.

| | Type of Study | PEDro | | | | | | | | | | | | Conflict of Interests |
|---|---|---|---|---|---|---|---|---|---|---|---|---|---|---|
| | | 1 | 2 | 3 | 4 | 5 | 6 | 7 | 8 | 9 | 10 | 11 | TOTAL | NO |
| [25] | Cross-sectional-study | + | - | + | + | - | - | - | + | + | + | + | 7/10 | NO |
| [23] | Cross-sectional study | + | - | + | + | - | - | - | - | + | + | + | 6/10 | NO |
| [24] | Parallel Randomized Trial | + | + | - | + | - | - | - | + | + | + | + | 7/10 | N/A |
| [27] | Cross-sectional-study | + | - | - | + | - | - | - | - | + | + | + | 5/10 | NO |
| [26] | Control-trial | + | - | - | + | - | - | - | + | + | + | + | 6/10 | NO |
| [28] | Control-trial | + | - | - | + | - | - | - | + | + | + | + | 6/10 | N/A |

1: Eligibility criteria were specified; 2: subjects were randomly allocated to groups; 3: allocation was concealed; 4: the groups were similar at baseline regarding the most important prognostic indicators; 5: blinding of all subjects; 6: blinding of all therapists who administered the therapy; 7: blinding of all assessors who measured at least one key outcome; 8: >85% outcomes of the subjects initially allocated to groups; 9: data for at least one key outcome by "intention to treat"; 10: between-group statistical comparisons; 11: point measures and measures of variability; N/A: not available; + sign means that it meets the quality criteria; - sign means that it does not meet the quality criteria.

## 4. Discussion

After analyzing the different studies, we observed that the practice of physical exercise and diet must be understood together to perform at one's maximum. As shown in Figure 4, the percentage of subjects who performed different endurance tests was evaluated as a function of their diet, and it was observed that in the tests of less than 21 km, the vegans were the ones who performed the largest number of tests, both male and female athletes (14% and 10%, respectively); in half marathons, male vegans (32%) and female vegetarians (43%) obtained the greatest percentage; and, finally, in marathon or ultra marathon events, male and female omnivores were the ones who performed the largest number of tests (60% and 37%, respectively) [27].

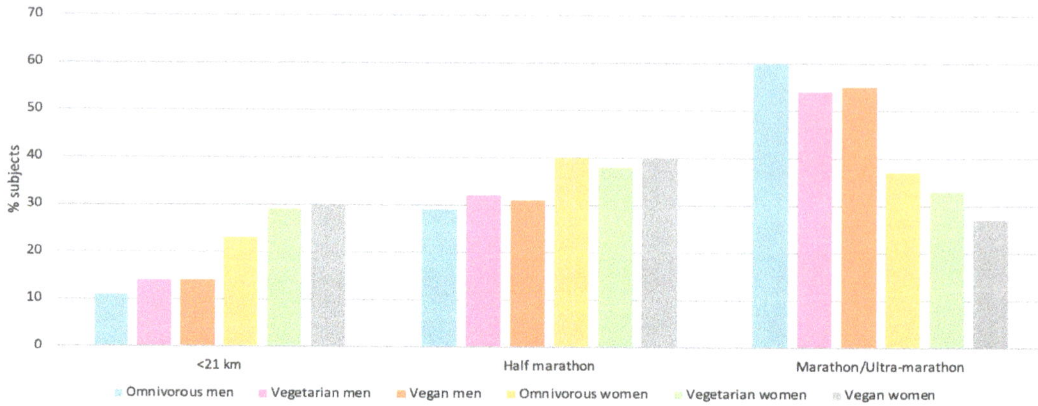


**Figure 4.** Percent of subjects performing different endurance modalities as a function of diet [27].

### 4.1. Physical Health

Through the quality-of-life questionnaire (WHOQOL-BREF), there is a difference in some variables related to health depending on diet and type of exercise. The results show that omnivorous women and men have better physical health, but the differences are not significant, so to say that both are adequate to maintain good physical health is not entirely accurate (Figure 5). Physical health is greater in women who run half marathons, followed by those who participate in marathons or ultra marathons, and, finally, those who run 10 km races. However, in men, physical fitness decreases gradually as the distance increases [25].

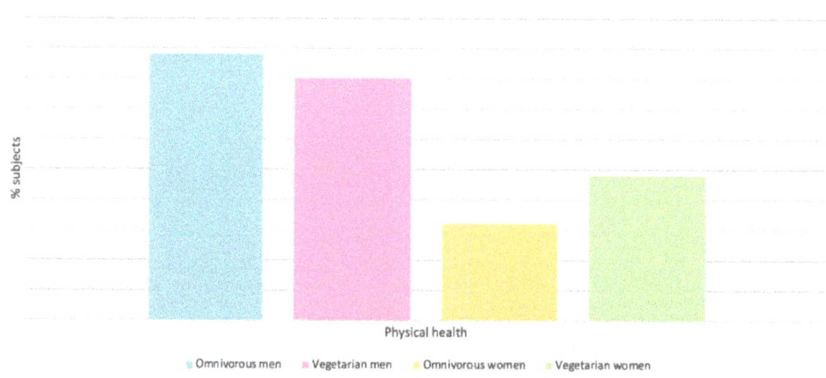


**Figure 5.** Physical health % of different subjects as a function of diet [25].

Vegetarian diets can help athletes protect themselves from degenerative and inflammatory diseases, as well as improve their body composition [29].

Other parameters related to health in the sports environment have also been studied, such as psychological well-being, the environment, and social relationships were also researched. In relation to psychological well-being and social relationships, athletes with an omnivorous diet report a higher level, although the differences are not significant. Finally, and in relation to the environment, the omnivorous subjects were also those who presented a better adaptation, with significant differences in women according to the sport modality, half marathon, and 10 km races, with the former presenting a greater adaptation to the environment [25].

### *4.2. Body Composition*

Body composition is a factor that is directly related to athletic performance, although there are no ideal values, since they vary depending on the sport (Figure 6) [23].

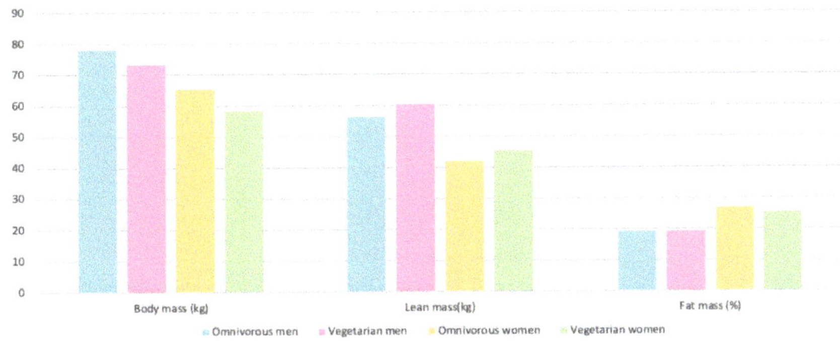


**Figure 6.** Body composition of subjects according to diet [23].

#### 4.2.1. Body Mass

Vegetarian athletes had body weights that were 11% higher compared to omnivores. This suggests that the body weight of vegetarians who are athletes is significantly greater than that of those who consume an omnivorous diet [23,30].

Lactovegetarians, on the other hand, had body weights that were 7.3% lower compared to omnivores. Lactovegetarians are vegetarians who consume dairy products, and they had a lower body weight compared to omnivores.

Vegetarian athletes were 11.1% more likely to fall into the "normal weight" category according to the criteria established by the World Health Organization (WHO), which defines normal weight as having a Body Mass Index (BMI) between 18.5 and 25 kg/m$^2$ [31]. This suggests that vegetarian athletes were more likely to maintain a normal weight compared to omnivores.

#### 4.2.2. Lean Mass

Muscle mass was 7% lower in vegetarian athletes compared to omnivores [23]. In male endurance athletes, muscle mass was also lower in those on an ovolactovegetarian diet compared to omnivores, specifically by 1.6% [30].

#### 4.2.3. Fat Mass

In relation to fat mass in athletes, it depends on sex and diet. In men, there are no significant differences in the percentage of fat mass, while in women, omnivorous athletes had 1.4% more fat mass according to their body weight [23].

The athlete's body composition is a factor that varies according to the competitive period that he/she is in. Both body weight and fat mass decrease as the season progresses, although skeletal muscle mass remains stable in relation to body weight. This may be due to training and competition, as well as energy intake and distribution [32].

### *4.3. Performance*

On diet and exercise compliance, vegetarians had a high adherence rate of 55%, while omnivores had an adherence rate of only 32%. Sometimes, this may be because high-performance athletes are hesitant to follow these types of nutritional guidelines that would allow them to achieve the desired performance for competition [24].

4.3.1. Endurance exercise

As shown in Figure 7, vegetarian subjects performed 20% more physical activity than omnivores [23]. In these studies, the maximum oxygen consumption was measured, being 13% in vegetarian women [23] and 12% in vegetarians [24]. As indicated by several authors in the literature, this variable is clearly marked as a performance marker in performance athletes, so that improvements of approximately 12% in this modality can clearly mark the result in these tests [23,24].

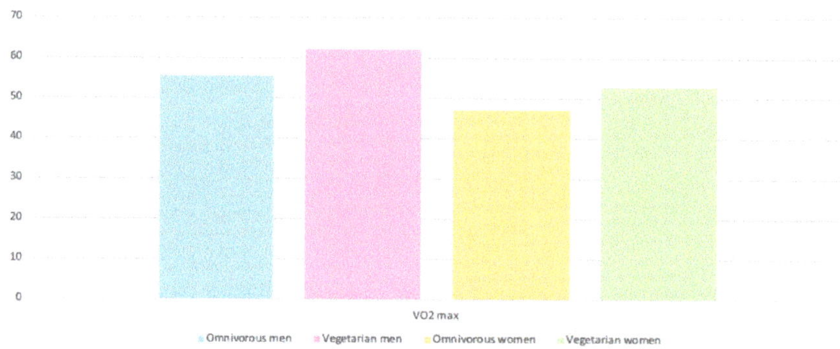


**Figure 7.** VO2 max of the subjects according to the type of diet [23].

In relation to energy expenditure, it increased by 50 kcal/week and decreased by 80 kcal/week in omnivorous athletes, even though they performed the same exercise protocol [24].

In an incremental cycloergometer test, vegetarian athletes obtained improvements of 3.5 mL/kg/min with respect to VO2máx and a higher VO2máx in a test at submaximal intensities with respect to omnivorous athletes, and, in the submaximal endurance test performed on a cycloergometer at 70% maintaining 70–80 rpm, improvements of 6.1 min were obtained in vegetarian athletes [26]. Possibly, these improvements in the VO2máx variable are related to the improvement of body composition parameters obtained thanks to this type of diet [22,26,30,31].

Improvements in endurance sports in vegetarian athletes may be due to effects on the number of mitochondria, capillary density, and hemoglobin concentration; however, specific studies in which these parameters are measured and evaluated would be necessary to indicate the origin of the improvements [33].

4.3.2. Strength Training

In relation to strength, no significant differences were shown in the quadriceps extension and shoulder press exercises, using the 1 RM technique [26]. As for muscle power, improvements of 21 W in muscle power were obtained in a one-hour test at 60% maximum HR in ovolactovegetarian athletes compared to omnivores [24]. However, there were no significant differences between the groups in average or maximal power in a four-sprint test with a cycloergometer, but maximal power was significantly higher in the first two sprints [28]. Specific research is needed in which tests and/or protocols for the improvement of strength parameters are carried out and can be evaluated.

### *4.4. Metabolism*

Another variable that was measured and is related to performance is macronutrient oxidation. Although there were no significant differences in fats or proteins, there were differences in carbohydrates, remaining in vegetarians at 0.3 mL/kg/min and decreasing in omnivores from 0.3 mL/kg/min to 0.1 mL/kg/min [24]. Furthermore, there were no significant differences in the respiratory quotient [24].

However, a review of studies comparing athletes on omnivorous or vegetarian diets found that there were no significant differences between the groups, and that the exercise protocols were very different [34].

#### 4.4.1. Energy Intake

Daily calorie intake varies according to the type of diet of the subjects, with the lowest to highest intakes being those of vegans (2383 kcal), vegetarians (2722 kcal), pesco-vegetarians (2744 kcal), semi-vegetarians (2849 kcal), and, finally, omnivores (2985 kcal) (Figure 8) [31].

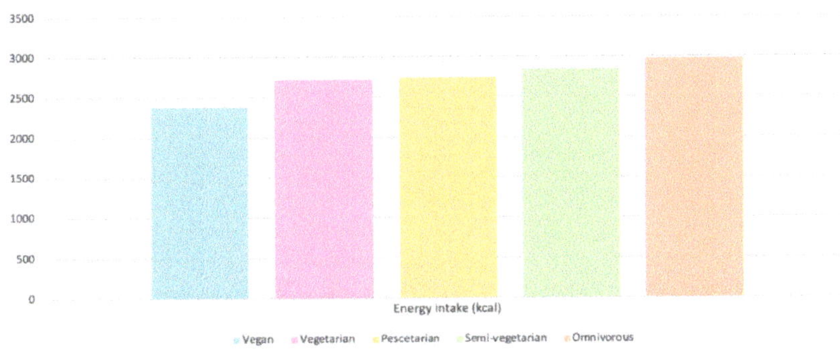


**Figure 8.** Energy intake as a function of diet [31].

In relation to athletes, energy consumption varies depending on the time of the season, being higher during the competitive period corresponding to months 6 and 9 [32].

#### 4.4.2. Macronutrient Intake

Vegetarians consume a higher amount of carbohydrates (343 g), compared to omnivores, who consume at least 322 g [31]. The same was observed in other studies, with vegetarians consuming 5%, 7.7%, and 17.9% more than omnivores, respectively [23,26,28] (Figures 9 and 10). The energy intake per week is higher in vegetarian women than in omnivorous women (21 kcal/kg/week), and in vegetarian men than in omnivorous men (17 kcal/kg/week) [23].

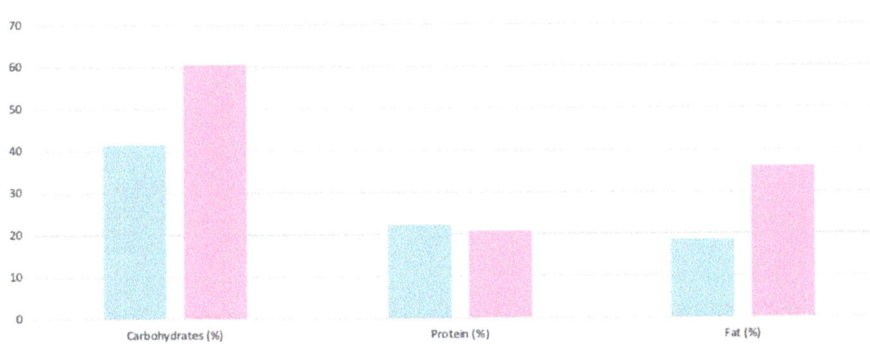


**Figure 9.** Macronutrient intake as a function of diet [26].

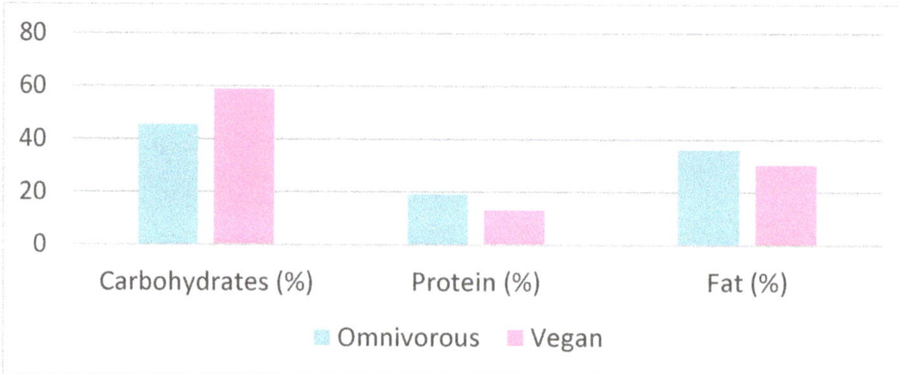


**Figure 10.** Macronutrient intake as a function of diet [28].

The Association of Sports Medicine and the College of Dietitian Nutritionists of Canada recommend a carbohydrate intake of 5–10 g/kg/day for athletes, depending on the volume and intensity of training, as well as the competition period.

The intake protein was 93 g in vegetarians and 112 g in omnivores [31]. Protein intake was 12% in vegetarians and 17% in omnivores, with significant differences in both cases. [23] (Figure 11). However, there are many food products suitable for vegetarians that contain high amounts of protein (Figure 12). In relation to protein intake, omnivores consume 9.2% more protein than vegetarians [26]. In relation to endurance athletes, the recommended intake is between 1.2 and 1.7 g/kg/day [35]. Protein intake during the first three months of the season represents 20.37% of the total energy intake, and, in months 6 and 9, it increases to 21.7%, which corresponds to 2.2 g/kg/day [32].

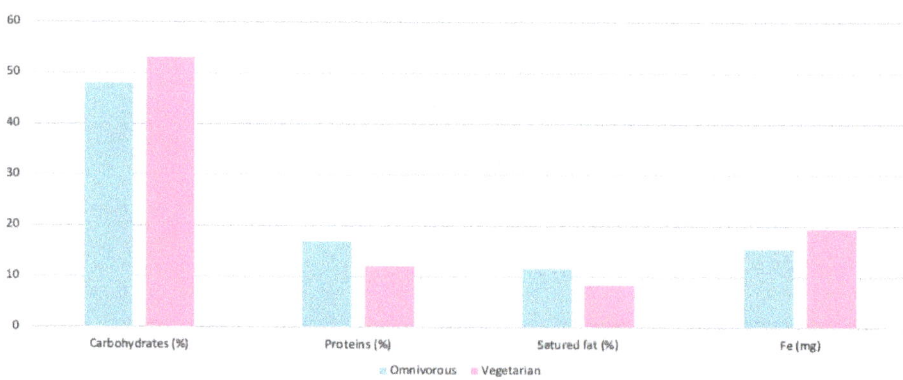


**Figure 11.** Macronutrient and iron intake by diet [23].

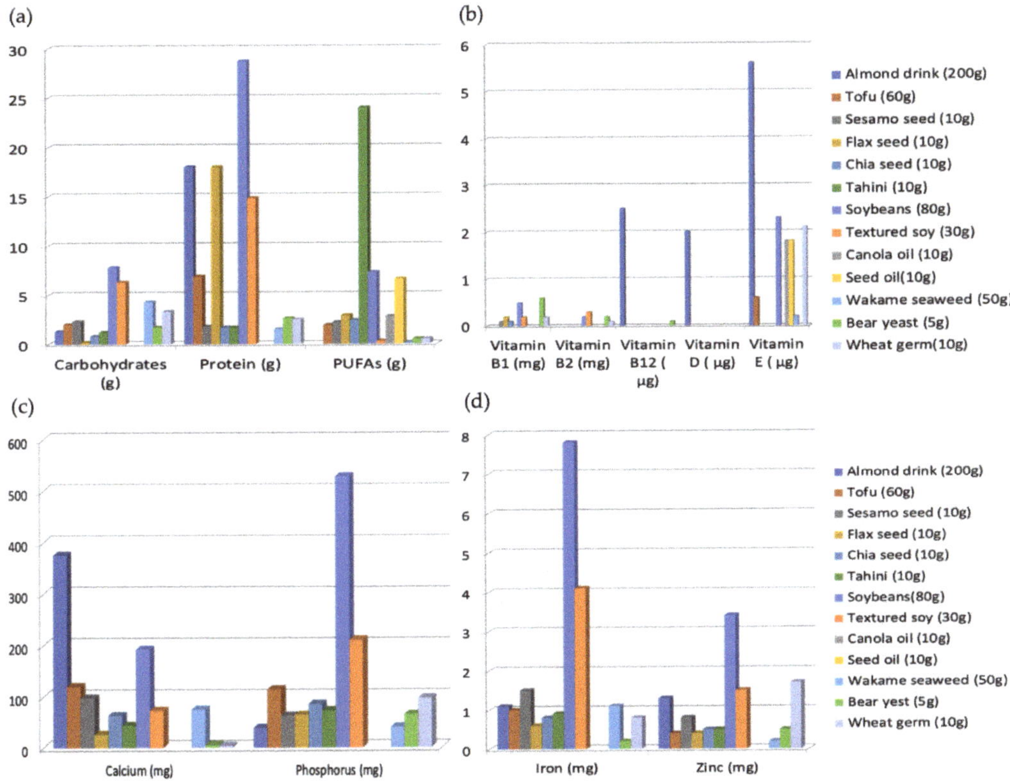


**Figure 12.** Quantity of macronutrient vitamins and minerals in different foods suitable for vegetarians and vegans [36]: (**a**) macronutrients; (**b**) vitamins; (**c**) calcium and phosphorous; (**d**) iron and zinc.

Protein intake is lower in vegetarian athletes, but there are many foods suitable for athletes who follow this type of diet, for example, textured soybeans contain 28.7 g/80 g, almond drink 18 g/200 g, or flax seeds 18 g/10 g, among many others [36].

The consumption of saturated fats represents 8.3% in vegetarians and 11.6% in omnivores [23] (Figure 11). Total fats were assessed and accounted for 31% in vegetarians and 36% in omnivores [31]. Furthermore, total and saturated fat consumption is higher in omnivores than in vegetarians, 7.1% and 136.5%, respectively [26,28] (Figures 9 and 10). The amount required for endurance athletes is 2 g/kg/day or 1.6 g/kg/day [32,35]. The average intake of essential fatty acids in endurance athletes is increased by 4% during the third and sixth months of the season [32].

Although it is widely believed that a vegetarian athlete hardly consumes any fat there are many vegetarian foods with a high fat content such as tahini, 24 g/10 g, soybeans 7.3 g/80 g, and olive oil 90 g/100 mL [36].

### 4.4.3. Micronutrient Intake

We will consider the following minerals: iron (Fe) and calcium (Ca), which have been analyzed in the different studies. For endurance athletes, iron consumption is higher in vegetarians (19.4 mg) than in omnivores (15.4 mg), which represents a significant difference [23] (Figure 11). Whereas red meat is generally thought to be the most iron-containing food, there are iron-rich foods that are suitable for vegetarians (Figure 12). Some of the foods that can be consumed by vegetarian athletes and that contain a significant amount of iron are texturized soybeans, 4.1 mg/30 g, soybeans 7.8 mg/80 g, or wakame seaweed 1.1 mg/50 g [36].

Calcium consumption is higher in vegetarians than in omnivores, with a significant difference of 266 mg per day [31]. Vitamin B12 intake is also noteworthy, with omnivores consuming 2.86 mcg more than vegetarians [26]. Although we normally think of dairy products when we talk about calcium, it is true that there are other beverages or foods that have an equal or greater amount, as is the case with almond drink, 376 mg/200 g, or tofu with 120 mg/60 g [36].

We analyzed cyanocobalamin (vitamin B12), which is the most frequently deficient in vegetarian athletes. This vitamin is not generally present in foods of vegetable origin; however, athletes can obtain it through meat analogs or algae and enriched foods, covering up to 100% of the requirements [36].

A well-planned vegetarian diet with the right combination of foods, which satisfies nutritional requirements, can be optimal for athletes to achieve high performance [37–40].

An interesting future line of research would be to determine whether the vegetarian diet is optimal for improving performance in strength sports and to evaluate the diets of vegetarian athletes to determine whether they achieve the dietary reference intakes (RDI) of different micronutrients.

## 5. Conclusions

In relation to performance, athletes on a vegetarian diet obtained significantly higher values of relative oxygen consumption and maximum power, compared to omnivores. However, no significant differences were found in strength-related parameters.

Physical fitness was higher in vegetarian women, although no significant differences were shown. Finally, and in relation to dietary intake, vegetarian or vegan athletes consumed significantly more carbohydrates and less protein and saturated fat. Therefore, it is important for athletes to plan a diet that meets their nutritional needs according to the type of sport, as well as the period of the season they are in.

**Supplementary Materials:** The following supporting information can be downloaded at: https://www.mdpi.com/article/10.3390/nu15214703/s1, Suplementary Material S1: PRISMA Checklist [41].

**Author Contributions:** Conceptualization, J.L.M.-M., P.G.-F., E.Ú.-D. and B.P.-R.; methodology, J.H.-L., E.Ú.-D. and J.P.H.-P.; software, J.H.-L. and P.G.-F.; validation, J.L.M.-M. and B.P.-R.; writing—original draft preparation, E.Ú.-D., J.H.-L. and J.P.H.-P.; writing—review and editing, B.P.-R., P.G.-F. and J.L.M.-M. All authors have read and agreed to the published version of the manuscript.

**Funding:** This research received no external funding.

**Conflicts of Interest:** The authors declare no conflict of interest.

## References

1. Agnoli, C.; Baroni, L.; Bertini, I.; Ciappellano, S.; Fabbri, A.; Papa, M.; Pellegrini, N.; Sbarbati, R.; Scarino, M.L.; Siani, V.; et al. Position paper on vegetarian diets from the working group of the Italian Society of Human Nutrition. *Nutr. Metab. Cardiovasc. Dis.* **2017**, *27*, 1037–1052. [CrossRef]
2. Kaushik, N.K.; Aggarwal, A.; Singh, M.; Deswal, S.; Kaushik, P. Vegetarian Diets: Health Benefits and Associated Risks. *IAIM* **2015**, *2*, 206–210. Available online: http://iaimjournal.com/wp-content/uploads/2015/03/34-Vegetarian-Diets.pdf (accessed on 4 October 2023).
3. Lynch, H.; Johnston, C.; Wharton, C. Plant-based diets: Considerations for environmental impact, protein quality, and exercise performance. *Nutrients* **2018**, *10*, 1841. [CrossRef]
4. Craig, W.J. Health effects of vegan diets. *Am. J. Clin. Nutr.* **2009**, *89*, 1627S–1633S. [CrossRef]
5. Rojas Allende, D.; Figueras Díaz, F.; Durán Agüero, S. Ventajas y desventajas nutricionales de ser vegano o vegetariano. *Rev. Chil. Nutr.* **2017**, *44*, 218–225. [CrossRef]
6. Key, T.J.; Appleby, P.N.; Rosell, M.S. Health effects of vegetarian and vegan diets. *Proc. Nutr. Society.* **2006**, *65*, 35–41. [CrossRef]
7. Shaw, K.A.; Zello, G.A.; Rodgers, C.D.; Warkentin, T.D.; Baerwald, A.R.; Chilibeck, P.D. Benefits of a plant-based diet and considerations for the athlete. *Eur. J. Appl. Physiol.* **2022**, *122*, 1163–1178. [CrossRef]
8. Barr, S.I.; Rideout, C.A. Nutritional considerations for vegetarian athletes. *Nutrition* **2004**, *20*, 696–703. [CrossRef]
9. Diets, V. News from the Association. *J. Neonatal Nurs.* **2009**, *15*, 189–190.

10. Saz-Peiró, P.; del Ruste, M.M.; Saz-Tejero, S. La dieta vegetariana y su aplicación terapéutica. *Med. Natur.* **2013**, *7*, 13–27.
11. Torres Flores, F.; Mata Ordóñez, F.; Pavia Rubio, E.; Ríos Quirce, C.; Sánchez-Oliver, A.J. Dieta vegetariana y rendimiento deportivo. *EmásF Rev. Digit. De Educ. Física* **2017**, *46*, 27–38. Available online: https://dialnet.unirioja.es/descarga/articulo/5963359.pdf (accessed on 4 October 2023).
12. Thomas, D.T.; Erdman, K.A.; Burke, L.M. Position of the Academy of Nutrition and Dietetics, Dietitians of Canada, and the American College of Sports Medicine: Nutrition and Athletic Performance. *J. Acad. Nutr. Diet.* **2016**, *116*, 501–528. [CrossRef]
13. Thomas, D.T.; Burke, L.M.; Erdman, K.A. Nutrition and Athletic Performance. *Med. Sci. Sports Exerc.* **2016**, *48*, 543–568. [PubMed]
14. Onzari, M. Introducción a la nutrición deportiva. In *Fundamentos de Nutrición en el Deporte*, 3rd ed.; El Ateneo: Buenos Aires, Argentina, 2021; pp. 15–27. Available online: https://editorialelateneo.com.ar/descargas/FUND. NUTRICIÓN EN EL DEPORTE (1er cap).pdf (accessed on 4 October 2023).
15. Bytomski, J.R. Fueling for Performance. *Sports Health* **2018**, *10*, 47–53. [CrossRef]
16. Herring, S.A.; Ben Kibler, W.; Putukian, M.; Brien, S.O.; York, N.; Jaffe, R.; Wilmington, D.E.; Lori Boyajian-O_Neill, D.O.; Overland Park, K.S.; Vincent Disabella, D.O.; et al. Selected Issues for Nutrition and the Athlete. *Med. Sci. Sports Exerc.* **2013**, *45*, 2378–2386.
17. Nieman, D.C. Physical fitness and vegetarian diets: Is there a relation? *Am. J. Clin. Nutr.* **1999**, *70*, 570S–575S. [CrossRef]
18. Fuhrman, J.; Ferreri, D.M. Fueling the vegetarian (vegan) athlete. *Curr. Sports Med. Rep.* **2010**, *9*, 233–241. [CrossRef]
19. Mayoral, J. La alimentación natural y deporte. *Nat. Food Sports* **2000**, *60*, 38–42. Available online: https://dialnet.unirioja.es/descarga/articulo/4989590.pdf (accessed on 4 October 2023).
20. Yepes-Nuñez, J.J.; Urrútia, G.; Romero-García, M.; Alonso-Fernández, S. The PRISMA 2020 statement: An updated guideline for reporting systematic reviews. *Rev. Esp. Cardiol.* **2021**, *74*, 790–799.
21. Wolfenden, L.; Barnes, C.; Jones, J.; Finch, M.; Wyse, R.J.; Kingsland, M.; Tzelepis, F.; Wiggers, J.; Williams, A.J.; Seward, K.; et al. Strategies to improve the implementation of healthy eating, physical activity and obesity prevention policies, practices or programmes within childcare services. *Cochrane Database Syst. Rev.* **2020**, *2020*, CD011779. [CrossRef]
22. Verhagen, A.P.; De Vet, H.C.W.; De Bie, R.A.; Kessels, A.G.H.; Boers, M.; Bouter, L.M.; Knipschild, P.G. The Delphi list: A criteria list for quality assessment of randomized clinical trials for conducting systematic reviews developed by Delphi consensus. *J. Clin. Epidemiol.* **1998**, *51*, 1235–1241. [CrossRef] [PubMed]
23. Lynch, H.M.; Wharton, C.M.; Johnston, C.S. Cardiorespiratory fitness and peak torque differences between vegetarian and omnivore endurance athletes: A cross-sectional study. *Nutrients* **2016**, *8*, 726. [CrossRef] [PubMed]
24. Veleba, J.; Matoulek, M.; Hill, M.; Pelikanova, T.; Kahleova, H. A vegetarian vs. conventional hypocaloric diet: The effect on physical fitness in response to aerobic exercise in patients with type 2 diabetes. A parallel randomized study. *Nutrients* **2016**, *8*, 671. [CrossRef] [PubMed]
25. Boldt, P.; Knechtle, B.; Nikolaidis, P.; Lechleitner, C.; Wirnitzer, G.; Leitzmann, C.; Rosemann, T.; Wirnitzer, K. Quality of life of female and male vegetarian and vegan endurance runners compared to omnivores—Results from the NURMI study (step 2). *J. Int. Soc. Sports Nutr.* **2018**, *15*, 33. [CrossRef]
26. Boutros, G.H.; Landry-Duval, M.A.; Garzon, M.; Karelis, A.D. Is a vegan diet detrimental to endurance and muscle strength? *Eur. J. Clin. Nutr.* **2020**, *74*, 1550–1555. [CrossRef]
27. Wirnitzer, K.; Motevalli, M.; Tanous, D.; Wirnitzer, G.; Leitzmann, C.; Wagner, K.H.; Rosemann, T.; Knechtle, B. Training and racing behaviors of omnivorous, vegetarian, and vegan endurance runners—Results from the nurmi study (Step 1). *Nutrients* **2021**, *13*, 3521. [CrossRef]
28. Pfeiffer, A.; Tomazini, F.; Bertuzzi, R.; Lima-Silva, A.E. Sprint Interval Exercise Performance in Vegans. *J. Am. Nutr. Assoc.* **2022**, *41*, 399–406. [CrossRef]
29. Oral, O.; Rezaee, Z.; Nomikos, G.N.; Tatlibal, P. Vegetarian diets and their impact on athletes. *Sci. Chron. Epistimonika Chron.* **2022**, *27*, 530–540.
30. Campbell, W.W.; Barton, M.L.; Cyr-Campbell, D.; Davey, S.L.; Beard, J.L.; Parise, G.; Evans, W.J. Effects of an omnivorous diet compared with a lactoovovegetarian diet on resistance-training-induced changes in body composition and skeletal muscle in older men. *Am. J. Clin. Nutr.* **1999**, *70*, 1032–1039. [CrossRef]
31. Clarys, P.; Deliens, T.; Huybrechts, I.; Deriemaeker, P.; Vanaelst, B.; De Keyzer, W.; Hebbelinck, M.; Mullie, P. Comparison of nutritional quality of the vegan, vegetarian, semi-vegetarian, pesco-vegetarian and omnivorous diet. *Nutrients* **2014**, *6*, 1318–1332. [CrossRef]
32. Pérez, F.J.G.; Vicho, G.B.; Dorado, A.C.; Marín, D.M.; Gil, M.C.R.; Mariño, M.M. Análisis nutricional en atletas de fondo y medio fondo durante una temporada deportiva. *Nutr. Hosp.* **2016**, *33*, 1136–1141.
33. West, S.; Monteyne, A.J.; van der Heijden, I.; Stephens, F.B.; Wall, B.T. Nutritional Considerations for the Vegan Athlete. *Adv. Nutr.* **2023**, *14*, 774–795. [CrossRef] [PubMed]
34. Craddock, J.C.; Probst, Y.C.; Peoples, G.E. Vegetarian and omnivorous nutrition-comparing physical performance. *Int. J. Sport Nutr. Exerc. Metab.* **2016**, *26*, 212–220. [CrossRef] [PubMed]
35. Phillips, S.M.; van Loon, L.J.C. Dietary protein for athletes: From requirements to optimum adaptation. *J. Sports Sci.* **2011**, *29* (Suppl. S1), 37–41. [CrossRef] [PubMed]
36. Menal-Puey, S.; Morán Del Ruste, M.; Marques-Lopes, I. Nutritional composition of common vegetarian food portions. *Nutr. Hosp.* **2016**, *33*, 386–394. [CrossRef]

37. Ahmed, A.; Afzaal, M.; Ali, S.W.; Muzammil, H.S.; Masood, A.; Saleem, M.A.; Saeed, F.; Hussain, M.; Rasheed, A.; Jbawi, E.A. Effect of vegan diet (VD) on sports performance: A mechanistic review of metabolic cascades. *Int. J. Food Prop.* **2022**, *25*, 2022–2043. [CrossRef]
38. Rogerson, D. Vegan diets: Practical advice for athletes and exercisers. *J. Int. Soc. Sports Nutr.* **2017**, *14*, 36. [CrossRef]
39. Śliż, D.; Parol, D.; Wełnicki, M.; Chomiuk, T.; Grabowska, I.; Dąbrowska, D.; Król, W.; Price, S. Macronutrient intake, carbohydrate metabolism and cholesterol in Polish male amateur athletes on a vegan diet. *Nutr. Bull.* **2021**, *46*, 120–127. [CrossRef]
40. Pohl, A.; Schünemann, F.; Bersiner, K.; Gehlert, S. The impact of vegan and vegetarian diets on physical performance and molecular signaling in skeletal muscle. *Nutrients* **2021**, *13*, 3884. [CrossRef]
41. Page, M.J.; McKenzie, J.E.; Bossuyt, P.M.; Boutron, I.; Hoffmann, T.C.; Mulrow, C.D.; Shamseer, L.; Tetzlaff, J.M.; Akl, E.A.; Brennan, S.E.; et al. The PRISMA 2020 statement: An updated guideline for reporting systematic reviews. *BMJ* **2021**, *372*, n1. [CrossRef]

nutrients

MDPI

Review

# Vegetarian Nutrition in Chronic Kidney Disease

**Yoko Narasaki [1,2,*], Kamyar Kalantar-Zadeh [2,3,4], Connie M. Rhee [1,4,5], Giuliano Brunori [6,7] and Diana Zarantonello [6]**

1 Department of Medicine, David Geffen School of Medicine at UCLA, Los Angeles, CA 90073, USA
2 Tibor Rubin Veterans Affairs Long Beach Healthcare System, Long Beach, CA 90822, USA
3 The Lundquist Institute at Harbor-UCLA Medical Center, Torrance, CA 90502, USA
4 Division of Nephrology, Hypertension, and Kidney Transplantation, University of California Irvine, Orange, CA 92868, USA
5 Nephrology Section, Veterans Affairs Greater Los Angeles Healthcare System, Los Angeles, CA 90073, USA
6 Department of Nephrology, Santa Chiara Hospital, APSS, 31822 Trento, Italy
7 CISMed, University of Trento, 38122 Trento, Italy
* Correspondence: ynarasaki@mednet.ucla.edu

**Abstract:** There is rising interest globally with respect to the health implications of vegetarian or plant-based diets. A growing body of evidence has demonstrated that higher consumption of plant-based foods and the nutrients found in vegetarian and plant-based diets are associated with numerous health benefits, including improved blood pressure, glycemic control, lipid levels, body mass index, and acid–base parameters. Furthermore, there has been increasing recognition that vegetarian and plant-based diets may have potential salutary benefits in preventing the development and progression of chronic kidney disease (CKD). While increasing evidence shows that vegetarian and plant-based diets have nephroprotective effects, there remains some degree of uncertainty about their nutritional adequacy and safety in CKD (with respect to protein-energy wasting, hyperkalemia, etc.). In this review, we focus on the potential roles of and existing data on the efficacy/effectiveness and safety of various vegetarian and plant-based diets in CKD, as well as their practical application in CKD management.

**Keywords:** nutrition; vegetarian diet; plant-based diet; chronic kidney disease

## 1. Introduction

There is rising interest worldwide regarding the health implications of vegetarian or plant-based diets, including reductions in animal-based food intake and/or fully excluding animal-based products from the diet [1]. A growing body of evidence has demonstrated that higher consumption of plant-based foods and the nutrients found within plant-based diets are associated with numerous health benefits, including improved blood pressure, glycemic control, lipid levels, body mass index (BMI), and acid–base parameters, as well as lower risk of complications such as diabetes [2], cardiovascular disease [3], and death [4]. Furthermore, there has been increasing recognition that plant-based diets have a potential salutary role in the management of chronic kidney disease (CKD). For example, the low-protein vegan diet (0.7 g/kg of body weight/day of protein), the low-protein supplemented vegan diet (0.6 g/kg of body weight/day of protein supplemented with essential amino acids (EAAs) and keto acids (KAs), i.e., one tablet per 10 kg of body weight), and the very-low-protein diet (0.3 g/kg of body weight/day of protein supplemented with EAAs and KAs, i.e., one tablet for every 5 kg of body weight) are vegan/vegetarian diets that have been proposed as possible kidney-conservative treatments [5]. A tablet of Ketosteril®, which is used globally, contains L-lysine (105 mg), L-threonine (53 mg), L-histidine (38 mg), L-tyrosine (30 mg), L-tryptophan (23 mg), hydroxy-methionine (59 mg), calcium-keto-valine (86 mg), calcium-keto-phenylalanine (68 mg), calcium-keto-leucine (101 mg), and calcium-keto-isoleucine (67 mg) [6]. Moreover the "Plant-Dominant Low-Protein Diet" (PLADO) [7] and

"Plant-Focused Nutrition in Patients With Diabetes and CKD Diet" (PLAFOND) [8] are two subtypes of plant-based diets that have been established for people with CKD as a means to reduce the progression of kidney disease (Table 1). A sizeable body of research has shown that vegetarian diets have nephroprotective effects, although there remains some degree of uncertainty about safety with respect to the high contents of minerals such as phosphorus and potassium, along with the potential risks of hyperphosphatemia and/or hyperkalemia that may ensue with greater plant-based food consumption. In this review, we focus on the potential roles of and existing data on vegan, lacto-ovo vegetarian, and PLADO diets in CKD, as well as the practical application of these diets in CKD management.

**Table 1.** Different types of plant-based low-protein diets.

| Diet | CKD Stage | Protein | Carbohydrates |
| --- | --- | --- | --- |
| LPD vegan | 3–4 | 0.7 g/kg/day (100% from grain and legumes) | From cereals |
| LPDs vegan | 3–4<br>Indicated in pregnant women with advanced CKD [9], in people at high risk of malnutrition, or in people who do not tolerate legumes [10] | 0.6 g/kg/day (100% from cereals and legumes) + EAAs/KAs (1 tablet every 10 kg of body weight) | From cereals |
| PLADO diet | 3–5 | 0.6 g/kg/day (with >50% plant-based sources) | From whole cereals |
| PLAFOND diet | 3–5<br>Diabetic nephropathy | 0.6 to <0.8 g/kg/day (with >50% plant-based sources) | From whole cereals |
| VLPDs | 4–5 | 0.3–0.4 g/kg/day + EAAs/KAs (1 tablet every 5 kg of body weight) | Especially from low-protein substitutes |

LPD: low-protein diet; LPDs: low-protein diet supplemented; PLADO: Plant-Dominant Low-Protein Diet; PLAFOND: patient-centered plant-focused LPD for the nutritional management of CKD/DM; VLPDs: very-low-protein diet supplemented. EAAs/KAs: essential amino acids/keto acids.

## 2. Overview of Vegetarian and Plant-Based Diets

Vegetarian or plant-based diets are types of diets composed of a larger proportion of foods from plant-based sources as opposed to animal-based sources. There are various forms of vegetarian diets, such that some types fully exclude all animal products (i.e., vegan diets), whereas other types include dairy products such as milk and cheese, eggs, and honey (i.e., lacto-ovo vegetarian diets) or may even include small amounts of fish and seafood (i.e., pescatarian), as well as meat and poultry (i.e., semi-vegetarian or flexitarian) [11]. The phrases "vegetarian" and "plant-based diet" are often used without differentiation, but the terminology "vegetarian" is commonly used to refer to lacto-ovo vegetarians, while the terminology "plant-based diet" is used to refer to dietary patterns with a greater proportion of foods derived from plant-based sources but may not mean that they are devoid of animal-based foods. In other words, a plant-based diet is a hybrid form of a diet rich in plant-based foods. A person who consumes a plant-based diet eats healthy plant-based foods (i.e., fresh/whole/unprocessed/unrefined foods and beverages) and avoids unhealthy plant-based foods (i.e., processed/refined/sugar-sweetened foods and beverages) [12]. Two types of plant-based diets that have specifically been designed for the non-dialysis-dependent CKD (NDD-CKD) population include the (1) Plant-Dominant Low-Protein Diet (PLADO), consisting of a dietary protein intake of 0.6–0.8 g/kg/day, with >50% from plant-based sources [7], and the (2) Plant-Focused Nutrition in CKD and Diabetes Diet (PLAFOND), consisting of a dietary protein intake of 0.6–0.8 g/kg/day from >50% plant-based sources [8]. Low-protein diets are supported by clinical practice guidelines to ameliorate the progression of CKD, and they are considered to be the centerpiece of conservative and preservative kidney disease management strategies as a means to delay or avert the need for dialysis [7,8]. Irrespective of the specific type of plant-based diet, such diets typically consist of a greater proportion of healthy plant-based foods (i.e., whole grains, cereals, nuts, fruits, and vegetables) and favorable nutrient profiles (i.e., dietary fiber, unsaturated fatty acids, folate, magnesium, vitamin C, vitamin E, carotenoids, phytochemicals, and low bioavailability of phosphorus and potassium) (Figure 1) [11]. Dietary phosphorus and potassium from unprocessed plant-based foods have lower bioavailability and, therefore, confer lower loads of phosphorus and potassium, respectively, compared to animal-based foods and processed foods, which is in part due to concomitantly higher glucose and dietary fiber contents. Additionally, phosphorus in plant-based foods is present in the form of phytate, which generally has limited bioavailability in the human digestive system. There is more discussion on this topic in the latter part of this review.

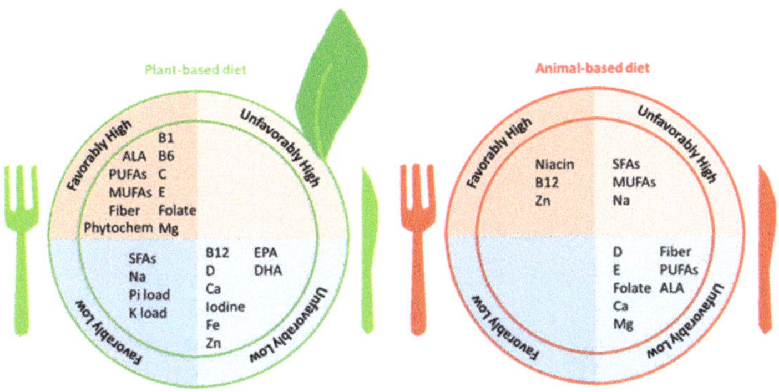


**Figure 1.** Characteristics of nutrients and components in plant-based vs. animal-based diets. Abbreviations: ALA, α-linolenic acid; B1, vitamin B1; B6, vitamin B6; B12, vitamin B12, Ca, calcium; D, vitamin D; DHA, docosahexaenoic acid; EPA, eicosapentaenoic acid; Fe, iron; K, potassium; Mg, magnesium; MUFAs, monounsaturated fatty acids; phytochem, phytochemicals; Pi, phosphorus; PUFAs, total polyunsaturated fatty acids; SFAs, saturated fatty acids; Zn, zinc.

In the general population, the popularity of plant-based diets is in part due to their perceived health benefits related to the control of diabetes, obesity, hypertension, and hyperlipidemia. More recently, there has been interest in the role of plant-based diets in preventing the development of de novo CKD, attenuating CKD progression, and mitigating CKD-related complications (Figure 2).

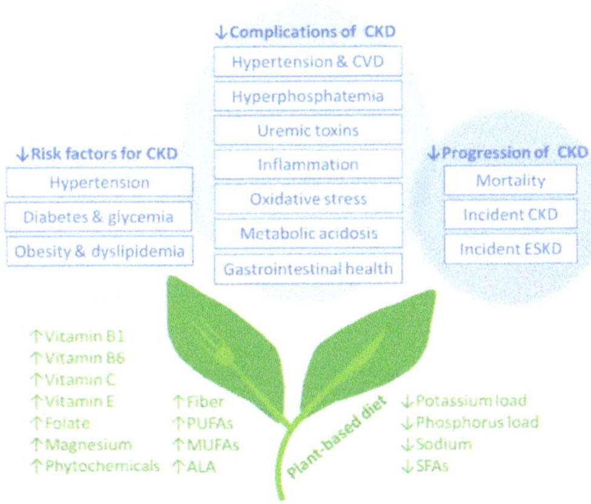


**Figure 2.** Plant-based diets and health benefits in chronic kidney disease. Abbreviations: ALA, α-linolenic acid; CKD, chronic kidney disease; CVD, cardiovascular disease; ESKD, end-stage kidney disease; MUFAs, monounsaturated fatty acids; PUFAs, total polyunsaturated fatty acids; SFAs, saturated fatty acids.

## 3. Vegetarian Diets and Risk Factors for Incident CKD

### *3.1. Hypertension in Non-CKD Populations*

Hypertension and CKD are closely interrelated, such that sustained hypertension can lead to incident CKD and CKD progression, which can in turn result in worse blood pressure (BP) control [13]. Randomized controlled trials have shown the benefits of plant-based diets for BP control. In a study of 59 normotensive participants without underlying CKD, consumption of a vegetarian diet for a six-week period lowered their mean systolic BP by 6.8 mmHg when measured at the laboratory, and by 4.9 mmHg when measured at home [14]. Another study in 58 participants with mild untreated hypertension, comparing ovo-lacto-vegetarian vs. omnivorous diets, showed that the ovo-lacto-vegetarian diet resulted in a reduction in BP by an average of 5.5 mmHg [15]. The Dietary Approach to Stop Hypertension (DASH) trial, a landmark randomized controlled trial examining the effects of a largely plant-based diet on BP control, showed that the DASH diet reduced BP by an average of 5.5 mmHg compared to the control diet [16]. A meta-analysis of seven clinical trials with an aggregate of 313 participants, which excluded the DASH diet trials, also confirmed the benefits of plant-based diets for BP, such that consumption of vegetarian diets reduced systolic BP by a mean of 4.8 mmHg compared to omnivorous diets [17].

### *3.2. Diabetes Mellitus in Non-CKD Populations*

Vegetarian diets have been reported as an effective intervention for the prevention and treatment of diabetes mellitus, the dominant etiology of CKD globally. It has been shown that the prevalence of type 2 diabetes in people consuming vegetarian diets is lower than that among non-vegetarians, even after adjusting for BMI [18]. A meta-analysis of nine large prospective studies with a total of 307,099 participants reported an inverse association between higher adherence to a plant-based dietary pattern and the risk of type 2 diabetes [19]. This association was strengthened in healthy plant-based diet patterns, i.e., consumption of more healthy plant-based foods (e.g., whole grains, fruits, vegetables, nuts, legumes, vegetable oils, tea, and coffee) vs. unhealthy foods (e.g., fruit juices, refined grains, fried potatoes or potato chips, desserts, and sweetened beverages).

Several potential mechanisms explain the relationship between plant-based diets and lower risk of diabetes mellitus. For example, the foods in healthy plant-based diets individually and jointly reduce the risk of diabetes by improving insulin sensitivity and BP [17,20], mitigating long-term weight gain, and ameliorating systemic inflammation [21]. Moreover, plant-based diets may reduce the risk of type 2 diabetes by ameliorating excessive weight gain. Multiple interventional and observational studies have shown that plant-based diets provide favorable weight control and/or weight loss in the short term and weight loss and/or prevention of weight gain in the long term [22–24]. Plant-based diets may also improve circulating levels of adiposity-related biomarkers, including leptin, adiponectin, high-sensitivity C-reactive protein, and interleukin-6 [25,26].

## 4. Vegetarian Diets and CKD Complications

### *4.1. Hypertension in CKD Populations*

Different components of vegetarian diets contribute to directly or indirectly lowering BP levels in people with CKD, through various pathways. First, lower consumption of sodium in plant-based vs. animal-based diets can prevent and control hypertension. Unprocessed plant-based foods generally have less sodium than animal-based foods and processed foods. Indeed, data from the National Health and Nutrition Examination Survey (NHANES) showed that vegetarians ate less sodium, as ascertained using 24 h dietary recall, compared to non-vegetarians (2347 $\pm$ 80 mg vs. 3621 $\pm$ 27 mg) [27]. A meta-analysis that included 21 studies among people with earlier stages of CKD, dialysis patients, and kidney transplant recipients reported that salt reduction reduced systolic and diastolic BP in the short term (i.e., 1 to 36 weeks) [28]. This study also reported that salt reduction resulted in lower albuminuria levels. Another meta-analysis also showed that salt restriction was associated with lower systolic BP, diastolic BP, and proteinuria levels among 738 people with stages 1–4 CKD [29], and another pooled analysis showed that reduction of salt intake resulted in lower systolic and diastolic BP among 101,077 people with CKD [30].

Second, higher potassium intake from plant-based diets may help reduce BP. It is well established that higher dietary potassium intake lowers BP in the general population. While studies examining the effects of dietary potassium on BP in people with CKD are sparse, limited data suggest potential benefits. In an animal study of rats with CKD, it was demonstrated that potassium supplementation lowered BP among rats with slightly higher serum potassium levels compared to rats on a low-potassium diet [31]. In a non-randomized study of 11 people with stage 3 CKD, receipt of the DASH diet (dietary potassium intake of 4.7 g/day) over two weeks resulted in no differences in clinical and mean 24 h ambulatory BP, whereas it resulted in lower nighttime systolic BP levels compared to BP levels during the baseline period while on a control diet (dietary potassium intake of 2.4 g/day) in the absence of hyperkalemia [32]. Randomized trials in people with stages 3–4 CKD have also shown that receipt of diets that are higher in fruits and vegetables resulted in lower systolic BP after one year [33] or three years [34], although narrowly missing statistical significance after a shorter follow-up period of four weeks [35].

Third, all plant-based foods contain dietary fiber, a carbohydrate that is indigestible by digestive tract enzymes (Table 2) [35]. Dietary fiber intake improves BP by modifying arterial contraction due to its effect on arterial smooth muscle, influencing the activity of the angiotensin-converting enzyme (ACE) or retaining minerals such as potassium and magnesium in its matrix [36,37]. In addition to BP control, there are a variety of health benefits of dietary fiber that affect CKD outcomes. For example, dietary fiber intake can improve glycemic control by delaying gastric emptying, reducing postprandial glucose absorption, providing a lower glycemic response, producing greater satiety, and improving insulin sensitivity [8,38]. Moreover, dietary fiber intake also contributes to improving dyslipidemia. Dietary soluble fiber with high viscosity decreases cholesterol absorption, binds to bile acids, and increases their fecal excretion. Bacterial fermentation in the colon can inhibit cholesterol production in the liver by producing short-chain fatty acids (SCFAs) [39]. SCFAs also exert trophic action on the mucosa and strengthen the defense function of the intestinal barrier by counteracting bacterial translocation and low-grade chronic inflammation [40]. Moreover, fiber intake reduces serum urea levels by promoting a fecal route of excretion for nitrogenous waste, and it can reduce serum levels of AGEs (advanced glycation end products) [35]. Lastly, greater dietary fiber intake may lead to improvements in constipation, increased satiety, reduced energy intake, weight control, and slower absorption of some nutrients in the intestine, leading to reduced inflammation [36].

Fourth, more balanced intake of macronutrients (including dietary protein, fat, and carbohydrates) conferred by a plant-based diet can contribute to better BP control. Results from observational studies indicate an inverse association between dietary plant protein intake and BP [41], and both prospective studies and randomized controlled trials have shown similar relationships between plant and animal protein intake with respect to BP [42]. The effects of plant vs. animal protein on BP control remain to be established. Additionally, vegetarian diets usually provide low intake of saturated fatty acids and omega-3 polyunsaturated fatty acids (PUFAs). In a cross-sectional study of 26 vegetarians vs. 26 non-vegetarians, matched according to age, sex, and BMI, the vegetarians had higher plant-based fat consumption than the non-vegetarians, which may lead to higher resting energy expenditure (REE) in vegetarians and potentially contribute to better body weight and BP control [43].

**Table 2.** Importance of dietary fiber in human health.

| Property | Function | Health Benefits |
|---|---|---|
| **Bulk** | • Adds bulk to diet<br>  ○ Satiety effect<br>• Adds bulk to stool<br>  ○ Improves GI motility<br>    ■ Increases bowel movement<br>    ■ Reduces intestinal transit time<br>  ○ Increases fecal bulk<br>  ○ Increases stool frequency | • Regulates energy intake<br>• Lowers blood pressure<br>• Promotes weight loss<br>• Alleviates constipation |
| **Viscosity** | • Inhibits intestinal digestion and absorption<br>  ○ Inhibits glucose absorption<br>    ■ Traps carbohydrates<br>    ■ Slows glucose absorption<br>  ○ Inhibits cholesterol absorption<br>    ■ Traps bile acids and extracts to feces<br>    ■ Increases the synthesis of bile acids from cholesterol<br>  ○ Traps carcinogenic substances | • Improves glycemic control<br>  ○ Lowers postprandial serum glucose levels<br>• Improves cholesterol control<br>  ○ Lowers serum total and LDL cholesterol<br>• Contributes to cancer prevention |
| **Fermentability** | • Alters intestinal microbiota composition and function<br>  ○ Increases gut-microbiome-induced production of SCFAs | • Anti-inflammation<br>• Anti-obesity<br>• Anti-diabetes<br>• Anticancer<br>• Hepatoprotection<br>• Cardiovascular protection<br>• Neuroprotection<br>• Constipation treatment<br>• Inflammatory bowel disease treatment<br>• Immunoregulation |

Abbreviations: GI, gastrointestinal; LDL, low-density lipoprotein; SCFAs, short-chain fatty acids.

### 4.2. Hyperphosphatemia in CKD Populations

In people with advanced CKD, decreased phosphorus excretion by the kidneys, coupled with disordered mineral metabolism, engenders hyperphosphatemia, leading to vascular calcification and stiffness, altered cardiac structure and function, kidney osteodystrophy, and increased mortality [44]. Therefore, in the traditional dietary management of advanced CKD patients, dietary phosphorous has been restricted and plant-based foods have been avoided due to concerns regarding high contents of minerals such as phosphorus. However, increasing evidence suggests that greater intake of plant-based foods may lead to better phosphorus control. The amount of phosphorus contained in food vs. phosphorus absorbed by the body is not always consistent. Given that phosphorus in plant-based foods is often in the form of phytate (which humans have limited ability to digest, given the absence of the phytase enzyme), phosphorus found in plant-based foods usually has lower absorbability and/or bioavailability (20 to 40% bioavailability) compared with animal foods, which often have phosphorus in the form of caseins (40 to 60% bioavailability), and processed foods, in which phosphorus is usually present as food additives (~100% bioavailability) [45,46]. Indeed, both animal and human studies show reduced phosphorus loads when consuming plant-based vs. animal-based diets, despite both diets having the same amounts of phosphorus. In a rat model of CKD–mineral bone disease (CKD–MBD), administration of a plant-based diet led to a reduced phosphorus load, such that rats fed grain-based diets showed similar serum phosphorus levels, calcium levels, and intact parathyroid hormone (PTH) levels, yet lower urinary phosphorus excretion and serum fibroblast growth factor 23 (FGF-23) levels vs. rats fed the same amount of phosphorous from casein-based diets [47]. In a crossover trial of people with stage 3–4 CKD, receipt of a vegetarian diet for one week led to lower serum phosphorus, phosphaturia, and FGF-23 levels compared to a meat-based diet with the same phosphorus content [48]. A randomized controlled trial in which participants underwent partial replacement of animal protein with plant protein also led to reduced serum phosphorus levels [49].

### 4.3. Uremic Toxins, Inflammation, and Oxidative Stress in CKD

Given the concomitant rich consumption of dietary fiber, along with their lower contents of carnitine, choline, phosphatidylcholine, tyrosine, and tryptophan, plant-based diets lead to less generation of uremic toxins (i.e., trimethylamine n-oxide (TMAO), indoxyl sulfate, and p-cresyl sulfate), as well as reducing inflammation and oxidative stress [50,51]. In a randomized controlled study of 32 non-dialysis-dependent CKD patients, one week of a supplemented very-low-protein diet of plant-based origin (0.3 g/kg body weight/day) led to reduced indoxyl sulfate levels [52]. In a randomized controlled study of 40 hemodialysis patients who received higher vs. lower dietary fiber intake for six weeks, those who received higher dietary fiber intake had reduced free plasma levels of indoxyl sulfate and p-cresyl sulfate [53]. Data from the NHANES III cohort included 14,543 participants, in whom it was observed that dietary fiber intake was negatively associated with serum C-reactive protein (CRP) levels, such that each 10 g/day increase in total fiber intake was associated with an 11% and 38% decline in the odds of elevated serum CRP levels in the CKD and non-CKD groups, respectively [54]. In a rat model of CKD, consumption of high-amylose maize resistant starch for three weeks also ameliorated inflammation and oxidative stress [55].

Dietary fiber confers a number of advantages for sustainable human health [56]. The bulking effect from the food is important to control the events in the digestive tract, including improved gastrointestinal motility (i.e., increased bowel movements and reduced intestinal transit time), increased fecal bulk, and greater stool frequency. Dietary fiber adds bulk not only to stool, but also to the overall diet, which provides a satiety effect and regulates energy intake. This bulking property of dietary fiber can also reduce BP, promote weight loss, and alleviate constipation [57]. The viscosity effect of dietary fiber can also improve glycemic and cholesterol control, and it may additionally contribute to cancer prevention. Increasing viscosity during digestion due to soluble dietary fiber results in the trapping of carbohydrates, slowing of glucose absorption, and lowering of postprandial blood glucose levels. Soluble fiber also helps to reduce total and LDL cholesterol levels by binding bile acids in the small intestine following extraction from the body through feces, as well as increasing the synthesis of bile acids from cholesterol. Dietary fiber also traps carcinogenic substances and may prevent the development of cancer [57]. Fermentable dietary fiber is the substrate for bacterial metabolism and stimulates the production of short-chain fatty acids (SCFAs) through intestinal fermentation, primarily acetate, propionate, and butyrate, leading to its protective effects against inflammation, obesity, diabetes, cancer, and cardiovascular disease, along with immune regulation and a number of other health benefits [58,59]. The mechanisms underlying the association between dietary fiber intake and lower uremic toxin levels, as well as urea and creatinine concentrations, are interrelated, such that greater dietary fiber intake (1) decreases toxin absorption and increases their fecal excretion by improving intestinal motility, (2) reduces the permeability of toxins by improving the integrity of tight junctions in the colonic epithelium by producing SCFAs, and (3) facilitates the growth of a more favorable microbiome.

### 4.4. Metabolic Acidosis

A large proportion of people with CKD suffer from metabolic acidosis and its adverse consequences, including muscle wasting, bone loss, impaired insulin sensitivity, chronic inflammation, and progression of kidney disease [60]. While alkali therapy is typically conducted to correct metabolic acidosis in CKD patients by administering sodium bicarbonate, a series of trials have shown that plant-based diets could also be used to treat metabolic acidosis. In a randomized controlled trial of 71 people with stage 4 CKD, people assigned to greater fruit and vegetable intake over the course of one year had higher plasma $CO_2$ levels and lower urinary indices of kidney injury [33]. Another randomized controlled trial of 108 people with stage 3 CKD also confirmed similar effects of fruit and vegetable intake on metabolic acidosis parameters, such that daily administration of two to four cups of fruits and vegetables over a period of three years resulted in higher $CO_2$ levels, lower net acid excretion, lower urinary albumin–creatinine ratios, and preserved kidney function [34]. According to this evidence, the KDOQI guidelines also support prescribing more fruits and vegetables for stage 1–4 CKD patients in order to decrease their body weight, blood pressure, and net acid production [36].

## 5. Vegetarian Diets, Incident CKD, and CKD Progression

### *5.1. Incident CKD and CKD Progression*

Several studies have shown favorable associations of plant-based diets with CKD outcomes, including incident CKD (i.e., development of albuminuria and/or eGFR decline) and CKD progression. With respect to the outcome of incident CKD, among participants in the Tehran Lipid and Glucose Study (TLGS), those in the highest quartile of plant protein intake exhibited a 30% lower risk of developing CKD than those in the lowest group of plant protein intake, while those in the highest quartile of animal protein intake had a 37% higher risk of de novo CKD than those in the lowest group of animal protein intake [61]. In the Multi-Ethnic Study of Atherosclerosis (MESA), a dietary pattern with higher intake of whole grains, fruits, vegetables, and low-fat dairy foods was associated with a 20% lower risk of CKD, whereas nondairy animal food intake was associated with an 11% higher urinary albumin-to-creatinine ratio [62]. In a large longitudinal observational study of the Atherosclerosis Risk in Communities (ARIC) cohort, which included 11,952 adults with normal kidney function at baseline, various sources of dietary protein intake had differential associations with the risk of CKD [63]. During a median follow-up of 23 years, there was a higher risk of incident CKD in those consuming greater amounts of protein from red and processed meat sources. Compared to those in the lowest quintiles of red and processed meat consumption, those in the highest quintile of intake had a 23% higher risk of incident CKD. Moreover, this study showed favorable associations of vegetable sources of proteins, such that those in the highest quintile of vegetable protein intake had a 24% reduced risk of incident CKD compared to those in the lowest quintile of intake. Furthermore, when one serving per day of nuts or legumes was used to substitute one serving per day of red and processed meat, a reduced risk of incident CKD was observed.

With respect to the outcome of CKD progression, in a prospective cohort study of approximately 1600 women from the Nurses' Health Study (NHS), among those with mild CKD, greater intake of both total protein and nondairy animal protein was associated with a decline in eGFR over a follow-up period of 11 years (i.e., each increment of +10 g/day of total protein intake and nondairy animal protein intake was associated with an eGFR decline of −7.72 and −1.21 mL/min per 1.73 $m^2$, respectively) [64]. Existing clinical trial data have also shown that partial replacement of animal protein with plant protein leads to reductions in albuminuria [49,65,66]. Finally, a recent systematic review suggested that a vegetarian diet improves renal filtration function in CKD patients [67].

### *5.2. Progression of ESKD*

End-stage kidney disease (ESKD) necessitating long-term dialysis or kidney transplantation is another highly relevant outcome with respect to studying the impact of vegetarian diets on kidney health. There are mixed data, such that some studies have provided evidence that vegetarian diets are associated with a lower risk of incident ESKD [68,69], whereas others have not observed a nephroprotective relationship [70,71]. A report from the Singapore Chinese Health Study showed the deleterious impact of high red meat intake on progression to ESKD, and it also showed that substituting one serving of red meat with one serving of soy/legumes was associated with a lower risk of incident ESKD [69]. In contrast, a meta-analysis showed no statistically significant association between healthy dietary patterns (i.e., those higher in fruits and vegetables, fish, legumes, cereals, whole grains, and fiber; and lower in red meat, salt, and refined sugars) and risk of ESKD, due to the competing risk of death and the relatively small number of events [70]. Similarly, among 3972 people with CKD from the Reasons of Geographic and Racial Differences in Stroke (REGARDS) study, there were no significant associations between dietary patterns and the risk of incident ESKD in multivariable models adjusted for age, race, sex, geographic region of residence, and caloric intake, nor in models further adjusted for socioeconomic and lifestyle factors, comorbidities, and baseline kidney function [71]. One possible explanation for the lack of a nephroprotective association between plant-based diets and ESKD in these studies may relate to inadequate power due to the relatively modest number of ESKD events.

## 6. Practical Application of Vegetarian Diets in CKD

### *6.1. Protein-Energy Wasting*

People with CKD are more predisposed to malnutrition–wasting conditions, including protein-energy wasting (PEW), which adversely impacts their health and survival [72]. The prevalence of PEW is increasingly higher with incrementally lower levels of kidney function, and more than half of people treated with maintenance dialysis therapy may suffer from this complication [73]. Thus, there has been concern about the potential nutritional adequacy of vegetarian diets in people with CKD, particularly with respect to energy and protein contents. However, a number of studies in experimental animal models [47,74,75] and human studies [76] have shown that vegetarian diets are indeed nutritionally adequate in CKD. For example, in a study of 239 people with advanced CKD, it was shown that vegetarian diets with very low protein contents (dietary protein intake of 0.3 g/kg/day) supplemented with keto analogues provided satisfactory nutritional status (i.e., BMI and serum albumin levels remained stable over a mean duration of 29.6 months) [70]. Another study of people with diabetes with elevated proteinuria levels demonstrated that consumption of a predominantly vegetable-protein diet (dietary protein intake of 0.7 g/kg/day) over eight weeks resulted in no considerable differences in body weight or triceps skinfold thickness [77]. Moreover, among people with diabetes, transitioning from a diet with a dietary protein intake of 1.0 to 1.3 g/kg/day to a vegan diet with a dietary protein intake of 0.7 g/kg/day was not associated with substantial changes in serum total protein or serum albumin levels [78]. Moreover a randomized controlled trial recently compared 43 people receiving a low-protein diet with soy protein (60% soy protein and 40% other vegetable proteins) plus KAs vs. 42 people who received a conventional low-protein diet and found that receipt of a low-protein diet with vegetable proteins and KAs was associated with a slower loss of lean mass [79]. Hence, growing research shows that people with CKD who consume vegetarian diets, including those on maintenance dialysis, are not at higher risk of PEW, although further investigation in this area is needed [80].

### *6.2. Overall Nutritional Adequacy*

While plant-based diets are generally considered to be healthier, there are concerns as to whether these diets have adequate contents of nutrients that are typically found in animal-based foods (Table 3). However, ensuring nutritional adequacy is an issue not only in CKD populations consuming plant-based diets, but also in those consuming animal-based diets; hence, it is important to provide optimal education, food fortification, and adequate supplementation to achieve optimal nutritional/nutrient status among people with CKD.

**Table 3.** Common concerns/myths and existing evidence with respect to plant-based diets.

| Topic | Concern/Myth | Evidence |
|---|---|---|
| **Nutritional adequacy** | Plant-based diets lack adequate contents of nutrients largely found in animal-based foods | • Dietary energy intake is similar across dietary patterns, and protein intake seems to be lower in people following plant-based diets compared to those following animal-based diets, but still well within the recommended intake levels [81]<br>• There are nutrient inadequacies across all dietary patterns, including plant-based diets and animal-based diets |
| **Protein adequacy** | Plant-based diets provide inferior protein quantity compared to animal-based diets | • Plant-based diets are not low-protein diets per se<br>• Large-population-based data have not shown differences in dietary protein intake across plant-based vs. animal-based diets [82] |
| | Plant-based diets provide inferior protein quality compared to animal-based diets | • Although individual plant proteins (except for soy protein) have insufficient levels of one or more indispensable amino acids, consumption of different sources of plant proteins over the course of the day can help to meet the requirements for indispensable amino acids and allow them to be complete proteins and provide health benefits [83] |
| | Plant proteins are inferior to animal proteins in terms of lean body mass and strength | • There is a lower percentage of leucine in plant proteins (e.g., soy protein: ~8%) than in animal proteins (e.g., whey protein: ~12%)<br>• Muscle protein synthesis (MPS) [84]<br>○ Soy protein promotes greater MPS at rest and post-exercise (vs. casein protein)<br>○ Soy protein promotes comparable MPS at rest and 20% lower MPS post-exercise (vs. whey protein)<br>• No differences between soy protein and animal proteins for improvements in bench press strength, squat/leg press strength, or lean body mass [85] |
| **Hormonal abnormalities** | Isoflavones from soy have potential adverse effects (e.g., thyroid dysfunction, breast cancer) | • Concerns have been raised largely based on in vitro cell cultures or rodent studies involving large doses of isoflavones<br>• Studies have not observed adverse hormonal effects from physiological amounts of soy foods in the diet [86] |
| **Hyperkalemia** | Plant-based diets cause hyperkalemia | • The occurrence of hyperkalemia is quite rare [87]<br>• The majority of hyperkalemic episodes seem to be related to the consumption of plant-based foods containing higher bioavailable potassium contents (e.g., juices, sauces, or dried fruits) compared with whole foods or unprocessed plant-based foods [88] |

Abbreviations: MPS, muscle protein synthesis.

In one systematic review [81], while dietary protein intake was lower in people consuming plant-based diets compared to those consuming animal-based diets, the overall dietary protein intake was well within the recommended intake levels for both groups, and dietary energy intake was comparable among those receiving plant-based vs. animal-based diets. Given that some nutrients are mainly present in and/or have greater bioavailability in plant-based or animal-based foods, some dietary patterns may lead to favorable intake of some nutrients yet inadequate intake of other nutrients. Plant-based diets typically have higher fiber, total PUFA, α-linolenic acid (ALA), vitamin B1, vitamin B6, vitamin C, vitamin E, folate, and magnesium contents, lower protein contents (albeit within recommended levels), and potentially lower eicosapentaenoic acid (EPA), docosahexaenoic acid (DHA), vitamin B12, vitamin D, calcium, iodine, iron (in women), and zinc contents. Taking vitamin B12 supplements or foods fortified with vitamin B12 is essential for people at risk of vitamin B12 deficiency, including those following vegan diets (owing to the absence of this vitamin in plant-based sources [89]) and people with CKD, who have reduced absorption of nutrients (age reduces absorption capacity), low intake of animal-based foods in a low-protein diet, and prescribed medications that can compromise the assimilation of vitamin B12 (e.g., proton-pump inhibitors and metformin) [90]. On the other hand, typical animal-based diets have higher protein, niacin, vitamin B12, and zinc contents, yet they may be inadequate with respect to fiber, total PUFA, ALA (in men), vitamin D, vitamin E, folate, calcium, and magnesium contents. Dietary monounsaturated fatty acids (MUFAs) can come from both plant-based and animal-based sources, but recent data have shown that MUFAs from plant-based foods have favorable associations with respect to lower risk of coronary heart disease [91] and mortality [92].

### 6.3. Protein Adequacy Overall and with Physical Activity

There has been a misconception that the nutritional quantity and quality of protein from plant-based diets are inferior to those of protein from animal-based foods. However, data from the general population do not support this impression. For example, landmark data from a cross-sectional analysis of 71,751 participants from the Adventist-Health-Study-2 showed that the median total protein intake did not differ among non-vegetarians (~75 g/day) vs. vegetarians (i.e., lacto-ovo vegetarians and vegans) (~71 g/day) [82]. A systematic review that included 141 observational and interventional studies, largely from Europe, South/East Asia, and North America, reported that the average dietary protein intake was lower in vegetarians and vegans compared to meat-eaters, but still within the recommended levels across these groups [81].

High-quality or complete protein sources for humans are dependent on whether the food contains adequate levels of indispensable amino acids to support human growth and/or is readily digested and absorbed [93]. According to the amino acid scoring system, which is currently the recommended method for evaluating dietary protein quality by the Food and Agricultural Organization of the United Nations (FAO) and the U.S. National Academy of Sciences, most animal proteins and soy proteins are generally considered to be complete protein sources [93]. Although individual plant proteins (except for soy protein) have insufficient levels of one or more indispensable amino acids, consumption of different sources of plant proteins over the course of the day can help to meet the requirements for indispensable amino acids, allowing them to be complete proteins and, hence, provide health benefits [83].

The topics of leucine content and muscle protein synthesis (MPS) have become popular in secular culture and among active individuals. Given the lower percentage of leucine in plant-based proteins (e.g., soy protein: ~8%) vs. animal proteins (e.g., whey protein: ~12%), there is a misconception that plant proteins are inferior to animal proteins with respect to attaining optimal lean body mass and muscle strength. Contrary to this hypothesis, a study examining differences in MPS at rest and following exercise followed by high-leucine/fast-digesting (hydrolyzed whey isolate), lower-leucine/intermediate-digesting (soy isolate), and high-leucine/slow-digesting (micellar casein) protein sources demonstrated that soy protein outperformed casein both at rest and post-exercise [84]. Neither soy nor caseins promoted greater post-exercise MPS than whey protein, and the post-exercise MPS fractional synthetic rate (%/h) for soy was still about 80% of that of whey. Moreover, MPS at rest after soy protein ingestion was similar to that after whey protein and higher than that after casein protein. Although some resistance training studies (duration 12–36 weeks) among young adults have reported better muscle mass and strength with fluid milk or whey protein [94,95], a meta-analysis of nine resistance training studies (duration 6 to 36 weeks) pooling together 266 participants, including both younger (18 to 38 years) and older (61 to 67 years) adults, showed no differences between soy protein and animal proteins with regards to improvements in bench press strength, squat/leg press strength, or lean body mass outcomes [85].

In terms of the effect of plant-based protein intake on risk of sarcopenia—the loss of skeletal muscle mass and physical function that occurs with advanced age—limited studies among non-CKD [96] and CKD populations [97] have reported that higher consumption of fruit and/or vegetables was correlated with a reduced risk of sarcopenia. Although these data and the comparable muscle-related benefits of plant-based protein compared to animal-based protein, as mentioned above, could mitigate concerns about developing sarcopenia following plant-based diets in people with advanced CKD, future studies evaluating the impact of plant-based diets vs. animal based-diets on muscle heath and sarcopenia, with consideration of overall diet quality and sufficient energy intake, are needed.

### 6.4. Soy Protein and Isoflavones

Given that soy protein contains isoflavones, which are compounds with a similar chemical structure to that of estrogen, it has been debated as to whether they provide health benefits or potential adverse effects (e.g., thyroid dysfunction, breast cancer). However, these concerns have largely stemmed from in vitro cell cultures or rodent studies involving large doses of isoflavones, and multiple lines of research over the past decade have not observed adverse hormonal effects from physiological amounts of soy foods in the diet [86].

### 6.5. Hyperkalemia

There has been a longstanding paradigm in the clinical management of CKD/ESKD patients to avoid plant-based diets and/or fruits due to concerns regarding the risk of hyperkalemia. In a case review of 27 people with underlying CKD, acute kidney injury, or unspecified kidney disease, the majority of hyperkalemic episodes were related to the consumption of plant-based foods with higher bioavailability of potassium (e.g., juices, sauces, or dried fruits) vs. whole foods or unprocessed plant-based foods [88]. Similar to the bioavailability of dietary phosphorus, potassium from unprocessed plant-based foods has lower bioavailability than that of animal-based foods and processed foods. In a crossover feeding trial of 11 healthy men and women, the bioavailability of potassium from unprocessed fruits and vegetables was no more than 60% and lower than that of animal-based foods and fruit juices [98]. Another crossover feeding trial including six volunteers found that processed foods with potassium-containing additives resulted in 90 to 100% potassium bioavailability [99]. A similarly high bioavailability of 50–60% was found in a study of the DASH diet among 11 men and women with CKD over two weeks [32]. A differential association of dietary potassium intake from plant-based and animal-based diets with mortality risk was also found in the NHANES cohort. This study reported that, compared with high dietary potassium intake from plant-based foods, participants with low potassium intake from animal-based foods and pairings of low potassium intake with high protein, low fiber, or high phosphorus consumption were each associated with a higher mortality risk among 3172 participants with impaired kidney function [100]. One possible reason for the lower bioavailability of potassium in plant-based foods may be the increased intercellular potassium uptake induced by the insulin response to concomitant glucose, as well as slower and attenuated rises in serum potassium levels due to high dietary fiber content (Figure 3). Indeed, data from prospective observational and experimental studies, along with cross-sectional analyses examining varying proportions of plant contents, show that the occurrence of hyperkalemia is quite rare with plant-based diets (Figure 4) [87].

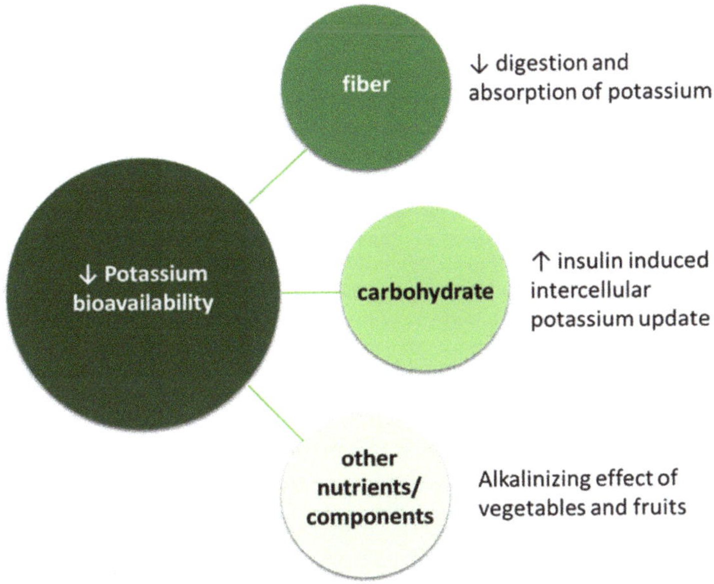


**Figure 3.** Potential mechanisms contributing to the lower bioavailability of potassium from plant-based foods. Abbreviations: K, potassium.

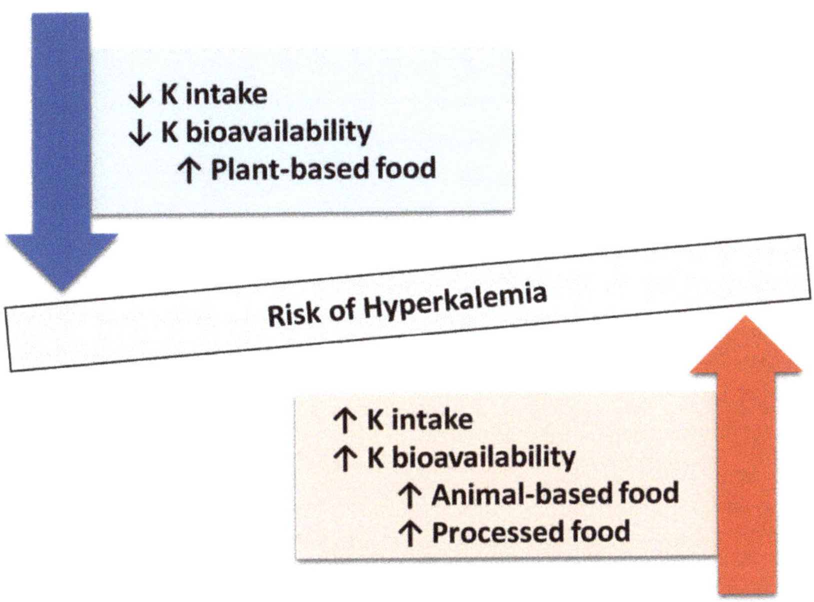


**Figure 4.** Potential dietary factors related to the risk of hyperkalemia. Lower absolute dietary potassium intake and/or having a diet with lower potassium bioavailability following consumption of healthy plant-based diets composed of unprocessed plant-based foods could result in a reduced risk of hyperkalemia. On the other hand, higher absolute dietary potassium intake and/or having a diet with higher potassium bioavailability following consumption of animal-based foods and processed foods could result in increased risk of hyperkalemia. Abbreviations: K, potassium.

### 6.6. *All-Cause Mortality*

Growing data show that plant-based diets are associated with greater survival in the general population, as well as in CKD patients. In an analysis of 1065 people with eGFR < 60 mL/min/1.73 $m^2$ from the NHANES study, each 33% increase in the proportion of plant protein to total protein intake was associated with a 23% lower mortality risk after a mean follow-up of 8.4 years [101]. Another analysis of the NHANES cohort also reported that higher total dietary protein intake of $\geq$1.4 g/kg actual body weight/day and the highest two tertiles of protein intake from animal-based foods were associated with a higher mortality risk among 1994 participants with impaired kidney function [102]. A study of 3972 people with CKD from the REGARDS study observed independent associations of southern and plant-based pattern scores with mortality risk after a mean 6.4 years of follow-up [71]. These results are in agreement with a meta-analysis of studies including 15,285 adults with CKD from seven cohorts, which showed that healthy dietary patterns (i.e., higher intake of fruit and vegetables, legumes, cereals, whole grains, and fiber) were associated with a lower risk of death [70].

## 7. Conclusions

In summary, incorporating vegetarian and plant-based diets using a personalized approach in the clinical management of CKD/ESKD not only provides health benefits to people with kidney disease, but also has the potential to maintain their nutritional status at optimal levels while avoiding the risk of PEW.

**Author Contributions:** Conceptualization, Y.N., K.K.-Z., C.M.R., G.B. and D.Z.; Writing—Original Draft Preparation, Y.N.; Writing—Review and Editing, Supervision, C.M.R., K.K.-Z., G.B. and D.Z.; Project Administration, D.Z. and G.B.; Funding Acquisition, D.Z. and G.B. All authors have read and agreed to the published version of the manuscript.

**Funding:** The authors are supported by research grants from the NIH/NIDDK: R01-DK122767 (C.M.R.), R01-DK124138 (C.M.R., K.K.-Z.), R01-DK132869 (C.M.R., K.K.-Z.), R01-DK132875 (K.K.-Z., C.M.R.), and the Japan Society for the Promotion of Science Overseas Research Fellowship (Y.N.).

**Institutional Review Board Statement:** Not applicable.

**Informed Consent Statement:** Not applicable.

**Data Availability Statement:** Not applicable.

**Conflicts of Interest:** The authors declare no conflicts of interest.

## References

1. Medawar, E.; Huhn, S.; Villringer, A.; Veronica Witte, A. The effects of plant-based diets on the body and the brain: A systematic review. *Transl. Psychiatry* **2019**, *9*, 226. [CrossRef] [PubMed]
2. Satija, A.; Bhupathiraju, S.N.; Rimm, E.B.; Spiegelman, D.; Chiuve, S.E.; Borgi, L.; Willett, W.C.; Manson, J.E.; Sun, Q.; Hu, F.B. Plant-Based Dietary Patterns and Incidence of Type 2 Diabetes in US Men and Women: Results from Three Prospective Cohort Studies. *PLoS Med.* **2016**, *13*, e1002039. [CrossRef] [PubMed]
3. Satija, A.; Bhupathiraju, S.N.; Spiegelman, D.; Chiuve, S.E.; Manson, J.E.; Willett, W.; Rexrode, K.M.; Rimm, E.B.; Hu, F.B. Healthful and Unhealthful Plant-Based Diets and the Risk of Coronary Heart Disease in U.S. Adults. *J. Am. Coll. Cardiol.* **2017**, *70*, 411–422. [CrossRef] [PubMed]
4. Baden, M.Y.; Liu, G.; Satija, A.; Li, Y.; Sun, Q.; Fung, T.T.; Rimm, E.B.; Willett, W.C.; Hu, F.B.; Bhupathiraju, S.N. Changes in Plant-Based Diet Quality and Total and Cause-Specific Mortality. *Circulation* **2019**, *140*, 979–991. [CrossRef] [PubMed]
5. Bellizzi, V.; Cupisti, A.; Locatelli, F.; Bolasco, P.; Brunori, G.; Cancarini, G.; Caria, S.; De Nicola, L.; Di Iorio, B.R.; Di Micco, L.; et al. Low-protein diets for chronic kidney disease patients: The Italian experience. *BMC Nephrol.* **2016**, *17*, 77. [CrossRef] [PubMed]
6. Garneata, L.; Stancu, A.; Dragomir, D.; Stefan, G.; Mircescu, G. Ketoanalogue-Supplemented Vegetarian Very Low-Protein Diet and CKD Progression. *J. Am. Soc. Nephrol.* **2016**, *27*, 2164–2176. [CrossRef] [PubMed]
7. Kalantar-Zadeh, K.; Joshi, S.; Schlueter, R.; Cooke, J.; Brown-Tortorici, A.; Donnelly, M.; Schulman, S.; Lau, W.L.; Rhee, C.M.; Streja, E.; et al. Plant-Dominant Low-Protein Diet for Conservative Management of Chronic Kidney Disease. *Nutrients* **2020**, *12*, 1931. [CrossRef] [PubMed]

8. Kalantar-Zadeh, K.; Rhee, C.M.; Joshi, S.; Brown-Tortorici, A.; Kramer, H.M. Medical nutrition therapy using plant-focused low-protein meal plans for management of chronic kidney disease in diabetes. *Curr. Opin. Nephrol. Hypertens.* **2022**, *31*, 26–35. [CrossRef]
9. Reyes-López, M.A.; Piccoli, G.B.; Leone, F.; Orozco-Guillén, A.; Perichart-Perera, O. Nutrition care for chronic kidney disease during pregnancy: An updated review. *Eur. J. Clin. Nutr.* **2020**, *74*, 983–990. [CrossRef]
10. Piccoli, G.B.; Vigotti, F.N.; Leone, F.; Capizzi, I.; Daidola, G.; Cabiddu, G.; Avagnina, P. Low-protein diets in CKD: How can we achieve them? A narrative, pragmatic review. *Clin. Kidney J.* **2015**, *8*, 61–70. [CrossRef]
11. Gluba-Brzózka, A.; Franczyk, B.; Rysz, J. Vegetarian Diet in Chronic Kidney Disease-A Friend or Foe. *Nutrients* **2017**, *9*, 374. [CrossRef]
12. Foundation, N.K. Plant-Based Diet or Vegetarian Diet—What is the Difference? Available online: https://www.kidney.org/atoz/content/plant-based-diet-or-vegetarian-diet-difference (accessed on 13 December 2023).
13. Ku, E.; Lee, B.J.; Wei, J.; Weir, M.R. Hypertension in CKD: Core Curriculum 2019. *Am. J. Kidney Dis.* **2019**, *74*, 120–131. [CrossRef] [PubMed]
14. Rouse, I.L.; Beilin, L.J.; Armstrong, B.K.; Vandongen, R. Blood-pressure-lowering effect of a vegetarian diet: Controlled trial in normotensive subjects. *Lancet* **1983**, *1*, 5–10. [CrossRef] [PubMed]
15. Margetts, B.M.; Beilin, L.J.; Vandongen, R.; Armstrong, B.K. Vegetarian diet in mild hypertension: A randomised controlled trial. *Br. Med. J. (Clin. Res. Ed.)* **1986**, *293*, 1468–1471. [CrossRef] [PubMed]
16. Appel, L.J.; Moore, T.J.; Obarzanek, E.; Vollmer, W.M.; Svetkey, L.P.; Sacks, F.M.; Bray, G.A.; Vogt, T.M.; Cutler, J.A.; Windhauser, M.M.; et al. A clinical trial of the effects of dietary patterns on blood pressure. DASH Collaborative Research Group. *N. Engl. J. Med.* **1997**, *336*, 1117–1124. [CrossRef] [PubMed]
17. Yokoyama, Y.; Nishimura, K.; Barnard, N.D.; Takegami, M.; Watanabe, M.; Sekikawa, A.; Okamura, T.; Miyamoto, Y. Vegetarian diets and blood pressure: A meta-analysis. *JAMA Intern. Med.* **2014**, *174*, 577–587. [CrossRef] [PubMed]
18. Tonstad, S.; Butler, T.; Yan, R.; Fraser, G.E. Type of vegetarian diet, body weight, and prevalence of type 2 diabetes. *Diabetes Care* **2009**, *32*, 791–796. [CrossRef] [PubMed]
19. Qian, F.; Liu, G.; Hu, F.B.; Bhupathiraju, S.N.; Sun, Q. Association Between Plant-Based Dietary Patterns and Risk of Type 2 Diabetes: A Systematic Review and Meta-analysis. *JAMA Intern. Med.* **2019**, *179*, 1335–1344. [CrossRef]
20. Kahleova, H.; Tura, A.; Hill, M.; Holubkov, R.; Barnard, N.D. A Plant-Based Dietary Intervention Improves Beta-Cell Function and Insulin Resistance in Overweight Adults: A 16-Week Randomized Clinical Trial. *Nutrients* **2018**, *10*, 189. [CrossRef]
21. Kahleova, H.; Matoulek, M.; Malinska, H.; Oliyarnik, O.; Kazdova, L.; Neskudla, T.; Skoch, A.; Hajek, M.; Hill, M.; Kahle, M.; et al. Vegetarian diet improves insulin resistance and oxidative stress markers more than conventional diet in subjects with Type 2 diabetes. *Diabet. Med. A J. Br. Diabet. Assoc.* **2011**, *28*, 549–559. [CrossRef]
22. Huang, R.Y.; Huang, C.C.; Hu, F.B.; Chavarro, J.E. Vegetarian Diets and Weight Reduction: A Meta-Analysis of Randomized Controlled Trials. *J. Gen. Intern. Med.* **2016**, *31*, 109–116. [CrossRef] [PubMed]
23. Mozaffarian, D.; Hao, T.; Rimm, E.B.; Willett, W.C.; Hu, F.B. Changes in diet and lifestyle and long-term weight gain in women and men. *N. Engl. J. Med.* **2011**, *364*, 2392–2404. [CrossRef] [PubMed]
24. Smith, J.D.; Hou, T.; Ludwig, D.S.; Rimm, E.B.; Willett, W.; Hu, F.B.; Mozaffarian, D. Changes in intake of protein foods, carbohydrate amount and quality, and long-term weight change: Results from 3 prospective cohorts. *Am. J. Clin. Nutr.* **2015**, *101*, 1216–1224. [CrossRef] [PubMed]
25. Baden, M.Y.; Satija, A.; Hu, F.B.; Huang, T. Change in Plant-Based Diet Quality Is Associated with Changes in Plasma Adiposity-Associated Biomarker Concentrations in Women. *J. Nutr.* **2019**, *149*, 676–686. [CrossRef] [PubMed]
26. Eichelmann, F.; Schwingshackl, L.; Fedirko, V.; Aleksandrova, K. Effect of plant-based diets on obesity-related inflammatory profiles: A systematic review and meta-analysis of intervention trials. *Obes. Rev.* **2016**, *17*, 1067–1079. [CrossRef]
27. Bowman, S.A. A Vegetarian-Style Dietary Pattern Is Associated with Lower Energy, Saturated Fat, and Sodium Intakes; and Higher Whole Grains, Legumes, Nuts, and Soy Intakes by Adults: National Health and Nutrition Examination Surveys 2013-2016. *Nutrients* **2020**, *12*, 2668. [CrossRef]
28. McMahon, E.J.; Campbell, K.L.; Bauer, J.D.; Mudge, D.W.; Kelly, J.T. Altered dietary salt intake for people with chronic kidney disease. *Cochrane Database Syst. Rev.* **2021**, *6*, Cd010070. [CrossRef]
29. Garofalo, C.; Borrelli, S.; Provenzano, M.; De Stefano, T.; Vita, C.; Chiodini, P.; Minutolo, R.; De Nicola, L.; Conte, G. Dietary Salt Restriction in Chronic Kidney Disease: A Meta-Analysis of Randomized Clinical Trials. *Nutrients* **2018**, *10*, 732. [CrossRef]
30. Shi, H.; Su, X.; Li, C.; Guo, W.; Wang, L. Effect of a low-salt diet on chronic kidney disease outcomes: A systematic review and meta-analysis. *BMJ Open* **2022**, *12*, e050843. [CrossRef]
31. Wang, W.; Soltero, L.; Zhang, P.; Huang, X.R.; Lan, H.Y.; Adrogue, H.J. Renal inflammation is modulated by potassium in chronic kidney disease: Possible role of Smad7. *Am. J. Physiol. Ren. Physiol.* **2007**, *293*, F1123–F1130. [CrossRef]
32. Tyson, C.C.; Lin, P.H.; Corsino, L.; Batch, B.C.; Allen, J.; Sapp, S.; Barnhart, H.; Nwankwo, C.; Burroughs, J.; Svetkey, L.P. Short-term effects of the DASH diet in adults with moderate chronic kidney disease: A pilot feeding study. *Clin. Kidney J.* **2016**, *9*, 592–598. [CrossRef] [PubMed]
33. Goraya, N.; Simoni, J.; Jo, C.H.; Wesson, D.E. A comparison of treating metabolic acidosis in CKD stage 4 hypertensive kidney disease with fruits and vegetables or sodium bicarbonate. *Clin. J. Am. Soc. Nephrol.* **2013**, *8*, 371–381. [CrossRef] [PubMed]

34. Goraya, N.; Simoni, J.; Jo, C.H.; Wesson, D.E. Treatment of metabolic acidosis in patients with stage 3 chronic kidney disease with fruits and vegetables or oral bicarbonate reduces urine angiotensinogen and preserves glomerular filtration rate. *Kidney Int.* **2014**, *86*, 1031–1038. [CrossRef] [PubMed]
35. Turban, S.; Juraschek, S.P.; Miller, E.R., 3rd; Anderson, C.A.M.; White, K.; Charleston, J.; Appel, L.J. Randomized Trial on the Effects of Dietary Potassium on Blood Pressure and Serum Potassium Levels in Adults with Chronic Kidney Disease. *Nutrients* **2021**, *13*, 2678. [CrossRef] [PubMed]
36. Ikizler, T.A.; Burrowes, J.D.; Byham-Gray, L.D.; Campbell, K.L.; Carrero, J.J.; Chan, W.; Fouque, D.; Friedman, A.N.; Ghaddar, S.; Goldstein-Fuchs, D.J.; et al. KDOQI Clinical Practice Guideline for Nutrition in CKD: 2020 Update. *Am. J. Kidney Dis.* **2020**, *76*, S1–S107. [CrossRef] [PubMed]
37. Sánchez-Muniz, F.J. Dietary fibre and cardiovascular health. *Nutr. Hosp.* **2012**, *27*, 31–45. [CrossRef] [PubMed]
38. Tuttle, K.R.; Bakris, G.L.; Bilous, R.W.; Chiang, J.L.; de Boer, I.H.; Goldstein-Fuchs, J.; Hirsch, I.B.; Kalantar-Zadeh, K.; Narva, A.S.; Navaneethan, S.D.; et al. Diabetic kidney disease: A report from an ADA Consensus Conference. *Diabetes Care* **2014**, *37*, 2864–2883. [CrossRef]
39. Trautwein, E.A.; McKay, S. The Role of Specific Components of a Plant-Based Diet in Management of Dyslipidemia and the Impact on Cardiovascular Risk. *Nutrients* **2020**, *12*, 2671. [CrossRef]
40. Montemurno, E.; Cosola, C.; Dalfino, G.; Daidone, G.; De Angelis, M.; Gobbetti, M.; Gesualdo, L. What would you like to eat, Mr CKD Microbiota? A Mediterranean Diet, please! *Kidney Blood Press. Res.* **2014**, *39*, 114–123. [CrossRef]
41. Altorf-van der Kuil, W.; Engberink, M.F.; Brink, E.J.; van Baak, M.A.; Bakker, S.J.; Navis, G.; van't Veer, P.; Geleijnse, J.M. Dietary protein and blood pressure: A systematic review. *PLoS ONE* **2010**, *5*, e12102. [CrossRef]
42. Tielemans, S.M.; Altorf-van der Kuil, W.; Engberink, M.F.; Brink, E.J.; van Baak, M.A.; Bakker, S.J.; Geleijnse, J.M. Intake of total protein, plant protein and animal protein in relation to blood pressure: A meta-analysis of observational and intervention studies. *J. Hum. Hypertens.* **2013**, *27*, 564–571. [CrossRef] [PubMed]
43. Montalcini, T.; De Bonis, D.; Ferro, Y.; Carè, I.; Mazza, E.; Accattato, F.; Greco, M.; Foti, D.; Romeo, S.; Gulletta, E.; et al. High Vegetable Fats Intake Is Associated with High Resting Energy Expenditure in Vegetarians. *Nutrients* **2015**, *7*, 5933–5947. [CrossRef] [PubMed]
44. Narasaki, Y.; Rhee, C.M. Dietary Therapy for Managing Hyperphosphatemia. *Clin. J. Am. Soc. Nephrol.* **2020**, *16*, 9–11. [CrossRef] [PubMed]
45. Kalantar-Zadeh, K.; Gutekunst, L.; Mehrotra, R.; Kovesdy, C.P.; Bross, R.; Shinaberger, C.S.; Noori, N.; Hirschberg, R.; Benner, D.; Nissenson, A.R.; et al. Understanding sources of dietary phosphorus in the treatment of patients with chronic kidney disease. *Clin. J. Am. Soc. Nephrol.* **2010**, *5*, 519–530. [CrossRef] [PubMed]
46. Narasaki, Y.; Yamasaki, M.; Matsuura, S.; Morinishi, M.; Nakagawa, T.; Matsuno, M.; Katsumoto, M.; Nii, S.; Fushitani, Y.; Sugihara, K.; et al. Phosphatemic Index Is a Novel Evaluation Tool for Dietary Phosphorus Load: A Whole-Foods Approach. *J. Ren. Nutr.* **2020**, *30*, 493–502. [CrossRef]
47. Moe, S.M.; Chen, N.X.; Seifert, M.F.; Sinders, R.M.; Duan, D.; Chen, X.; Liang, Y.; Radcliff, J.S.; White, K.E.; Gattone, V.H., 2nd. A rat model of chronic kidney disease-mineral bone disorder. *Kidney Int.* **2009**, *75*, 176–184. [CrossRef]
48. Moe, S.M.; Zidehsarai, M.P.; Chambers, M.A.; Jackman, L.A.; Radcliffe, J.S.; Trevino, L.L.; Donahue, S.E.; Asplin, J.R. Vegetarian compared with meat dietary protein source and phosphorus homeostasis in chronic kidney disease. *Clin. J. Am. Soc. Nephrol.* **2011**, *6*, 257–264. [CrossRef]
49. Azadbakht, L.; Esmaillzadeh, A. Soy-protein consumption and kidney-related biomarkers among type 2 diabetics: A crossover, randomized clinical trial. *J. Ren. Nutr.* **2009**, *19*, 479–486. [CrossRef]
50. Cases, A.; Cigarrán-Guldrís, S.; Mas, S.; Gonzalez-Parra, E. Vegetable-Based Diets for Chronic Kidney Disease? It Is Time to Reconsider. *Nutrients* **2019**, *11*, 1263. [CrossRef]
51. Koppe, L.; Fouque, D.; Soulage, C.O. The Role of Gut Microbiota and Diet on Uremic Retention Solutes Production in the Context of Chronic Kidney Disease. *Toxins* **2018**, *10*, 155. [CrossRef]
52. Marzocco, S.; Dal Piaz, F.; Di Micco, L.; Torraca, S.; Sirico, M.L.; Tartaglia, D.; Autore, G.; Di Iorio, B. Very low protein diet reduces indoxyl sulfate levels in chronic kidney disease. *Blood Purif.* **2013**, *35*, 196–201. [CrossRef] [PubMed]
53. Sirich, T.L.; Plummer, N.S.; Gardner, C.D.; Hostetter, T.H.; Meyer, T.W. Effect of increasing dietary fiber on plasma levels of colon-derived solutes in hemodialysis patients. *Clin. J. Am. Soc. Nephrol.* **2014**, *9*, 1603–1610. [CrossRef] [PubMed]
54. Krishnamurthy, V.M.R.; Wei, G.; Baird, B.C.; Murtaugh, M.; Chonchol, M.B.; Raphael, K.L.; Greene, T.; Beddhu, S. High dietary fiber intake is associated with decreased inflammation and all-cause mortality in patients with chronic kidney disease. *Kidney Int.* **2012**, *81*, 300–306. [CrossRef] [PubMed]
55. Vaziri, N.D.; Liu, S.M.; Lau, W.L.; Khazaeli, M.; Nazertehrani, S.; Farzaneh, S.H.; Kieffer, D.A.; Adams, S.H.; Martin, R.J. High amylose resistant starch diet ameliorates oxidative stress, inflammation, and progression of chronic kidney disease. *PLoS ONE* **2014**, *9*, e114881. [CrossRef] [PubMed]
56. Dahl, W.J.; Stewart, M.L. Position of the Academy of Nutrition and Dietetics: Health Implications of Dietary Fiber. *J. Acad. Nutr. Diet.* **2015**, *115*, 1861–1870. [CrossRef] [PubMed]
57. Dhingra, D.; Michael, M.; Rajput, H.; Patil, R.T. Dietary fibre in foods: A review. *J. Food Sci. Technol.* **2012**, *49*, 255–266. [CrossRef] [PubMed]

58. Veronese, N.; Solmi, M.; Caruso, M.G.; Giannelli, G.; Osella, A.R.; Evangelou, E.; Maggi, S.; Fontana, L.; Stubbs, B.; Tzoulaki, I. Dietary fiber and health outcomes: An umbrella review of systematic reviews and meta-analyses. *Am. J. Clin. Nutr.* **2018**, *107*, 436–444. [CrossRef]
59. Xiong, R.G.; Zhou, D.D.; Wu, S.X.; Huang, S.Y.; Saimaiti, A.; Yang, Z.J.; Shang, A.; Zhao, C.N.; Gan, R.Y.; Li, H.B. Health Benefits and Side Effects of Short-Chain Fatty Acids. *Foods* **2022**, *11*, 2863. [CrossRef]
60. de Brito-Ashurst, I.; Varagunam, M.; Raftery, M.J.; Yaqoob, M.M. Bicarbonate supplementation slows progression of CKD and improves nutritional status. *J. Am. Soc. Nephrol.* **2009**, *20*, 2075–2084. [CrossRef]
61. Yuzbashian, E.; Asghari, G.; Mirmiran, P.; Hosseini, F.S.; Azizi, F. Associations of dietary macronutrients with glomerular filtration rate and kidney dysfunction: Tehran lipid and glucose study. *J. Nephrol.* **2015**, *28*, 173–180. [CrossRef]
62. Nettleton, J.A.; Steffen, L.M.; Palmas, W.; Burke, G.L.; Jacobs, D.R., Jr. Associations between microalbuminuria and animal foods, plant foods, and dietary patterns in the Multiethnic Study of Atherosclerosis. *Am. J. Clin. Nutr.* **2008**, *87*, 1825–1836. [CrossRef] [PubMed]
63. Haring, B.; Selvin, E.; Liang, M.; Coresh, J.; Grams, M.E.; Petruski-Ivleva, N.; Steffen, L.M.; Rebholz, C.M. Dietary Protein Sources and Risk for Incident Chronic Kidney Disease: Results From the Atherosclerosis Risk in Communities (ARIC) Study. *J. Ren. Nutr.* **2017**, *27*, 233–242. [CrossRef] [PubMed]
64. Knight, E.L.; Stampfer, M.J.; Hankinson, S.E.; Spiegelman, D.; Curhan, G.C. The Impact of Protein Intake on Renal Function Decline in Women with Normal Renal Function or Mild Renal Insufficiency. *Ann. Intern. Med.* **2003**, *138*, 460–467. [CrossRef] [PubMed]
65. Teixeira, S.R.; Tappenden, K.A.; Carson, L.; Jones, R.; Prabhudesai, M.; Marshall, W.P.; Erdman, J.W., Jr. Isolated soy protein consumption reduces urinary albumin excretion and improves the serum lipid profile in men with type 2 diabetes mellitus and nephropathy. *J. Nutr.* **2004**, *134*, 1874–1880. [CrossRef] [PubMed]
66. Azadbakht, L.; Atabak, S.; Esmaillzadeh, A. Soy protein intake, cardiorenal indices, and C-reactive protein in type 2 diabetes with nephropathy: A longitudinal randomized clinical trial. *Diabetes Care* **2008**, *31*, 648–654. [CrossRef] [PubMed]
67. Świątek, Ł.; Jeske, J.; Miedziaszczyk, M.; Idasiak-Piechocka, I. The impact of a vegetarian diet on chronic kidney disease (CKD) progression—A systematic review. *BMC Nephrol.* **2023**, *24*, 168. [CrossRef]
68. Kelly, J.T.; Carrero, J.J. Dietary Sources of Protein and Chronic Kidney Disease Progression: The Proof May Be in the Pattern. *J. Ren. Nutr.* **2017**, *27*, 221–224. [CrossRef] [PubMed]
69. Lew, Q.-L.J.; Jafar, T.H.; Koh, H.W.L.; Jin, A.; Chow, K.Y.; Yuan, J.-M.; Koh, W.-P. Red meat intake and risk of ESRD. *J. Am. Soc. Nephrol.* **2017**, *28*, 304–312. [CrossRef]
70. Kelly, J.T.; Palmer, S.C.; Wai, S.N.; Ruospo, M.; Carrero, J.J.; Campbell, K.L.; Strippoli, G.F. Healthy Dietary Patterns and Risk of Mortality and ESRD in CKD: A Meta-Analysis of Cohort Studies. *Clin. J. Am. Soc. Nephrol.* **2017**, *12*, 272–279. [CrossRef]
71. Gutiérrez, O.M.; Muntner, P.; Rizk, D.V.; McClellan, W.M.; Warnock, D.G.; Newby, P.K.; Judd, S.E. Dietary patterns and risk of death and progression to ESRD in individuals with CKD: A cohort study. *Am. J. Kidney Dis.* **2014**, *64*, 204–213. [CrossRef]
72. Kalantar-Zadeh, K.; Ikizler, T.A.; Block, G.; Avram, M.M.; Kopple, J.D. Malnutrition-inflammation complex syndrome in dialysis patients: Causes and consequences. *Am. J. Kidney Dis.* **2003**, *42*, 864–881. [CrossRef] [PubMed]
73. Levey, A.S.; Coresh, J.; Bolton, K.; Culleton, B.; Harvey, K.S.; Ikizler, T.A.; Johnson, C.A.; Kausz, A.; Kimmel, P.L.; Kusek, J. K/DOQI clinical practice guidelines for chronic kidney disease: Evaluation, classification, and stratification. *Am. J. Kidney Dis.* **2002**, *39*, S1–S266.
74. Ogborn, M.R.; Bankovic-Calic, N.; Shoesmith, C.; Buist, R.; Peeling, J. Soy protein modification of rat polycystic kidney disease. *Am. J. Physiol.* **1998**, *274*, F541–F549. [CrossRef] [PubMed]
75. Trujillo, J.; Ramírez, V.; Pérez, J.; Torre-Villalvazo, I.; Torres, N.; Tovar, A.R.; Muñoz, R.M.; Uribe, N.; Gamba, G.; Bobadilla, N.A. Renal protection by a soy diet in obese Zucker rats is associated with restoration of nitric oxide generation. *Am. J. Physiol. Ren. Physiol.* **2005**, *288*, F108–F116. [CrossRef] [PubMed]
76. Mitch, W.E.; Remuzzi, G. Diets for patients with chronic kidney disease, should we reconsider? *BMC Nephrol.* **2016**, *17*, 80. [CrossRef] [PubMed]
77. Jibani, M.M.; Bloodworth, L.L.; Foden, E.; Griffiths, K.D.; Galpin, O.P. Predominantly vegetarian diet in patients with incipient and early clinical diabetic nephropathy: Effects on albumin excretion rate and nutritional status. *Diabet. Med. A J. Br. Diabet. Assoc.* **1991**, *8*, 949–953. [CrossRef] [PubMed]
78. Barsotti, G.; Morelli, E.; Cupisti, A.; Meola, M.; Dani, L.; Giovannetti, S. A low-nitrogen low-phosphorus Vegan diet for patients with chronic renal failure. *Nephron* **1996**, *74*, 390–394. [CrossRef]
79. Milovanova, L.Y.; Volkov, A.V.; Milovanova, S.Y.; Taranova, M.V.; Nezhdanov, K.S. Soy Protein as a Part of a Low-protein Diet is a New Direction in Cardio- and Nephroprotection in Patients With 3b-4 Stages of Chronic kidney Disease. *J. Ren. Nutr.* **2023**, *33*, 435–442. [CrossRef]
80. Wu, T.T.; Chang, C.Y.; Hsu, W.M.; Wang, I.K.; Hsu, C.H.; Cheng, S.H.; Liang, C.C.; Chang, C.T.; Huang, C.C. Nutritional status of vegetarians on maintenance haemodialysis. *Nephrology* **2011**, *16*, 582–587. [CrossRef]
81. Neufingerl, N.; Eilander, A. Nutrient Intake and Status in Adults Consuming Plant-Based Diets Compared to Meat-Eaters: A Systematic Review. *Nutrients* **2021**, *14*, 29. [CrossRef]
82. Rizzo, N.S.; Jaceldo-Siegl, K.; Sabate, J.; Fraser, G.E. Nutrient profiles of vegetarian and nonvegetarian dietary patterns. *J. Acad. Nutr. Diet.* **2013**, *113*, 1610–1619. [CrossRef] [PubMed]

83. Young, V.R.; Pellett, P.L. Plant proteins in relation to human protein and amino acid nutrition. *Am. J. Clin. Nutr.* **1994**, *59*, 1203s–1212s. [CrossRef] [PubMed]
84. Tang, J.E.; Moore, D.R.; Kujbida, G.W.; Tarnopolsky, M.A.; Phillips, S.M. Ingestion of whey hydrolysate, casein, or soy protein isolate: Effects on mixed muscle protein synthesis at rest and following resistance exercise in young men. *J. Appl. Physiol.* **2009**, *107*, 987–992. [CrossRef] [PubMed]
85. Messina, M.; Lynch, H.; Dickinson, J.M.; Reed, K.E. No Difference Between the Effects of Supplementing With Soy Protein Versus Animal Protein on Gains in Muscle Mass and Strength in Response to Resistance Exercise. *Int. J. Sport. Nutr. Exerc. Metab.* **2018**, *28*, 674–685. [CrossRef] [PubMed]
86. Additives, E.P.o.F.; Food, N.S.a.t. Risk assessment for peri-and post-menopausal women taking food supplements containing isolated isoflavones. *EFSA J.* **2015**, *13*, 4246.
87. Joshi, S.; McMacken, M.; Kalantar-Zadeh, K. Plant-Based Diets for Kidney Disease: A Guide for Clinicians. *Am. J. Kidney Dis.* **2021**, *77*, 287–296. [CrossRef]
88. Te Dorsthorst, R.P.M.; Hendrikse, J.; Vervoorn, M.T.; van Weperen, V.Y.H.; van der Heyden, M.A.G. Review of case reports on hyperkalemia induced by dietary intake: Not restricted to chronic kidney disease patients. *Eur. J. Clin. Nutr.* **2019**, *73*, 38–45. [CrossRef]
89. Melina, V.; Craig, W.; Levin, S. Position of the Academy of Nutrition and Dietetics: Vegetarian Diets. *J. Acad. Nutr. Diet.* **2016**, *116*, 1970–1980. [CrossRef]
90. Zarantonello, D.; Brunori, G. The Role of Plant-Based Diets in Preventing and Mitigating Chronic Kidney Disease: More Light than Shadows. *J. Clin. Med.* **2023**, *12*, 6137. [CrossRef]
91. Zong, G.; Li, Y.; Sampson, L.; Dougherty, L.W.; Willett, W.C.; Wanders, A.J.; Alssema, M.; Zock, P.L.; Hu, F.B.; Sun, Q. Monounsaturated fats from plant and animal sources in relation to risk of coronary heart disease among US men and women. *Am. J. Clin. Nutr.* **2018**, *107*, 445–453. [CrossRef]
92. Guasch-Ferré, M.; Zong, G.; Willett, W.C.; Zock, P.L.; Wanders, A.J.; Hu, F.B.; Sun, Q. Associations of Monounsaturated Fatty Acids From Plant and Animal Sources With Total and Cause-Specific Mortality in Two US Prospective Cohort Studies. *Circ. Res.* **2019**, *124*, 1266–1275. [CrossRef] [PubMed]
93. Hertzler, S.R.; Lieblein-Boff, J.C.; Weiler, M.; Allgeier, C. Plant Proteins: Assessing Their Nutritional Quality and Effects on Health and Physical Function. *Nutrients* **2020**, *12*, 3704. [CrossRef] [PubMed]
94. Hartman, J.W.; Tang, J.E.; Wilkinson, S.B.; Tarnopolsky, M.A.; Lawrence, R.L.; Fullerton, A.V.; Phillips, S.M. Consumption of fat-free fluid milk after resistance exercise promotes greater lean mass accretion than does consumption of soy or carbohydrate in young, novice, male weightlifters. *Am. J. Clin. Nutr.* **2007**, *86*, 373–381. [CrossRef] [PubMed]
95. Volek, J.S.; Volk, B.M.; Gómez, A.L.; Kunces, L.J.; Kupchak, B.R.; Freidenreich, D.J.; Aristizabal, J.C.; Saenz, C.; Dunn-Lewis, C.; Ballard, K.D.; et al. Whey protein supplementation during resistance training augments lean body mass. *J. Am. Coll. Nutr.* **2013**, *32*, 122–135. [CrossRef] [PubMed]
96. Kim, J.; Lee, Y.; Kye, S.; Chung, Y.S.; Kim, K.M. Association of vegetables and fruits consumption with sarcopenia in older adults: The Fourth Korea National Health and Nutrition Examination Survey. *Age Ageing* **2015**, *44*, 96–102. [CrossRef] [PubMed]
97. Inoshita, H.; Asaoka, D.; Matsuno, K.; Yanagisawa, N.; Suzuki, Y.; Miyauchi, K. Cross-Sectional Study on the Association between Dietary Patterns and Sarcopenia in Elderly Patients with Chronic Kidney Disease Receiving Conservative Treatment. *Nutrients* **2023**, *15*, 4994. [CrossRef] [PubMed]
98. Naismith, D.J.; Braschi, A. An investigation into the bioaccessibility of potassium in unprocessed fruits and vegetables. *Int. J. Food Sci. Nutr.* **2008**, *59*, 438–450. [CrossRef] [PubMed]
99. Braschi, A.; Gill, L.; Naismith, D.J. Partial substitution of sodium with potassium in white bread: Feasibility and bioavailability. *Int. J. Food Sci. Nutr.* **2009**, *60*, 507–521. [CrossRef]
100. Narasaki, Y.; You, A.S.; Malik, S.; Moore, L.W.; Bross, R.; Cervantes, M.K.; Daza, A.; Kovesdy, C.P.; Nguyen, D.V.; Kalantar-Zadeh, K.; et al. Dietary potassium intake, kidney function, and survival in a nationally representative cohort. *Am. J. Clin. Nutr.* **2022**, *116*, 1123–1134. [CrossRef]
101. Chen, X.; Wei, G.; Jalili, T.; Metos, J.; Giri, A.; Cho, M.E.; Boucher, R.; Greene, T.; Beddhu, S. The Associations of Plant Protein Intake With All-Cause Mortality in CKD. *Am. J. Kidney Dis.* **2016**, *67*, 423–430. [CrossRef]
102. Narasaki, Y.; Okuda, Y.; Moore, L.W.; You, A.S.; Tantisattamo, E.; Inrig, J.K.; Miyagi, T.; Nakata, T.; Kovesdy, C.P.; Nguyen, D.V.; et al. Dietary protein intake, kidney function, and survival in a nationally representative cohort. *Am. J. Clin. Nutr.* **2021**, *114*, 303–313. [CrossRef] [PubMed]

*nutrients*

MDPI

*Article*

# Impact of Reducing Intake of Red and Processed Meat on Colorectal Cancer Incidence in Germany 2020 to 2050—A Simulation Study

**Tobias Niedermaier [1,*,†], Thomas Gredner [1,†], Michael Hoffmeister [1], Ute Mons [1,2,3] and Hermann Brenner [1,4,5]**

1 Division of Clinical Epidemiology and Aging Research, German Cancer Research Center (DKFZ), 69120 Heidelberg, Germany
2 Cancer Prevention Unit, German Cancer Research Center (DKFZ), 69120 Heidelberg, Germany
3 Department of Cardiology, Faculty of Medicine and University Hospital Cologne, University of Cologne, 50931 Cologne, Germany
4 Division of Preventive Oncology, German Cancer Research Center (DKFZ) and National Center for Tumor Diseases (NCT), 69120 Heidelberg, Germany
5 German Cancer Consortium (DKTK), German Cancer Research Center (DKFZ), 69120 Heidelberg, Germany
* Correspondence: t.niedermaier@dkfz-heidelberg.de
† These authors contributed equally to this work.

**Abstract:** Background: According to the International Agency for Research on Cancer (IARC), there is sufficient evidence for the carcinogenicity of processed meat consumption in humans, specifically regarding colorectal cancer (CRC) risk. Evidence for the carcinogenicity of red meat consumption is more limited but points in the same direction. Methods: A macro-simulation approach was used to calculate age- and sex-specific potential impact fractions in a 30-year period (2020–2050). Aims: We estimated numbers and proportions of future CRC cases preventable under different scenarios of reducing the intake of processed and red meat in the German population. Results: Eliminating processed meat intake could reduce the burden of CRC by approximately 205,000 cases in Germany (9.6%) in 2020–2050, 2/3 among males (145,000) and 1/3 among females (60,000). Without red meat intake, approximately 63,000 CRC cases could be avoided (2.9%), 39,000 among males and 24,000 among females. Reductions in the mean consumption of both processed and red meat by one or two servings (each 11 or 22 g) per day would be expected to reduce CRC case numbers by 68,000 (3.1%) and 140,000 (6.5%), respectively. Conclusion: A reduction in red and processed meat intake might substantially reduce the incidence of CRC in Germany. The means of achieving such a reduction might include price and taxation policies, food labeling, and clearer risk communication aiming to reduce individual intake.

**Keywords:** potential impact fraction; red meat; processed meat; colorectal cancer; policy intervention

## 1. Introduction

Colorectal cancer (CRC) ranks second among the most common cancer-related causes of death, and third among the most common cancers, with approximately 870,000 and 1.1 million new cases among women and men worldwide, respectively, in 2020 [1]. In Germany, CRC is the third most common cancer in terms of incidence, with approximately 60,000 incident cases annually, and the second most common cancer in terms of mortality, with approximately 25,000 deaths per year. Furthermore, it involves substantial treatment costs [2]. The International Agency for Research on Cancer (IARC) concluded in 2018 that there was "sufficient evidence in humans for the carcinogenicity of consumption of processed meat" (Group 1) with respect to CRC [3]. This classification is based on "sufficient evidence" from epidemiological studies. Similarly, red meat was classified as a likely cancer risk factor (Group 2A, probably carcinogenic to humans). This classification is based on "limited evidence" from epidemiological studies (confounding could not be ruled out).

The intake of red or processed meat is high in Germany: According to a nationally representative survey from 2008 to 2011 (German Health Interview and Examination Survey for Adults—DEGS1) [4], the median daily intake is approximately 38 g of red meat and of 46 g of processed meat. The IARC recommends limiting the daily intake of red or processed meat. Every 100 g of red meat intake or 50 g of processed meat intake per day have been associated with an increase in CRC risk by 12% and 16%, respectively [5]. More than a quarter of the adult population consumes more than 108 g of red or processed meat per day (756 g per week) [4], which by far exceeds the recommendation of the German Nutrition Society of 300–600 g per week [6]. A previous study estimated that of all incident CRC cases in 2018, 11.4% could be attributed to processed meat consumption, and 0.7% to red meat consumption [7].

Reducing the amount of red and processed meat consumed is, thus, expected to have a relevant potential to reduce the incidence of CRC in Germany. In this study, we estimated the potential impact of a reduction in or elimination of red or processed meat intake on numbers of CRC cases in the German population from 2020 until 2050.

## 2. Materials and Methods

We applied a macro-simulation approach in which age- and sex-specific potential impact fractions (PIFs) were calculated, based on expected numbers of CRC cases in Germany and preventable CRC cases if changes in dietary habits occurred, i.e., if consumption of red and/or processed meat was reduced or eliminated. Similar to population-attributable fractions (PAFs), PIFs reflect a proportional decline in disease (here: CRC) risk following a partial or complete removal of exposure to one or more cancer risk factors [8]. The following input parameters were used in the simulation model:

### *2.1. Red and Processed Meat Intake*

We used self-reported information on the amount and frequency of red and processed meat intake from the DEGS1 survey, a nationally representative survey in which health status and health behavior were assessed among 8152 adults aged 18 to 79 years from Germany in 2008 to 2011. The validated food frequency questionnaire in DEGS1 with 53 items included information on the frequency of different types of red meat (including hamburgers, kebab, all types of pork, beef, and deer) and processed meat (sausages or ham) and the amount of the respective type of meat (number of servings per day). Portion sizes in grams were taken from a Master thesis conducted at the Robert Koch Institute (RKI) [9], from which we derived intake in grams per day.

### *2.2. Expected Numbers of CRC Cases without Intervention*

Data on CRC incidence in Germany was taken from the German Centre for Cancer Registry Data (ZfKD), Robert Koch Institute, Berlin [10]. Expected numbers of CRC cases without any intervention were estimated assuming age- and sex-specific incidence rates to remain constant at the levels observed in 2017/2018 and forecasts of the sex- and age-specific population figures (variant 1 assuming moderate changes in fertility, life expectancy, and net immigration) made by the Federal Statistical Office [11].

### *2.3. Risk Estimates*

Relative risks (RRs) for the association between red or processed meat intake and risk of CRC were obtained from a published report by the World Cancer Research Fund (WCRF)/International Agency for the Research on Cancer (IARC) [5], according to which CRC risk is increased by 16% for every unit of 50 g of processed meat per day, and by 12% for every unit of 100 g of red meat per day.

Red or processed meat intake, respectively, were assumed to be reduced or eliminated over a 5-year period (2020–2024). CRC risk reductions following a reduction in red or processed meat intake were not assumed to take effect immediately. Instead, the concepts of latency times (LAT) and lag times (LAG) were applied [12]. During the LAT time, cancer risk remained constant after cancer risk factor exposure changed. During the subsequent LAG time, risk gradually changed (here: decreased) until the risk of individuals not exposed to the risk factor was reached (relative risk [RR] = 1). In our main analysis, we assumed a LAT time of 1 year and a LAG time of 9 years. In sensitivity analyses, the LAG time was varied between 5 and 15 years. Those durations are reasonable estimates based on the previously reported time for development from preclinical cancer to manifest CRC of approximately 5 years [13], plus approximately 5 years that are required for the development of CRC from adenomas [14–16].

### 2.4. Statistical Analysis

Let $RR_{rm}$ be the relative risk of CRC per 100 g red meat consumed per day, and $RR_{pm}$ be the relative risk per 50 g processed meat consumed per day.

According to the WCRF/AICR estimates [5], $RR_{pm}$ and $RR_{rm}$ were assumed to be 1.16 and 1.12, respectively. Let $M_{pm}$ and $M_{rm}$ be the mean consumption of processed or red meat in each individual, respectively. Assuming a log–linear relationship between consumption of red or processed meat and CRC risk, the RRs for individual consumption levels ($RR_{pm,\,i}$ and $RR_{rm,\,i}$) compared to no consumption were computed as follows:

$$RR_{rm,\,i} = \exp\,(M_{rm,\,i} \bullet \ln\,(RR_{rm})/100)$$

$$RR_{pm,\,i} = \exp\,(M_{pm,\,i} \bullet \ln\,(RR_{pm})/50)$$

For example, if an individual consumes 50 g of red meat, this individual $RR_{rm,\,i}$ would be $\exp(50 \bullet \ln(1.16)/100) = 1.08$. Then, the potential impact fraction (PIF) of the incidence resulting from the modification in the processed or red meat consumption was calculated, using the "RR shift" method [8]:

$$\text{PIF} = 1 - \sum_{\text{i}}^{\text{n}} \text{RR}_i(M_i^*) / \sum_{\text{i}}^{\text{n}} \text{RR}_i(M_i)$$

where $M_i$ is the consumption level of processed or red meat of individual $i$, $RR_i$ is the corresponding time-dependent CRC relative risk for that individual (which we assumed to be independent of age in the absence of age-dependent RRs), and $M_i^*$ is the modified consumption level of individual $i$ in a specific intervention scenario. If, for example, everyone consumed an amount of processed meat corresponding to an RR of 1.16 (=50 g), and that amount was reduced by 50%, the corresponding PIF would be 1 − (1.08/1.16) = 0.07, or 7%.

For our simulation scenarios, sex- and age-specific (5-year age groups) estimates of PIF were multiplied with predicted sex- and age-specific numbers of CRC cases in the absence of any specific intervention, assuming constant incidence rates over time at the level of 2020.

We examined the following interventions: reduction in mean red meat intake by one serving per week (75 g per week or approximately 10.7 g per day), reduction by two servings per week, and elimination of red meat intake. Analogous scenarios were examined for processed meat intake, assuming the same serving sizes. All analyses were performed with the statistical software R [17] version 4.1.3.

## 3. Results

Between 2008 and 2011, the age-standardized mean amount (frequency multiplied with the amount per serving) of red and processed meat intake in grams per day according to the nationally representative DEGS1 survey was as follows: men, 47 g and 61 g, respectively; women, 29 g and 32 g, respectively (Table 1). The intake of red and processed meat was higher among males than among females in all age groups. More than 500 g of red meat per week was consumed by 5% of the females and 13% of the males, and more than 150 g of processed meat was consumed by 52% of women and 80% of men.

**Table 1.** Summary statistics of red and processed meat intake (grams/day) in Germany according to the DEGS1 survey among 8152 adults aged 18 to 79 conducted between 2008 and 2011, overall, by sex, and by 5-year age categories.

| | Males | Females | Overall | 18–24 | 25–29 | 30–34 | 35–39 | 40–44 | 45–49 | 50–54 | 55–59 | 60–64 | 65–69 | 70–74 | 75–79 |
|---|---|---|---|---|---|---|---|---|---|---|---|---|---|---|---|
| Red meat intake | | | | | | | | | | | | | | | |
| Minimum | 0 | 0 | 0 | 0 | 0 | 0 | 0 | 0 | 0 | 0 | 0 | 0 | 0 | 0 | 0 |
| 1st quartile | 11 | 11 | 11 | 11 | 11 | 11 | 13 | 11 | 11 | 11 | 11 | 11 | 11 | 11 | 11 |
| Median | 26 | 26 | 26 | 26 | 26 | 26 | 26 | 26 | 26 | 26 | 26 | 26 | 26 | 26 | 26 |
| Mean | 47 | 29 | 38 | 45 | 39 | 39 | 41 | 38 | 37 | 37 | 33 | 35 | 34 | 29 | 28 |
| 3rd quartile | 60 | 30 | 60 | 60 | 60 | 60 | 60 | 60 | 60 | 60 | 60 | 60 | 60 | 30 | 30 |
| 99th perc. | 240 | 120 | 189 | 240 | 240 | 240 | 240 | 120 | 120 | 120 | 120 | 120 | 120 | 120 | 120 |
| Processed meat intake | | | | | | | | | | | | | | | |
| Minimum | 0 | 0 | 0 | 0 | 0 | 0 | 0 | 0 | 0 | 0 | 0 | 0 | 0 | 0 | 0 |
| 1st quartile | 24 | 11 | 16 | 19 | 16 | 18 | 19 | 17 | 17 | 17 | 17 | 14 | 14 | 15 | 12 |
| Median | 47 | 23 | 33 | 42 | 37 | 38 | 40 | 36 | 35 | 34 | 32 | 27 | 29 | 27 | 26 |
| Mean | 61 | 32 | 46 | 55 | 50 | 55 | 54 | 47 | 47 | 46 | 44 | 39 | 39 | 35 | 36 |
| 3rd quartile | 78 | 42 | 59 | 74 | 66 | 66 | 73 | 63 | 62 | 60 | 55 | 52 | 54 | 48 | 45 |
| 99th perc. | 242 | 169 | 220 | 239 | 199 | 219 | 244 | 213 | 236 | 199 | 511 | 169 | 172 | 147 | 171 |
| Red and processed meat intake | | | | | | | | | | | | | | | |
| Minimum | 0 | 0 | 0 | 0 | 0 | 0 | 0 | 0 | 0 | 0 | 0 | 0 | 0 | 0 | 0 |
| 1st quartile | 54 | 28 | 37 | 41 | 35 | 39 | 44 | 40 | 41 | 40 | 37 | 36 | 35 | 35 | 32 |
| Median | 89 | 48 | 68 | 77 | 66 | 70 | 75 | 73 | 69 | 72 | 65 | 65 | 63 | 56 | 52 |
| Mean | 107 | 61 | 84 | 100 | 88 | 95 | 95 | 86 | 84 | 83 | 76 | 74 | 73 | 65 | 64 |
| 3rd quartile | 135 | 81 | 108 | 133 | 123 | 119 | 122 | 111 | 106 | 110 | 101 | 97 | 97 | 85 | 85 |
| 99th perc. | 415 | 233 | 340 | 478 | 410 | 341 | 378 | 309 | 356 | 323 | 275 | 231 | 278 | 203 | 235 |

Abbreviations: perc., percentile; DEGS1, first wave of the "study on health among adults in Germany".

Without any intervention, approximately 1.2 million CRC cases are expected to occur among men between 2020 and 2050, and approximately 940,000 cases among women, of which approximately 15% (men) and 9% (women) can statistically be attributed to the intake of processed and red meat (Table 2).

**Table 2.** Estimated number and proportion of colorectal cancer cases preventable under different theoretical scenarios of reducing red and processed meat intake over a 30-year period (2020–2050) in the German population, stratified by sex.

| Sex Analysis | Expected Number of Cancer Cases in the Absence of Changes | Total (#) and Relative (%) Number of Prevented Colorectal Cancer Cases Per Scenario | | | | | | | | | | | |
|---|---|---|---|---|---|---|---|---|---|---|---|---|---|
| | | -1 Serving Red Meat Per Day | | -2 Servings Red Meat Per Day | | Elimination of Red Meat Intake | | -1 Serving Processed Meat Per Day | | -2 Servings Processed Meat Per Day | | Elimination of Processed Meat Intake | |
| | | # | % | # | % | # | % | # | % | # | % | # | % |
| Men | | | | | | | | | | | | | |
| Main analysis [1] | 1,208,329 | 10,890 | 0.9 | 19,292 | 1.6 | 39,178 | 3.2 | 28,633 | 2.4 | 60,721 | 5.0 | 145,291 | 12.0 |
| Lag time: 5 years | | 11,718 | 1.0 | 20,763 | 1.7 | 42,183 | 3.5 | 30,809 | 2.5 | 65,334 | 5.4 | 156,403 | 12.9 |
| Lag time: 15 years | | 9611 | 0.8 | 17,019 | 1.4 | 34,541 | 2.9 | 25,268 | 2.1 | 53,586 | 4.4 | 128,182 | 10.6 |
| Women | | | | | | | | | | | | | |
| Main analysis [1] | 939,932 | 7641 | 0.8 | 12,925 | 1.4 | 23,611 | 2.5 | 20,381 | 2.2 | 46,975 | 5.0 | 60,273 | 6.4 |
| Lag time: 5 years | | 8224 | 0.9 | 13,927 | 1.5 | 25,446 | 2.7 | 21,960 | 2.3 | 50,607 | 5.4 | 64,978 | 6.9 |
| Lag time: 15 years | | 6732 | 0.7 | 11,387 | 1.2 | 20,800 | 2.2 | 17,989 | 1.9 | 41,401 | 4.4 | 53,073 | 5.6 |

[1] Red or processed meat intake, respectively, is assumed to be reduced or eliminated over a 5-year period (2020–2024). Assuming a lag period of 9 years and a latency period of 1 year if not stated otherwise.

Figure 1a shows the potential impact fractions (i.e., preventable proportions of cases) multiplied with expected case numbers, thus the expected preventable numbers of cases, for CRC in the investigated time frame in the scenario of reduced or eliminated red meat consumption. By assumption, annual preventable case numbers would gradually increase in the initial 10 years due to the assumed latency (1 year) and lag (9 years) time. Thereafter, numbers would remain largely constant and vary only due to projected differences in the expected case numbers resulting from demographic changes. A permanent decrease in red meat intake by only one serving per day could reduce the annual number of CRC cases by almost 500 among men and by more than 300 among women (Figure S1). Two servings less would correspond to almost twice those numbers. Eliminating the risk factor "red meat" could prevent more than 1700 cases among men and 1000 cases among women every year in the long term in Germany.

Figure 1b shows the corresponding numbers for processed meat. Numbers of preventable CRC cases per year would be much higher than for red meat because of the higher RR associated with processed meat intake compared to the same amount of red meat. More than 6000 cases among men and more than 2500 among women could eventually be prevented per year by eliminating processed meat consumption, with correspondingly lower reductions if consumption was reduced by only two or only one serving per day (Figure S2).

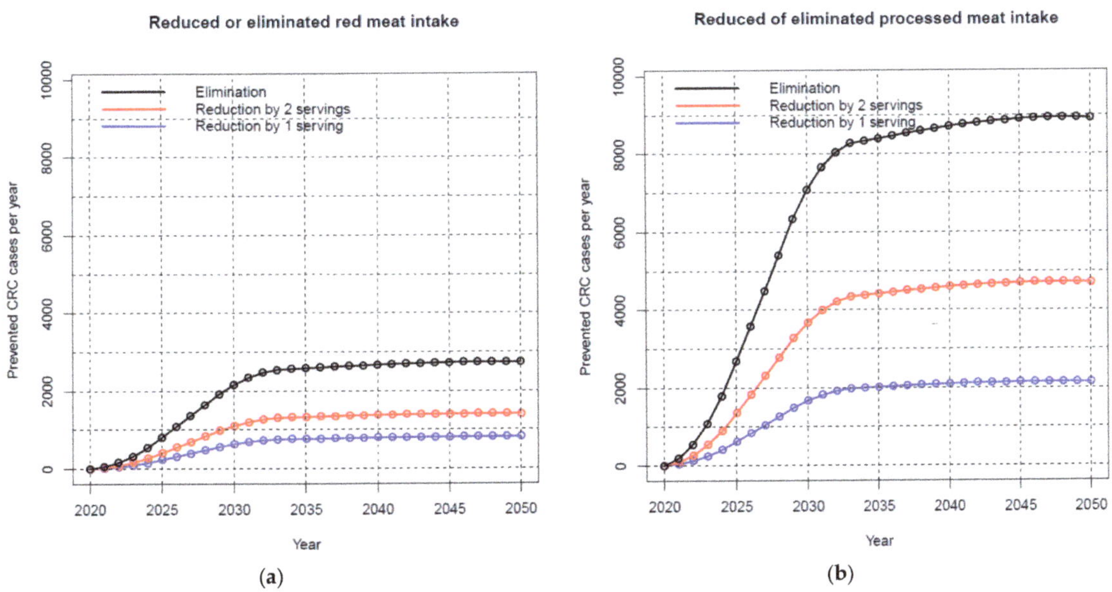


**Figure 1.** Prevented colorectal cancer cases per year in case of a reduction in consumption of (**a**) red meat and (**b**) processed meat (men and women combined). Abbreviations: CRC, colorectal cancer.

The cumulative effect of reduced red meat intake on CRC incidence is shown in Figure 2a and summarized in Table 2. Over the entire study period (until 2050), numbers of preventable CRC cases with eliminated red meat intake would sum up to almost 40,000 among men and more than 20,000 among women. Reduction would be larger among men than among women because of the higher CRC incidence and meat consumption among men. Reducing the amount of red meat consumed by one serving per day is expected to lower the number of CRC cases in that time frame by almost 19,000 among men and women combined. Two servings less of red meat intake could reduce the number of CRC cases by more than 19,000 among men alone, and almost 13,000 among women, i.e., by approximately 32,000 cases in total.

Reducing processed meat intake by one serving per day was estimated to decrease the number of incident CRC cases by almost 50,000, again with a higher number among men (almost 29,000) than among women (more than 20,000). Higher numbers of preventable CRC cases could be achieved if intake could be reduced by two servings per day (in total more than 100,000, approximately 61,000 among men and 47,000 among women). In the optimistic scenario of an elimination of processed meat intake, almost 206,000 cases of CRC could potentially be avoided until 2050, thereof approximately two thirds among men (Table 2, Figure 2b).

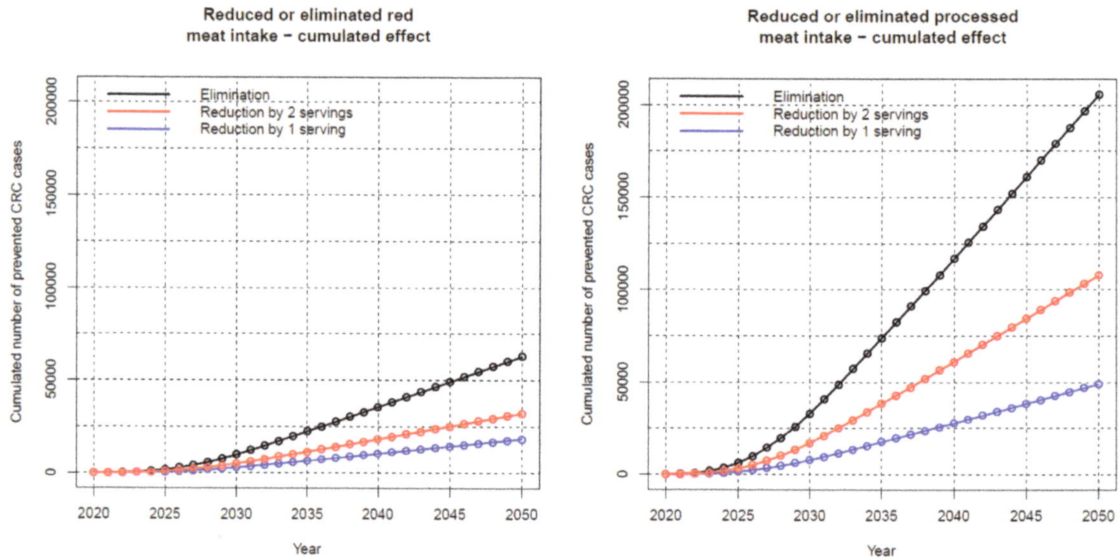


(a) (b)

**Figure 2.** Cumulative prevented colorectal cancer cases over time in case of a reduction in (**a**) red and (**b**) processed meat consumption (men and women combined). Abbreviations: CRC, colorectal cancer.

Sensitivity analyses using shorter or longer lag periods did not change the results materially. Estimated numbers of preventable CRC cases were slightly lower if a longer lag period of 15 years was assumed and slightly higher if a shorter lag period of 5 years was assumed (by approximately 10% each).

## 4. Discussion

In this study, we used a macro-simulation modeling approach to simulate the decrease in future incident CRC cases associated with a reduction in red and processed meat intake over a 30-year horizon. Different scenarios were investigated, from a reduction by one serving per day over two servings to a total elimination of red and processed meat intake. Overall, our simulation suggests that until 2050, up to almost 63,000 CRC cases (2.9% of all CRC cases) could be avoided if red meat intake were eliminated and almost 220,000 cases (9.6% of all CRC cases) if processed meat intake were decreased to zero. In the conservative scenario of a reduction by one serving per day, approximately 19,000 (red meat) and 49,000 (processed meat) CRC cases could be prevented. A reduction by two servings per day would result in those numbers approximately doubling.

Notably, "sufficient evidence for a causal link" between intake of processed meat (and "limited evidence" for a causal link between red meat) and CRC risk does not indicate particularly strong associations. Most likely, substantially more CRC cases could be prevented by increasing screening uptake and physical activity, and by a reduced prevalence of smoking, alcohol consumption, and overweight or obesity. Nevertheless, carcinogenesis is a multifactorial phenomenon, and awareness of certain types of meat being now considered established (processed meat) and suggested (red meat) CRC risk factors, respectively, should be increased.

Suggested mechanisms by which the intake of red and processed meat increase CRC risk include *N*-nitrose compounds [18,19] and lipid peroxidation [19]. Furthermore, heterocyclic aromatic amines (HAAs) are produced when cooking meat at high temperature [3]. Future studies might investigate whether CRC risk associated with red and processed meat intake differs and could potentially be reduced by different manufacturing techniques (e.g., reduction or avoidance of nitrous compounds in processed meat) or consumption (e.g., by cooking with lower temperatures, avoiding open fire, or removing burnt parts of red meat). Until the underlying mechanisms are clarified, the safest way of avoiding the excess CRC risk associated with processed and red meat intake is avoidance or at least reducing intake of those foods. In addition, this would also be in line with the planetary health diet as proposed by the EAT-Lancet Commission, which is mainly plant-based and flexitarian and recommends greatly limiting meat consumption to achieve a healthy and, at the same time, environmentally sustainable diet [20]. Meat production is more energy-intense than that of plant-based foods, and is the most important source of methane, which is a potent greenhouse gas [21].

Few other studies published between 2017 and 2019 [22–26] have investigated the burden of CRC related to red and/or processed meat consumption: de Vries et al. [22] estimated that eliminating red and processed meat intake could reduce CRC incidence in Colombia by approximately 13% (males, red meat), 10% (females, red meat), 14% (males, processed meat), and 13% (females, processed meat). Those numbers are higher compared to our study, apparently because of the higher intake of red and processed meat in Colombia compared to Germany. Similarly, a study from Denmark with methodology comparable to ours [23] and also using a 30-year time period (2016–2045) found that an elimination of red and processed meat (combined) could prevent almost 17,000 CRC cases, or almost 20% of all cases. Again, this percentage was higher than in our study (also when considering red and processed meat combined), apparently because red meat intake in Denmark is almost twice as high as in Germany. In Canada, 0.9% and 0.7% of all cancers in 2015 were attributed to red and processed meat intake, respectively [26], using comparable methods. A study from France [24] suggested that 19 disability-adjusted life years (DALYs) per 100,000 people were associated with red meat consumption for CRC. More DALYs (21/100,000) were expected to be contributed by the association between red meat consumption and cardiovascular disease. Finally, a cost-effectiveness study from the US [25] pointed to methods of how to potentially achieve the desired reduction in red and processed meat consumption. The authors suggested that an excise tax and warning labels would be highly cost-saving (not only cost-effective) and substantially reduce cancer burden.

Our study adds to the growing body of evidence on preventable cancer cases if recommendations regarding physical activity and body weight [7], smoking [27], alcohol consumption [28], and dietary habits [7] were adhered to. However, the aforementioned estimations of PIFs and population-attributable fractions (PAFs) did not consider correlations between risk factors. Attributable numbers of cancer cases (with different hypothetical interventions to decrease them) should, thus, instead be used to rank their relative importance and priority to address them, and not to sum them up across different risk factors. Additionally, from a public health perspective, the focus should be broadened from CRC risk as a relevant health outcome associated with red and processed meat intake to all relevant health outcomes, since red and processed meat intake have also been consistently suggested to increase risk of cardiovascular disease [29–31] and even all-cause mortality [29–31].

Similar to tobacco control policies, a combination of interventions would most likely be favorable in order to achieve a long-term decrease in red and processed meat intake, targeting both the supply and the demand side: First, risks of red and processed meat intake should be communicated clearly, specifically the difference between certainty of evidence and potential population impact (association strength and prevalence). Even though it is only partly under the control of the responsible authorities, misunderstandings such as those caused by the IARC/WCRF report, [5] that was widely—and falsely—understood as red and processed meat being similarly dangerous with respect to cancer risk as smoking, should be avoided. Nevertheless, the current fourth edition of the European Code Against Cancer [32] includes the avoidance of processed meat and the limitation of red meat intake as part of the recommendation for a healthy diet. Second, as demonstrated by tobacco control policies, price increases are highly effective in reducing demand. Taxation of red and processed meat beyond current levels of value-added tax would most likely also be very effective in reducing red and processed meat consumption [33]. Other types of "nudging" to decrease meat consumption (e.g., proposing "veggie days" in company canteens) are also an option, but entail the risk of exerting unintended opposite effects by causing psychological reactance.

Another approach could be to set the right incentives ("make the healthy choice the easy choice") [34]. This could include the span of policies similar to those used for tobacco control, e.g., taxation and warning labels, but also other measures such as food labeling are conceivable. For example, mandatory information about production facilities (space and average life-span per animal, use of antibiotics, etc.) on meat products could influence consumer perceptions and would probably reduce meat consumption. On the other hand, measures to improve the conditions under which meat is produced (e.g., more space per animal) would lower consumption by resulting in higher prices. A unit tax (e.g., per 100 g of meat) would likely be preferable over an ad valorem tax, because the latter might shift demand towards lower-priced low-quality meat, unless minimum prices are specified.

Red and processed meat intake are currently not the main drivers of cancer incidence worldwide and also not mentioned in the latest Global Burden of Disease Study 2019 study report [35]. Nevertheless, as the prevalence of other risk factors such as smoking decreases in Germany and many other countries, the relevance of red and processed meat intake is likely to remain substantial despite recent slight decreases in meat intake in Germany.

This study has several important strengths. It is—to our knowledge—the first study to model the potential impact of a reduced intake of red and processed meat on CRC incidence in Germany. We used nationally representative data on red and processed meat consumption. Strengths of associations were taken from the best currently available evidence (WCRF report). Lag and latency periods were considered in order to avoid an overestimation of effects. Sensitivity analyses assuming longer or shorter lag periods did not affect the results materially, suggesting that our findings are robust with respect to key modeling assumptions.

Our study also has limitations. Risks associated with red and processed meat intake are most likely substantially influenced by the way it is processed (temperature, duration, use of open fire, and use of nitrates and heme iron and lipids that are involved in lipid peroxidation), which could not be investigated in detail due to a lack of data. Our calculations, therefore, instead correspond to the estimated impact of a reduction in intake of "average" red and processed meat. Assumptions regarding latency and lag times from exposure to red and processed meat to CRC development had to be made since they are not precisely known. However, the impact of those assumptions was small. Finally, data on meat intake from the DEGS1 survey was self-reported, and was collected from 2008 to 2011, more than 10 years ago. Even though meat consumption has remained fairly stable in the past 10 years in Germany [36], recent slight decreases would imply that estimated numbers of future preventable CRC cases were slightly overestimated. Such a potential, though very small, of overestimation of potentially achievable effects would not affect our results qualitatively or any of its implications.

More studies and data are required to assess potential differences in impact on cancer incidence according to different ages at exposure and a reduction/elimination of exposure. For example, it is unclear if exposure to the risk factor "processed meat consumption" (and potentially red meat consumption) increases CRC risk at all ages similarly (in which case an exposure criterion analogous to smoking pack–years could be established) or if exposure is more relevant at younger or at older ages.

In future studies, it should be investigated in more detail if the risk increase associated with red and processed meat intake is modified by other CRC risk and protective factors such as smoking. Such information could be valuable for the calculation of individual CRC risk, for instance, in risk scores. Furthermore, potential substitution effects should also be carefully assessed. For example, the intake of red and processed meat would most likely not simply be reduced ceteris paribus (all else equal) as we assumed in our study, but go along with an increase in demand for other foods. Ideally, those would be "healthy foods" such as high-fiber vegetables and whole-grain products, and/or lead to a reduction in calorie intake and, thus, contribute to a reduction in overweight and obesity in the population. Increased vegetable and whole grain intake would further reduce CRC risk. In a pessimistic scenario, reduced intake of red and processed meat would be compensated by higher intake of energy-dense foods such as fried vegetables, sweets, etc., that would promote another common CRC risk factor (obesity). "Health-risk-adapted" taxation of foods could guide substitution in the desired direction, not only with respect to CRC risk.

Future studies should assess the means by which a reduction in red and processed meat intake could be achieved most efficiently (i.e., at the lowest costs from a societal perspective) in Germany, be it unit or ad valorem taxes and/or subsidies for more healthy alternatives. One possibility would be applying the regular value-added tax (currently 19%) to red and processed meat rather than the reduced rate (currently 7%) that applies to "essential goods". In return, more healthy foods that are associated with lower risk of CRC and other diseases such as fruits, vegetables, and whole-grain products could be exempt from taxation.

Given that producing and consuming red and processed meat is and almost certainly will always be legal in Germany, one could question the legitimacy of measures aiming to decrease consumption. However, similar measures have been undertaken for other non-essential and harmful products such as tobacco and alcohol. Considering the high treatment costs of CRC in Germany [37,38], the taxation of products increasing the risk of developing CRC or other cancers would rather reflect an internalization of externalities. To be clear: We do not propose that red and processed meat should be banned, which would be incompatible with a liberal democratic society. However, from a public and planetary health perspective, it seems justified to aim to change food taxation in order to shift demand, to some extent, in the direction of healthier foods and a diet with a smaller environmental footprint.

## 5. Conclusions

In summary, a reduction in red and processed meat intake would most likely have a modest, but non-negligible positive impact on CRC incidence in Germany, with approximately 205,000 (processed meat) and 63,000 (red meat) preventable cases in 2020–2050. The optimal way to achieve such a reduction (e.g., a combination of taxation and subsidies, among other measures) needs to be elucidated by further research. More education about the health risks associated with red and processed meat intake and further preventive efforts are warranted.

**Supplementary Materials:** The following supporting information can be downloaded at: https://www.mdpi.com/article/10.3390/nu15041020/s1, Figure S1: Prevented colorectal cancer cases per year in case of a reduction in red meat consump-tion, stratified by sex.; Figure S2: Prevented colorectal cancer cases per year in case of a reduction in processed meat consumption, stratified by sex.

**Author Contributions:** Conceptualization, H.B. and U.M.; methodology, T.G.; software, T.G.; validation, T.G. and T.N.; formal analysis, T.G.; investigation, T.G.; resources, H.B.; data curation, T.G.; writing—original draft preparation, T.N.; writing—review and editing, all authors; visualization, T.N.; supervision, H.B.; project administration, H.B.; funding acquisition, H.B. and U.M.; T.N., T.G., M.H., U.M. and H.B. have read and critically revised the manuscript. All authors have read and agreed to the published version of the manuscript.

**Funding:** The study was funded in part by the German Cancer Aid ("Deutsche Krebshilfe"), grant number 70112097. UM is funded by the Marga and Walter Boll Foundation, Kerpen, Germany.

**Institutional Review Board Statement:** Not applicable.

**Informed Consent Statement:** Not applicable.

**Data Availability Statement:** The data supporting the findings of this manuscript are publicly available as described in the section "Materials and Methods".

**Conflicts of Interest:** The authors declare no conflict of interest. The funders had no role in the design of the study; in the collection, analyses, or interpretation of data; in the writing of the manuscript; or in the decision to publish the results.

## References


1. Ferlay, J.; Soerjomataram, I.; Ervik, M.; Dikshit, R.; Eser, S.; Mathers, C.; Rebelo, M.; Parkin, D.M.; Forman, D.; Bray, F. *International Agency for Research on Cancer*; GLOBOCAN: Lyon, France; Available online: https://gco.iarc.fr/ (accessed on 25 April 2022).
2. Heisser, T.; Simon, A.; Hapfelmeier, J.; Hoffmeister, M.; Brenner, H. Treatment Costs of Colorectal Cancer by Sex and Age: Population-Based Study on Health Insurance Data from Germany. *Cancers* **2022**, *14*, 3836. [CrossRef] [PubMed]
3. Bouvard, V.; Loomis, D.; Guyton, K.Z.; Grosse, Y.; El Ghissassi, F.; Benbrahim-Tallaa, L.; Guha, N.; Mattock, H.; Straif, K.; Corpet, D. Carcinogenicity of consumption of red and processed meat. *Lancet Oncol.* **2015**, *16*, 1599–1600. [CrossRef] [PubMed]
4. Kamtsiuris, P.; Lange, M.; Hoffmann, R.; Rosario, A.S.; Dahm, S.; Kuhnert, R.; Kurth, B.M. Die erste Welle der Studie zur Gesundheit Erwachsener in Deutschland (DEGS1) [The first wave of the German Health Interview and Examination Survey for Adults]. *Bundesgesundheitsblatt Gesundh. Gesundh.* **2013**, *56*, 620–630. [CrossRef] [PubMed]
5. World Cancer Research Fund; American Institute for Cancer Research. Continuous Update Project Expert Report 2018. Diet, Nutrition, Physical Activity and Colorectal Cancer. Available online: http://dietandcancerreport.org (accessed on 30 March 2022).
6. Deutsche Gesellschaft für Ernährung e.V. Vollwertig Essen und Trinken Nach den 10 Regeln der DGE. Available online: https://www.dge.de/ernaehrungspraxis/vollwertige-ernaehrung/10-regeln-der-dge (accessed on 1 September 2022).
7. Behrens, G.; Gredner, T.; Stock, C.; Leitzmann, M.F.; Brenner, H.; Mons, U. Cancers Due to Excess Weight, Low Physical Activity, and Unhealthy Diet. *Dtsch. Arztebl. Int.* **2018**, *115*, 578–585. [CrossRef] [PubMed]
8. Barendregt, J.J.; Veerman, J.L. Categorical versus continuous risk factors and the calculation of potential impact fractions. *J. Epidemiol. Community Health* **2010**, *64*, 209–212. [CrossRef]
9. Kuhn, D.-A. *Entwicklung Eines Index zur Bewertung der Ernährungsqualität in der Studie zur Gesundheit Erwachsener in Deutschland (DEGS1)*; Robert Koch-Institut: Berlin, Germany, 2018.
10. Robert Koch Institut. German Centre for Cancer Registry Data (ZfKD). Available online: http://www.krebsdaten.de (accessed on 17 June 2022).
11. Federal Statistical Office (Destatis). Germany's Population by 2060: Results of the 14th Coordinated Population Projection. Wiesbaden: Destatis. Available online: https://www.destatis.de/EN/Themes/Society-Environment/Population/Population-Projection/_node.html#sprg479856 (accessed on 22 April 2022).
12. Soerjomataram, I.; de Vries, E.; Engholm, G.; Paludan-Müller, G.; Brønnum-Hansen, H.; Storm, H.H.; Barendregt, J.J. Impact of a smoking and alcohol intervention programme on lung and breast cancer incidence in Denmark: An example of dynamic modelling with Prevent. *Eur. J. Cancer* **2010**, *46*, 2617–2624. [CrossRef]
13. Brenner, H.; Altenhofen, L.; Katalinic, A.; Lansdorp-Vogelaar, I.; Hoffmeister, M. Sojourn time of preclinical colorectal cancer by sex and age: Estimates from the German national screening colonoscopy database. *Am. J. Epidemiol.* **2011**, *174*, 1140–1146. [CrossRef]
14. Haggar, F.A.; Boushey, R.P. Colorectal cancer epidemiology: Incidence, mortality, survival, and risk factors. *Clin. Colon Rectal Surg.* **2009**, *22*, 191–197. [CrossRef]
15. De Jong, A.E.; Morreau, H.; Nagengast, F.M.; Mathus-Vliegen, E.M.; Kleibeuker, J.H.; Griffioen, G.; Cats, A.; Vasen, H.F. Prevalence of adenomas among young individuals at average risk for colorectal cancer. *Off. J. Am. Coll. Gastroenterol. ACG* **2005**, *100*, 139–143. [CrossRef]
16. Davies, R.J.; Miller, R.; Coleman, N. Colorectal cancer screening: Prospects for molecular stool analysis. *Nat. Rev. Cancer* **2005**, *5*, 199–209. [CrossRef]
17. R Core Team. *R: A Language and Environment for Statistical Computing*; R Foundation for Statistical Computing: Vienna, Austria, 2022; Available online: http://www.R-project.org/ (accessed on 28 April 2022).
18. Kuhnle, G.G.; Bingham, S.A. Dietary meat, endogenous nitrosation and colorectal cancer. *Biochem. Soc. Trans.* **2007**, *35*, 1355–1357. [CrossRef] [PubMed]
19. Van den Bussche, J.; Hemeryck, L.Y.; Van Hecke, T.; Kuhnle, G.G.; Pasmans, F.; Moore, S.A.; Van de Wiele, T.; De Smet, S.; Vanhaecke, L. O(6)-carboxymethylguanine DNA adduct formation and lipid peroxidation upon in vitro gastrointestinal digestion of haem-rich meat. *Mol. Nutr. Food Res.* **2014**, *58*, 1883–1896. [CrossRef] [PubMed]
20. Willett, W.; Rockstrom, J.; Loken, B.; Springmann, M.; Lang, T.; Vermeulen, S.; Garnett, T.; Tilman, D.; DeClerck, F.; Wood, A.; et al. Food in the Anthropocene: The EAT-Lancet Commission on healthy diets from sustainable food systems. *Lancet* **2019**, *393*, 447–492. [CrossRef] [PubMed]
21. Godfray, H.C.J.; Aveyard, P.; Garnett, T.; Hall, J.W.; Key, T.J.; Lorimer, J.; Pierrehumbert, R.T.; Scarborough, P.; Springmann, M.; Jebb, S.A. Meat consumption, health, and the environment. *Science* **2018**, *361*, eaam5324. [CrossRef] [PubMed]
22. de Vries, E.; Quintero, D.C.; Henriquez-Mendoza, G.; Herran, O.F. Population attributable fractions for colorectal cancer and red and processed meats in Colombia-a macro-simulation study. *Colomb. Med.* **2017**, *48*, 64–69.
23. Lourenco, S.; Gunge, V.B.; Andersson, T.M.; Andersen, C.L.E.; Lund, A.Q.; Koster, B.; Hansen, G.L. Avoidable colorectal cancer cases in Denmark-The impact of red and processed meat. *Cancer Epidemiol.* **2018**, *55*, 1–7. [CrossRef]

24. De Oliveira Mota, J.; Boue, G.; Guillou, S.; Pierre, F.; Membre, J.M. Estimation of the burden of disease attributable to red meat consumption in France: Influence on colorectal cancer and cardiovascular diseases. *Food Chem. Toxicol.* **2019**, *130*, 174–186. [CrossRef]
25. Kim, D.D.; Wilde, P.E.; Michaud, D.S.; Liu, J.; Lizewski, L.; Onopa, J.; Mozaffarian, D.; Zhang, F.F.; Wong, J.B. Cost Effectiveness of Nutrition Policies on Processed Meat: Implications for Cancer Burden in the U.S. *Am. J. Prev. Med.* **2019**, *57*, e143–e152. [CrossRef]
26. Ruan, Y.; Poirier, A.E.; Hebert, L.A.; Grevers, X.; Walter, S.D.; Villeneuve, P.J.; Brenner, D.R.; Friedenreich, C.M.; Com, P.S.T. Estimates of the current and future burden of cancer attributable to red and processed meat consumption in Canada. *Prev. Med.* **2019**, *122*, 31–39. [CrossRef]
27. Gredner, T.; Niedermaier, T.; Brenner, H.; Mons, U. Impact of Tobacco Control Policies on Smoking-Related Cancer Incidence in Germany 2020 to 2050-A Simulation Study. *Cancer Epidemiol. Biomark. Prev.* **2020**, *29*, 1413–1422. [CrossRef]
28. Gredner, T.; Niedermaier, T.; Brenner, H.; Mons, U. Impact of reducing alcohol consumption through price-based policies on cancer incidence in Germany 2020–2050—A simulation study. *Addiction* **2021**, *116*, 1677–1688. [CrossRef] [PubMed]
29. Zhong, V.W.; Van Horn, L.; Greenland, P.; Carnethon, M.R.; Ning, H.; Wilkins, J.T.; Lloyd-Jones, D.M.; Allen, N.B. Associations of Processed Meat, Unprocessed Red Meat, Poultry, or Fish Intake With Incident Cardiovascular Disease and All-Cause Mortality. *JAMA Intern. Med.* **2020**, *180*, 503–512. [CrossRef] [PubMed]
30. Wang, X.; Lin, X.; Ouyang, Y.Y.; Liu, J.; Zhao, G.; Pan, A.; Hu, F.B. Red and processed meat consumption and mortality: Dose-response meta-analysis of prospective cohort studies. *Public Health Nutr.* **2016**, *19*, 893–905. [CrossRef] [PubMed]
31. Iqbal, R.; Dehghan, M.; Mente, A.; Rangarajan, S.; Wielgosz, A.; Avezum, A.; Seron, P.; AlHabib, K.F.; Lopez-Jaramillo, P.; Swaminathan, S.; et al. Associations of unprocessed and processed meat intake with mortality and cardiovascular disease in 21 countries [Prospective Urban Rural Epidemiology (PURE) Study]: A prospective cohort study. *Am. J. Clin. Nutr.* **2021**, *114*, 1049–1058. [CrossRef]
32. International Agency for Research on Cancer. European Code Against Cancer—12 Ways to Reduce Your Cancer Risk. Available online: https://cancer-code-europe.iarc.fr/index.php/en/ (accessed on 25 May 2022).
33. Schröck, R. Analyse der Preiselastizitäten der Nachfrage nach Biolebensmitteln unter Berücksichtigung Nicht Direkt Preisrelevanten Verhaltens der Verbraucher (Analysis of Price Elasticities for Organic Food Products in Consideration of Not Price-Related Consumer Behaviour); BÖLN-Bundesprogramm Ökologischer Landbau und Andere Formen Nachhaltiger Landwirtschaft: 2013. Available online: https://orgprints.org/id/eprint/22414/ (accessed on 25 April 2022).
34. Volpp, K.G.; Asch, D.A. Make the healthy choice the easy choice: Using behavioral economics to advance a culture of health. *QJM* **2017**, *110*, 271–275. [CrossRef]
35. Tran, K.B.; Lang, J.J.; Compton, K.; Xu, R.; Acheson, A.R.; Henrikson, H.J.; Kocarnik, J.M.; Penberthy, L.; Aali, A.; Abbas, Q.; et al. The global burden of cancer attributable to risk factors, 2010–19: A systematic analysis for the Global Burden of Disease Study 2019. *Lancet* **2022**, *400*, 563–591. [CrossRef]
36. Ahrens, S. Fleischverbrauch in Deutschland pro Kopf in den Jahren 1991 bis 2020. Available online: https://de.statista.com/statistik/daten/studie/36573/umfrage/pro-kopf-verbrauch-von-fleisch-in-deutschland-seit-2000/ (accessed on 1 May 2022).
37. Stintzing, S.; van Oostrum, I.; Pescott, C.P.; Ronga, P.; Heeg, B.; Heinemann, V. Cost-effectiveness of FOLFIRI + cetuximab vs FOLFIRI + bevacizumab in the first-line treatment of RAS wild-type metastatic colorectal cancer in Germany: Data from the FIRE-3 (AIO KRK-0306) study. *J. Med. Econ.* **2020**, *23*, 448–455. [CrossRef]
38. Haug, U.; Engel, S.; Verheyen, F.; Linder, R. Estimating colorectal cancer treatment costs: A pragmatic approach exemplified by health insurance data from Germany. *PLoS ONE* **2014**, *9*, e88407. [CrossRef]

*nutrients*

MDPI

*Article*

# Soy Milk Consumption in the United States of America: An NHANES Data Report

**Maximilian Andreas Storz [1,*], Maria Brommer [2], Mauro Lombardo [3] and Gianluca Rizzo [4]**

1 Department of Internal Medicine II, Centre for Complementary Medicine, Medical Center—University of Freiburg, Faculty of Medicine, University of Freiburg, 79106 Freiburg, Germany
2 Interdisciplinary Medical Intensive Care (IMIT), Medical Center—University of Freiburg, Faculty of Medicine, University of Freiburg, 79106 Freiburg, Germany
3 Department of Human Sciences and Promotion of the Quality of Life, San Raffaele Roma Open University, 00166 Rome, Italy; mauro.lombardo@uniroma5.it
4 Independent Researcher, Via Venezuela 66, 98121 Messina, Italy; drgianlucarizzo@gmail.com
* Correspondence: maximilian.storz@uniklinik-freiburg.de; Tel.: +49-157-5454-3852

**Abstract:** With the increasing adoption of plant-based diets in the United States, more and more individuals replace cow milk with plant-based milk alternatives. Soy milk is a commonly used cow milk substitute, which is characterized by a higher content of polyunsaturated fatty acids and fibers. Despite these favorable characteristics, little is known about the current prevalence of soy milk consumption the United States. We used data from the National Health and Nutrition Examination Surveys (NHANES) to assess soy milk usage in the United States and identified potential predictors for its consumption in the US general population. The proportion of individuals reporting soy milk consumption in the NHANES 2015–2016 cycle was 2%, and 1.54% in the NHANES 2017–2020 cycle. Non-Hispanic Asian and Black ethnicities (as well as other Hispanic and Mexican American ethnicities in the 2017–2020 cycle) significantly increased the odds for soy milk consumption. While a college degree and weekly moderate physical activity were associated with significantly higher odds for consuming soy milk (OR: 2.21 and 2.36, respectively), sex was not an important predictor. In light of the putative health benefits of soy milk and its more favorable environmental impact as compared to cow milk, future investigations should attempt to identify strategies that may help promote its consumption in selected populations.

**Keywords:** soybean milk; plant-based milks; milk substitutes; soy; consumption; consumer attitudes; prevalence; NHANES

## 1. Introduction

The plant-based diet is increasingly adopted by the general population in Western countries and has also attracted the interest of the scientific community and the food industry [1–3]. As a result, the market has increased the available amounts of innovative plant-based foods to meet this growing demand [4,5]. The interest in switching to plant-based alternatives is frequently derived from ethical aspects and advantages associated with health [6,7], and recently also from a greater sensitivity towards environmental aspects that have emerged from the scientific literature [8–10].

Adoption of vegetarian and vegan diets has shown a beneficial effect on cancer incidence [6], and has been associated with a reduction in cardiovascular morbidity and mortality in recent clinical studies [7,11]. These aspects are particularly relevant considering that around one third of cardiovascular and neoplastic diseases in the world could be prevented by increasing fruit and vegetable intake, according to the World Health Organization and the World Cancer Research Fund [12].

With the increase in the demand for plant-based foods, the consumption of alternatives to cow milk also raised, with a forecast increase of over 10% from 2000 to 2024 (globally), with the major trend observed for the Asia-Pacific region [13]. At the same time, research has also moved to bridge the gap between consumer needs (milk allergy, lactose intolerance, or vegan diet) and commercial options [14–16]. Although the term "milk" had already been regulated as an exclusive term for the mammary secretion of cows and other mammals by the Food and Drugs Administration (FDA) and the European Union [17,18], the FDA recently issued a recommendation regarding the labelling of plant-based dairy alternatives, defining the lawfulness of including the term "milk" [19]. The consumer is now thoroughly familiar with these foods so there is no longer need for the previous terminological restrictions, with the recommendation of clear labelling regarding the nutritional properties of the products. Accurate labelling and fortification of plant-products already available on the market would allow consumers to assess the adequacy of vitamins and other micronutrients usually lacking in these products if compared to cow milk [20].

Among plant-based drinks, one of the most commonly used as a substitute for cow milk is soy milk [21]. Soy is a widely used food in vegetarian diets [22]. Among its nutritional characteristics, soy milk is the only plant-based alternative to cow milk with a similar protein content [23]. Furthermore, it has a comparable Digestible Indispensable Amino Acid Score, demonstrating a good protein quality [24]. Additionally, soy milk is characterized by a higher content of polyunsaturated fatty acids, fibers, and by the absence of cholesterol [25]. These features may help reduce LDL levels [26]. The replacement of cow milk with soy milk could have an advantage in vegetarian diets as regards the absence of iron in the former and the possible presence of vegetable ferritin in the latter [27].

Soybean crops have a relevant environmental impact, with a variable effect on factors such as eutrophication, acidification, and global warming in different countries [28], and with a negative social impact on humans [29]. Nevertheless, soybean represents the main source of animal feed production [30]. Moreover, almost 80% of the world's soy production is destined for livestock, including milk and dairy production [31], with about 2% designated for soy milk for humans [32].

Used as an alternative to cow milk, soy milk represents a more sustainable solution in terms of environmental impact and can be consistent with food security objectives [33]. Even if the presence of isoflavones has raised health concerns, it could have an advantage in mitigating menopausal disorders, without critical hormonal and fertility disturbance [34,35]. Nonetheless, soy milk has shown beneficial antioxidant actions, mainly attributable to the content of isoflavones [36].

Based on comments submitted to the FDA, dietitians appear to have a more accurate understanding of plant-based substitutes than other healthcare professionals [37]. More than half of consumers do not believe that dairy products are nutritionally better than plant-based alternatives and think that the latter can be part of a healthy diet [37]. In a sensory evaluation study, soy milk was shown to be the most popular milk alternative across various groups of participants, including omnivores and vegans [38].

Soy milk is one of the most common plant-based alternatives to cow milk and the only plant-based dairy substitute in the Dietary Guidelines for Americans [39]. Yet, data on its consumption in the US is sparse. This cross-sectional study sought to investigate the prevalence of soy milk consumption in a large and nationally representative cohort of American adults (NHANES—National Health and Nutrition Examination Survey) and aimed at a better understanding of its association with correlated sociodemographic aspects.

## 2. Materials and Methods

### *2.1. Study Population and Design*

This analysis is based on data from the NHANES—an ongoing program of studies by the Centers for Disease Control and Prevention designed to comprehensively assess the health and nutritional status of the non-institutionalized U.S. population [40,41]. The NHANES' complex multistage, stratified, clustered, and probability sampling design allows for nationally representative health and nutritional status assessments. Key program characteristics (including recruitment methods, study size, and study execution details) have been described elsewhere in detail [39,40]. NHANES was approved by the National Center for Health Statistics (NCHS) and all study participants gave written and oral consent to the study [42].

For this analysis, we used data from two different NHANES cycles: (I) the NHANES 2015–2016 cycle, and (II) NHANES 2017–2020 (which is also called the pre-pandemic cycle) [43,44]. Both cycles were analyzed independently for methodological issues because some important variables that were included in the 2015–2016 cycle were no longer available in the NHANES pre-pandemic cycle.

### 2.2. Primary Outcome Variable

Data on soy milk consumption was obtained from the NHANES Diet Behavior and Nutrition questionnaire. This module provides personal interview data on various dietary behavior and nutrition related topics. Amongst others, it includes one question on milk product consumption in the past 30 days. Said question reads as follows:

*"In the past 30 days, how often did you have milk to drink or on your cereal?"*

Participants were instructed to include chocolate and other flavored milks as well as hot cocoa made with milk. Moreover, they were instructed not to count small amounts of milk added to coffee or tea. The question did not cover milk usage in cooking. Answer options included "never", "rarely—less than once a week", "sometimes—once a week or more, but less than once a day", "often—once a day or more", "varied", and "never". All participants that reported at least some occasional milk consumption were further asked:

*"What type of milk was it? Was it usually ..."?*

Subsequently, the NHANES inquired about several milk types, including (but not limited to) whole-milk, 1% fat milk, skim milk, and soy milk. Those participants who indicated soy milk consumption at least less than once a week were considered soy milk consumers. Those who denied soy milk consumption were considered non-consumers.

### 2.3. Covariates

Covariates for this analysis included sociodemographic data (gender, race/ethnicity, age, marital status, educational level, annual household income, household size, number of persons in the household, household food security category) as well as self-perceived general health status. Moreover, we included diabetes status (as assessed by the question: "*Have you ever been told by a doctor or health professional that you have diabetes or sugar diabetes?*"), smoking status (as assessed by the question "*Have you smoked at least 100 cigarettes in your entire life?*"), and physical activity (as assessed by the question "*In a typical week do you do any moderate-intensity sports, fitness, or recreational activities that cause a small increase in breathing or heart rate such as brisk walking, bicycling, swimming, or volleyball for at least 10 min continuously?*"). Apart from age (continuous variable) all other variables were treated as categorical variables.

### 2.4. Inclusion and Exclusion Criteria

We included all participants with the following criteria: age $\geq$ 20 years, available demographic data, and available milk intake data. Individuals with incomplete or missing data were not considered for this study.

### 2.5. Statistical Analysis

Statistical analysis was performed with Stata 14 statistical software (StataCorp. 2015. Stata Statistical Software: Release 14. College Station, TX, USA: StataCorp LP). The primary sampling unit variable for variance estimation and the pseudo-stratum variable as the stratification variable that were provided with both NHANES cycles were used for each analysis. To avoid missing standard errors because of strata with a single sampling unit, we used the "singleunit(scaled)" option in Stata, which is a scaled version of singleunit(certainty) and introduces a scaling factor that is derived from using the average of the variances from the strata with multiple sampling units for each stratum with a singleton primary sampling unit [45].

We used histograms and subpopulation summary statistics to check for normality of the data. Categorical variables were described with their weighted proportions and standard error in parenthesis. Normally distributed variables were described with their mean and standard error in parenthesis. All standard errors were estimated using Taylor series linearization to account for the complex NHANES sampling design. All weighting procedures were performed in accordance with the most recent applied survey data analysis techniques by Heeringa, West, and Berglund [46], and in compliance with the current National Center for Health Statistics (NCHS) data presentation standards for proportions [47]. All weighted proportions were manually screened for reliability using the user-written post-estimation Stata command "kg_nchs" [48]. Potentially unreliable proportions that did not meet the NCHS presentation standards were highlighted and clearly marked with superscript letters.

Stata's Rao–Scott test and multivariate logistic regression models were used to examine potential associations between self-reported soy milk intake and various predictor variables. Logistic regression models were constructed based on the recommendations of Heeringa, West, and Berglund [46]. In a first step, we conducted exploratory bivariate analyses to check the eligibility of potential candidate predictors of soy milk intake. Candidate predictors of scientific interest and a bivariate relationship of significance $p < 0.25$ with the response variable were included in the multivariate logistic models. Subsequently, we evaluated the contribution of each predictor to the multivariate model using Wald tests. All variables (except age) were entered as categorical variables into the regression models. At least two models were constructed for each cycle, based on the available cycle-specific predictors. A $p$-value $< 0.05$ was used as the cutoff for statistical significance.

## 3. Results

The total NHANES 2015–2016 sample for analysis comprised $n = 5264$ participants with a full data set, of which $n = 132$ reported soy milk consumption. This may be extrapolated to represent $n = 4{,}427{,}078$ US Americans. The NHANES 2017–2020 pre-pandemic cycle included $n = 8511$ participants with a full dataset, of which $n = 187$ reported soy milk consumption. This may be extrapolated to represent $n = 3{,}460{,}784$ US Americans. Figure 1 shows the participant inclusion flow chart for the 2015–2016 cycle on the left side and for the NHANES 2017–2020 pre-pandemic cycle on the right side.

The weighted proportion of individuals reporting soy milk consumption in the 2015–2016 cycle was 2%, whereas it was 1.54% in the NHANES 2017–2020 pre-pandemic cycle.

### 3.1. NHANES 2015–2016

The sample characteristics of the participants reporting soy milk consumption are shown in Table 1. The weighted percentage of females consuming soy milk tended to be higher as compared to males drinking soy milk (Table 1); however, the difference was not statistically significant. Almost 43% (weighted proportion) of soy milk consumers were of Non-Hispanic White origin. Non-Hispanic Blacks and Non-Hispanic Asians accounted for more than 17% each.

Significant differences between soy milk consumers and non-consumers were found with regard to educational level. A significantly higher weighted proportion of individuals reporting soy milk intake had a college degree or higher (46.96% vs. 32.18%, $p = 0.03$). No significant intergroup differences were found with regard to household size, household food security level, and annual income. A significantly higher proportion of soy milk consumers indicated moderate recreational activities as compared to non-consumers.

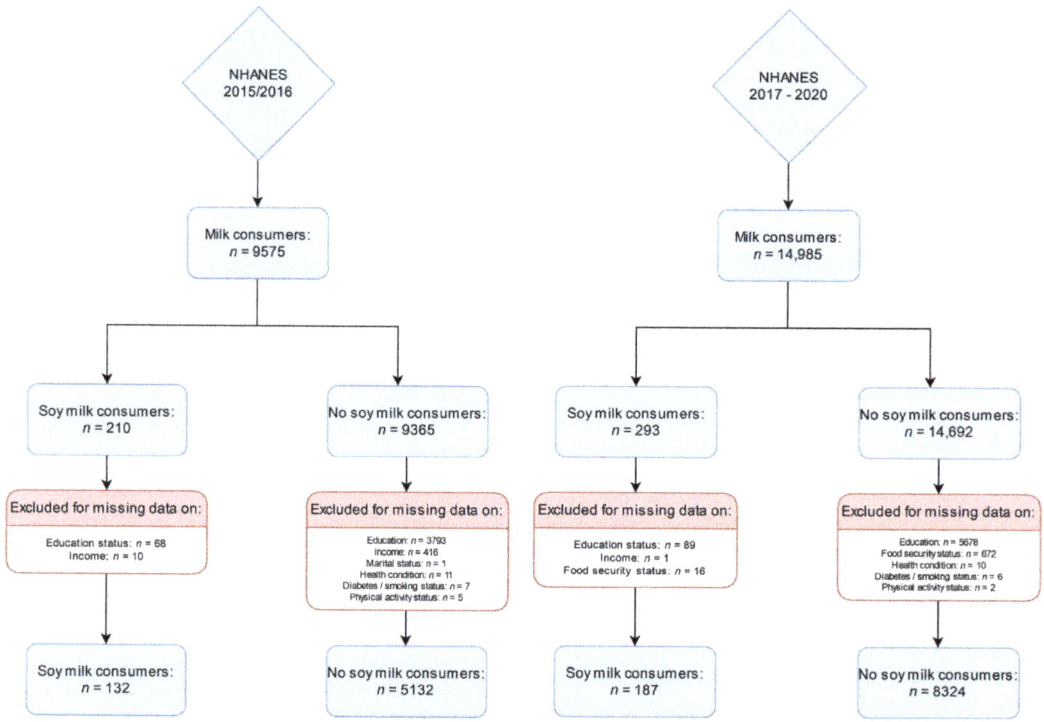


**Figure 1.** Participant inclusion flowchart for the NHANES 2015–2016 cycle (**left side**) and the NHANES 2017–2020 cycle (**right side**).

In a next step, we used multivariate logistic regression models to examine potential associations between soy milk intake status (dependent variable) and various predictor variables (Table 2). While female sex did not increase the odds for soy milk consumption, Non-Hispanic Black and Non-Hispanic Asian ethnicities significantly increased the odds (OR: 2.51 and 4.87, respectively) in model 1. In a second (model 2) households with six or more persons had significantly lower odds for soy milk consumption (Table 2). Notably, said model was overall no longer statistically significant. When adding physical activity in model 3, statistical significance was retained. Participants with moderate-intensity sports and recreational activities had significantly higher odds for soy milk consumption (OR: 2.36).

### *3.2. NHANES 2017–2020*

Sample characteristics of participants reporting soy milk consumption in the NHANES pre-pandemic cycle are shown in Table 3. The weighted percentage of females consuming soy milk was significantly higher in the NHANES 2017–2020 cycle: 63.45% vs. 36.55%. Only 34.55% (weighted proportion) of soy milk consumers were of Non-Hispanic White origin, whereas approximately 18.52% were Non-Hispanic Asians. Significant differences between both groups were also found with regard to educational level. The weighted proportion of individuals with a high school degree was substantially lower among soy milk consumers (16.01% vs. 27.10%, $p = 0.006$) while the weighted proportion of participants with (some) college degree tended to be higher. No significant differences were found with regard to household food security level, general (self-perceived health condition), and annual income. A significantly higher proportion of soy milk consumers indicated moderate recreational activities as compared to non-consumers. The weighted proportion of smokers also differed significantly between groups.

**Table 1.** Sample characteristics by soy milk consumption status: NHANES 2015–2016.

| | Soy Milk: Consumers $n$ = 132 | Soy Milk: Non-Consumers $n$ = 5132 | $p$-Value |
|---|---|---|---|
| **Sex** | | | |
| Male | 40.46% (5.80) | 48.04% (0.54) | $p = 0.217$ [b] |
| Female | 59.54% (5.80) | 51.96% (0.54) | |
| **Age (years)** | 46.40 (2.24) | 47.82 (0.55) | $p = 0.508$ [c] |
| **Race/ethnicity** | | | |
| Mexican American | 6.35% (2.53) [f] | 8.59% (2.05) | |
| Other Hispanic | 8.93% (3.22) [f] | 6.10% (1.34) | |
| Non-Hispanic White | 42.90% (7.76) [e,f] | 65.54% (3.89) | **$p < 0.001$** [b] |
| Non-Hispanic Black | 18.11% (4.27) | 10.88% (2.13) | |
| Non-Hispanic Asian | 17.06% (4.83) [e] | 5.34% (1.16) | |
| Other Race [a] | 6.64% (3.61) [f] | 3.56% (0.35) | |
| **Marital status** | | | |
| Married/Living with Partner | 60.07% (1.53) [f] | 64.69% (1.55) | |
| Widowed/Divorced/Separated | 15.48% (0.80) | 18.00% (1.19) | $p = 0.401$ [b] |
| Never married | 24.45% (6.34) | 17.31% (1.27) | |
| **Annual household income** | | | |
| <20,000 US$ | 9.97% (2.59) | 12.95% (1.23) | $p = 0.315$ [b] |
| >20,000 US$ | 90.03% (2.59) | 87.05% (1.23) | |
| **Education Level** | | | |
| Less than 9th grade | 5.25% (1.27) [f] | 5.66% (0.91) | |
| 9–11th grade | 4.89% (2.01) [f] | 8.35% (0.90) | $p = 0.124$ [b] |
| High school graduate/GED [d] | 16.32% (5.07) [f] | 20.97% (1.18) | |
| Some college or AA degree | 26.58% (4.73) | 32.84% (1.52) | |
| College graduate or above | 46.96% (5.09) [e] | 32.18% (3.09) | |
| **Food security category** | | | |
| Full food security | 70.91% (4.66) | 71.90% (2.16) | |
| Marginal food security | 15.32% (4.35) | 10.38% (1.00) | $p = 0.416$ [b] |
| Low food security | 8.19% (2.86) [f] | 10.73% (1.03) | |
| Very low food security | 5.58% (2.12) [f] | 7.00% (0.58) | |
| **Household size** | | | |
| One person | 9.77% (2.26) | 14.01% (0.81) | |
| Two persons | 43.98% (6.72) | 33.35% (1.71) | |
| Three persons | 20.19% (3.85) | 17.36% (1.38) | |
| Four persons | 10.67% (2.62) [e] | 17.33% (1.10) | $p = 0.101$ [b] |
| Five persons | 12.44% (4.03) [f] | 9.87% (0.69) | |
| Six persons | 1.96% (1.15) [e,f] | 4.45% (0.57) | |
| Seven persons or more | 0.99% (0.70) [e] | 3.63% (0.49) | |
| **General health condition** | | | |
| Excellent | 18.42% (0.87) | 14.63% (0.87) | |
| Very good | 32.71% (4.70) | 32.62% (1.44) | $p = 0.158$ [b] |
| Good | 35.63% (5.97) | 34.66% (1.04) | |
| Fair | 7.11% (1.50) [e,f] | 14.77% (1.09) | |
| Poor | 6.13% (2.01) [f] | 3.32% (0.38) | |
| **Diabetes status** | | | |
| Yes | 7.53% (2.60) [f] | 10.84% (0.80) | |
| No | 91.85% (2.82) | 87.15% (0.84) | $p = 0.224$ [b] |
| Borderline | 0.63% (0.43) [e,f] | 2.01% (0.30) | |
| **Smoking status** | | | |
| Yes | 46.37% (5.84) | 43.39% (1.05) | $p = 0.624$ [b] |
| No | 53.63% (5.84) | 56.61% (1.05) | |
| **Moderate recreational activities** | | | |
| Yes | 65.59% (5.32) [e] | 46.72% (1.79) | **$p = 0.005$** [b] |
| No | 34.41% (5.32) [e] | 53.28% (1.79) | |

Weighted proportions. Total number of unweighted observations: $n$ = 5264. Continuous variables shown as mean (standard error). Categorical variables shown as weighted proportion (standard error). [a] = includes multi-racial; [b] = based on Stata's design-adjusted Rao–Scott test, [c] = based on regression analyses followed by adjusted Wald tests, [d] = or equivalent, [e] = indicates significant differences in the weighted proportions, [f] = weighted proportions to be considered unreliable, as per recent NCHS Guidelines. Column percentages may not equal 100% due to rounding.

**Table 2.** Multivariate logistic regression models examining potential associations between soy milk consumption status and sex, race/ethnicity, and household size.

| Independent Variables | OR | CI | *p* | OR | CI | *p* | OR | CI | *p* |
|---|---|---|---|---|---|---|---|---|---|
| | | Model 1 | | | Model 2 | | | Model 3 | |
| **Sex** | | | | | | | | | |
| Female | 1.34 | [0.80, 2.25] | 0.242 | 1.36 | [0.81, 2.28] | 0.229 | 1.33 | [0.79, 2.24] | 0.258 |
| **Ethnicity** | | | | | | | | | |
| Mexican American | 1.14 | [0.49, 2.66] | 0.750 | 1.44 | [0.60, 3.44] | 0.392 | 1.29 | [0.54, 3.07] | 0.547 |
| Other Hispanic | 2.24 | [0.96, 5.23] | 0.061 | 2.59 | [1.15, 5.81] | **0.024** | 2.43 | [1.05, 5.63] | **0.039** |
| Non-Hispanic Black | 2.51 | [1.18, 5.40] | **0.022** | 2.81 | [1.38, 5.70] | **0.007** | 2.72 | [1.32, 5.60] | **0.010** |
| Non-Hispanic Asian | 4.87 | [2.45, 9.68] | **<0.001** | 5.48 | [2.74, 11.01] | **<0.001** | 5.27 | [2.59, 10.70] | **<0.001** |
| Other Race [a] | 2.87 | [0.76, 10.83] | 0.112 | 2.89 | [0.75,11.21] | 0.115 | 3.06 | [0.80,11.72] | 0.096 |
| **Household size** | | | | | | | | | |
| 1 person | | | | 0.51 | [0.24, 1.11] | 0.084 | | | |
| 3 persons | | | | 0.74 | [0.41, 1.34] | 0.292 | | | |
| 4 persons | | | | 0.40 | [0.20, 0.78] | **0.011** | | | |
| 5 persons | | | | 0.77 | [0.30, 1.93] | 0.547 | | | |
| 6 persons | | | | 0.26 | [0.08, 0.92] | **0.039** | | | |
| 7 persons or more | | | | 0.14 | [0.03, 0.67] | **0.017** | | | |
| **Moderate activity** | | | | | | | | | |
| Yes | | | | | | | 2.36 | [1.40, 3.99] | **0.003** |

Legend: [a] = includes multi-racial. A significant regression equation was found for model 1: $F(6,10) = 4.57$ (model 1) with a *p*-value of 0.017. When adding household size (model 2), the regression equation was no longer significant: $F(6,10) = 4.56$ with a *p*-value of 0.078. When adding physical activity to model 1 (model 3), a significant regression equation was found: $F(7,9) = 8.06$, *p*-value: 0.003. Reference categories were as follows: Male sex; Non-Hispanic White; Household size: two persons. Moderate recreational activities in a typical week: "no". OR = odds ratio. CI = confidence interval. The model is based on a total *n* of 5264 participants.

**Table 3.** Sample characteristics by soy milk consumption status: NHANES 2017–2020.

| | **Soy Milk: Consumers** *n* = 187 | **Soy Milk: Non-Consumers** *n* = 8324 | ***p*-Value** |
|---|---|---|---|
| **Sex** | | | |
| Male | 36.55% (5.33) [e] | 48.09% (0.80) | $p = 0.048$ [b] |
| Female | 63.45% (5.33) [e] | 51.91% (0. 80) | |
| **Age (years)** | 50.26 (2.05) | 48.37 (0.56) | $p = 0.373$ [c] |
| **Race/ethnicity** | | | |
| Mexican American | 16.40% (4.68) | 8.21% (1.12) | |
| Other Hispanic | 12.01% (3.41) | 7.40% (0.68) | |
| Non-Hispanic White | 34.55% (5.71) [e] | 63.69% (2.44) | $p < 0.001$ [b] |
| Non-Hispanic Black | 14.77% (3.22) | 11.24% (1.43) | |
| Non-Hispanic Asian | 18.52% (2.92) [e] | 5.52% (0.84) | |
| Other Race [a] | 3.75% (1.60) [f] | 3.95% (1.60) | |
| **Marital status** | | | |
| Married/Living with Partner | 56.74% (3.62) | 61.82% (1.34) | |
| Widowed/Divorced/Separated | 23.05% (4.07) | 18.92% (0.76) | $p = 0.430$ [b] |
| Never married | 20.21% (3.92) | 19.26% (1.09) | |
| **Education Level** | | | |
| Less than 9th grade | 5.81% (1.29) [f] | 3.64% (0.36) | |
| 9–11th grade | 6.95% (1.82) | 7.12% (0.33) | |
| High school graduate/GED [d] | 16.01% (3.61) [e] | 27.10% (1.38) | $p = 0.080$ [b] |
| Some college or AA degree | 32.09% (5.44) | 30.56% (0.92) | |
| College graduate or above | 39.13% (4.84) | 31.57% (2.14) | |

**Table 3.** *Cont.*

| | Soy Milk: Consumers $n = 187$ | Soy Milk: Non-Consumers $n = 8324$ | $p$-Value |
|---|---|---|---|
| **Food security category** | | | |
| Full food security | 65.45% (4.41) | 72.22% (1.14) | |
| Marginal food security | 14.61% (2.98) | 10.73% (0.58) | $p = 0.304$ [b] |
| Low food security | 11.70% (2.31) | 10.45% (0.61) | |
| Very low food security | 8.24% (2.13) | 6.59% (0.48) | |
| **General health condition** | | | |
| Excellent | 17.43% (3.79) | 13.94% (1.05) | |
| Very good | 24.71% (4.84) | 32.34% (0.87) | $p = 0.285$ [b] |
| Good | 40.38% (3.95) | 35.15% (0.96) | |
| Fair | 13.77% (3.40) | 16.01% (0.74) | |
| Poor | 3.70% (1.14) [f] | 2.57% (0.15) | |
| **Ratio of family income to poverty** | | | |
| <1 | 11.68% (2.24) | 11.82% (0.84) | |
| ≥1 and <2 | 19.61% (3.91) | 17.86% (0.87) | $p = 0.443$ [b] |
| ≥2 and <3 | 18.48% (3.44) | 14.19% (0.80) | |
| ≥3 | 50.23% (5.60) | 56.12% (1.57) | |
| **Diabetes status** | | | |
| Yes | 15.11% (2.96) | 11.61% (0.42) | $p = 0.289$ [b] |
| No | 81.86% (2.95) | 85.90% (0.41) | |
| Borderline | 3.03% (0.92) [f] | 2.49% (0.29) | |
| **Smoking status** | | | |
| Yes | 29.22% (4.25) [e] | 42.59% (1.22) | **$p = 0.010$** [b] |
| No | 70.78% (4.25) [e] | 57.41% (1.22) | |
| **Moderate recreational activities** | | | |
| Yes | 58.62% (4.21) [e] | 46.64% (1.17) | **$p = 0.009$** [b] |
| No | 41.38% (4.21) [e] | 53.36% (1.17) | |

Weighted proportions. Total number of unweighted observations: $n = 8511$. Continuous variables shown as mean (standard error). Categorical variables shown as weighted proportion (standard error). [a] = includes multi-racial; [b] = based on Stata's design-adjusted Rao–Scott test, [c] = based on regression analyses followed by adjusted Wald tests, [d] = or equivalent, [e] = indicates significant differences in the weighted proportions, [f] = weighted proportions to be considered unreliable, as peer recent NCHS Guidelines. Column percentages may not equal 100% due to rounding.

Again, we used multivariate logistic regression models to examine potential associations between soy milk intake status and various predictor variables (Table 4). Female sex did not increase the odds for soy milk consumption after adjustment for race/ethnicity and education level. Notably, Mexican American and Other Hispanic ethnicities significantly increased the odds (OR: 4.26 and 3.21, respectively). The same applied to Non-Hispanic Black and Non-Hispanic Asian ethnicities (OR: 2.62 and 5.60, respectively) in a second model adjusted for smoking status and moderate intensity activity. In both models, college graduates had a significantly higher OR for soy milk consumption (Table 4). The additional adjustment for physical activity did not significantly alter the findings from model 1. Participants with moderate-intensity sports and recreational activities had significantly higher odds for soy milk consumption (OR: 1.65).

**Table 4.** Multivariate logistic regression models examining potential associations between soy milk consumption status and sex, race/ethnicity, education level, and age.

| Independent Variables | OR | CI | $p$ | OR | CI | $p$ |
|---|---|---|---|---|---|---|
| | | Model 1 | | | Model 2 | |
| **Sex** | | | | | | |
| Female | 1.57 | [0.97, 2.56] | 0.067 | 1.55 | [0.96, 2.51] | 0.071 |
| **Ethnicity** | | | | | | |
| Mexican American | 4.26 | [2.07, 8.76] | **<0.001** | 4.16 | [2.52, 10.18] | **<0.001** |
| Other Hispanic | 3.21 | [1.61, 6.41] | **0.002** | 3.22 | [1.85, 6.91] | **0.002** |
| Non-Hispanic Black | 2.55 | [1.56, 4.17] | **0.001** | 2.62 | [1.69, 4.44] | **<0.001** |
| Non-Hispanic Asian | 5.70 | [3.82, 8.53] | **<0.001** | 5.60 | [4.23, 9.30] | **<0.001** |
| Other Race [a] | 1.85 | [0.73, 4.72] | 0.185 | 1.95 | [0.78, 4.99] | 0.150 |
| **Education level** | | | | | | |
| Less than 9th grade | 1.51 | [0.86, 2.65] | 0.143 | 1.60 | [0.93, 2.77] | 0.087 |
| 9–11th grade | 1.36 | [0.78, 2.35] | 0.265 | 1.47 | [0.85, 2.57] | 0.159 |
| Some college or AA degree | 1.83 | [0.93, 3.62] | 0.079 | 1.75 | [0.88, 3.47] | 0.105 |
| College graduate or above | 2.14 | [1.21, 3.80] | **0.011** | 1.84 | [1.01, 3.33] | **0.045** |
| **Moderate activity** | | | | | | |
| Yes | | | | 1.65 | [1.14, 2.40] | **0.011** |
| **Smoking** | | | | | | |
| Yes | | | | 0.82 | [0.51, 1.32] | 0.402 |

Legend: [a] = includes multi-racial. Significant regression equations were found for both models: F(10,16) = 21.98 (model 1) and F(12,14) = 21.16 (model 2), respectively, with a $p$-value < 0.001 for both. Reference categories were as follows: Male sex; Non-Hispanic White; High school graduate/GED; Moderate recreational activities in a typical week: "no"; Smoking: "no". OR = odds ratio. CI = confidence interval. The model is based on a total $n$ of 8511 participants.

## 4. Discussion

We used NHANES data to assess the prevalence of soy milk consumption in the Unites States and sought to identify potential sociodemographic predictors increasing the likelihood of its usage. The weighted proportion of individuals reporting soy milk intake in the NHANES 2015–2016 cycle was 2% and changed slightly to 1.54% in the NHANES 2017–2020 pre-pandemic cycle. Non-Hispanic Asian and Black ethnicities (as well as other Hispanic and Mexican American ethnicities in the 2017–2020 cycle) significantly increased the odds for soy milk consumption. College graduates also had significantly higher odds for consuming soy milk (OR: 2.14) in the pre-pandemic NHANES cycle. Our results also suggest that sex is apparently not an important predictor of soy milk consumption in this cross-sectional sample, while moderate physical activity was associated with higher odds.

Soy milk is one of the fastest growing categories in the U.S. plant-based non-dairy functional beverage market [49,50]. Cow milk allergies, lactose intolerance, calorie concerns, an unfavorable lipid profile, and a preference towards vegan diets for health and ethical reasons (including aspects such as environmental concerns and animal welfare) have increasingly influenced consumers across the globe towards choosing cow milk alternatives [50,51].

In addition to that, individuals are also increasingly concerned about potential negative health impacts of dairy products [52], including their high saturated fat content, their potential hormonal contamination [53], and, above all, their potential association with several diseases including various types of cancer [54–56]. However, recent systematic data highlighted some beneficial aspects of cow milk consumption in osteoporosis, cardiovascular diseases, and metabolic syndrome at various stages of life [57,58]. Nevertheless, concerns about acne, infant iron-deficiency anemia, prostate, colorectal and bladder cancers, and Parkinson's disease associated with cow milk consumption remain.

For the aforementioned reasons, soy milk is as a rapidly emerging competitor to dairy milk [49]. With regard to its nutritional profile, a 2018 review suggested that soy milk is the best alternative milk for replacing cow milk in the human diet [16]. Soy milk may also favorably affect circulating estrogen levels in premenopausal women, which could reduce the risk for breast cancer [59]. In men, soy milk consumption was associated with a reduction in prostate cancer risk [60].

Despite these putative benefits, data on soy milk intake is scarce. Sociodemographic predictors and drivers of soy milk have rarely been investigated. A study by Dharmasena and Capps suggested that age, employment status, education level, race, ethnicity, region, and presence of children in a household are significant drivers of the demand for soy milk [49]. While based on a larger sample, their study dates back to the year 2008 [49]. Using more recent data from the NHANES, we were able to confirm some of the previously identified sociodemographic predictors.

Our findings may provide valuable information about soy milk consumers and could be employed in possible public health strategies to enhance soy milk product usage and consumption. Marketing for soy products is said to require meticulous consumer segmentation in order to development food products that may appeal to different populations with various opinion and tastes [61,62]. Based on our results, individuals of Non-Hispanic White ethnicity could be such a group. The same may apply to individuals with a lower education level. Targeted marketing improving the nutritional knowledge about soy milk as a potential dairy substitute could enhance consumption in said prospective buyers.

*Strengths and Limitations*

The present study has various strengths and limitations that require further discussion. One major limitation is the cross-sectional nature of this analysis, which does not allow for any causal inference. Although we used a nationally-representative sample of United States Americans, the number of soy milk consumers was only modest, and some estimated reported proportions must be considered unreliable as per recent NCHS guidelines. We transparently flagged these proportions in the results section and clearly acknowledge this limitation. Furthermore, this analysis solely relied on data from the NHANES Diet Behavior & Nutrition module, it is not based on 24-h dietary recalls and does not inquire about reasons for (and barriers to) soy milk consumption. Such variables were unavailable in the employed NHANES cycles but would have significantly enriched our analysis. Finally, the NHANES "only" inquired about the usage of (soy) milk consumption as a drink or in combination with cereals. This excludes cooking and therefore some classical (vegan) meals that include soy milk, including but not limited to dairy-free macaroni and cheese, dairy-free lasagna, soy milk shakes as well as dairy-free pies, desserts, and cookies. As such, we may have underestimated the true prevalence of soy milk consumption. Nevertheless, we believe in the value of our data and call for additional studies in this particular field to enhance our understanding of soy milk consumption.

## 5. Conclusions

The weighted proportion of individuals reporting soy milk consumption in the NHANES ranged from approximately 1.54 to 2.0% in some of the latest NHNAES cycles. Several sociodemographic predictors of soy milk consumption (including race/ethnicity, household size, and educational level) were identified. Nevertheless, additional studies are warranted to gain a better understanding of drivers for (and barriers to) soy milk consumption in the United States. In light of the putative health benefits of soy milk and its more favorable environmental impact as compared to cow milk, future investigations should attempt to identify strategies that help promote its consumption.

**Author Contributions:** Conceptualization, M.A.S. and M.B.; methodology, M.A.S.; software, M.A.S.; validation, M.A.S.; formal analysis, M.A.S.; investigation, M.A.S. and M.B.; resources, M.A.S., M.L. and G.R.; data curation, M.A.S.; writing—original draft preparation, M.A.S. and G.R.; writing—review and editing, M.A.S., M.B., M.L. and G.R.; visualization, M.A.S.; supervision, M.A.S., M.L. and G.R.; project administration, M.A.S.; funding acquisition, M.A.S., M.L. and G.R. All authors have read and agreed to the published version of the manuscript.

**Funding:** The article processing charge was partly funded by the Baden-Wuerttemberg Ministry of Science, Research and Art and the University of Freiburg in the funding program Open Access Publishing.

**Institutional Review Board Statement:** The present study is a negligible risk research that involves existing collections of data that contain only non-identifiable data about human beings. It is a de-identified secondary analysis of freely available data. The research was performed in accordance with the Declaration of Helsinki and approved by the NCHS Research Ethics Review Board (https://www.cdc.gov/nchs/nhanes/irba98.htm; accessed on 15 May 2022). Protocol #2011-17 and Protocol #2018-01. NHANES was approved by the National Centre for Health Statistics research ethics review board, and informed consent was obtained for all participants.

**Informed Consent Statement:** Informed consent was obtained from all subjects involved in the study.

**Data Availability Statement:** Data are publicly available online (https://wwwn.cdc.gov/nchs/nhanes/Default.aspx; accessed on 2 July 2022). The datasets used and analyzed during the current study are available from the corresponding author upon reasonable request.

**Conflicts of Interest:** The authors declare no conflict of interest.

## References

1. Marrone, G.; Guerriero, C.; Palazzetti, D.; Lido, P.; Marolla, A.; Di Daniele, F.; Noce, A. Vegan Diet Health Benefits in Metabolic Syndrome. *Nutrients* **2021**, *13*, 817. [CrossRef] [PubMed]
2. Storz, M.A. What Makes a Plant-Based Diet? A Review of Current Concepts and Proposal for a Standardized Plant-Based Dietary Intervention Checklist. *Eur. J. Clin. Nutr.* **2022**, *76*, 789–800. [CrossRef] [PubMed]
3. Dressler, J.; Storz, M.A.; Müller, C.; Kandil, F.I.; Kessler, C.S.; Michalsen, A.; Jeitler, M. Does a Plant-Based Diet Stand Out for Its Favorable Composition for Heart Health? Dietary Intake Data from a Randomized Controlled Trial. *Nutrients* **2022**, *14*, 4597. [CrossRef] [PubMed]
4. Dedehayir, O.; Riverola, C.; Velasquez, S.; Smidt, M. Diffusion of Vegan Food Innovations: A Dual-Market Perspective. In *Responsible Consumption and Production*; Leal Filho, W., Azul, A.M., Brandli, L., Özuyar, P.G., Wall, T., Eds.; Encyclopedia of the UN Sustainable Development Goals; Springer International Publishing: Cham, Switzerland, 2019; pp. 1–9. ISBN 978-3-319-71062-4.
5. Nikbakht Nasrabadi, M.; Sedaghat Doost, A.; Mezzenga, R. Modification approaches of plant-based proteins to improve their techno-functionality and use in food products. *Food Hydrocoll.* **2021**, *118*, 106789. [CrossRef]
6. Dinu, M.; Abbate, R.; Gensini, G.F.; Casini, A.; Sofi, F. Vegetarian, Vegan Diets and Multiple Health Outcomes: A Systematic Review with Meta-Analysis of Observational Studies. *Crit. Rev. Food Sci. Nutr.* **2017**, *57*, 3640–3649. [CrossRef]
7. Kim, H.; Caulfield, L.E.; Garcia-Larsen, V.; Steffen, L.M.; Coresh, J.; Rebholz, C.M. Plant-Based Diets Are Associated With a Lower Risk of Incident Cardiovascular Disease, Cardiovascular Disease Mortality, and All-Cause Mortality in a General Population of Middle-Aged Adults. *J. Am. Heart Assoc.* **2019**, *8*, e012865. [CrossRef]
8. Carey, C.N.; Paquette, M.; Sahye-Pudaruth, S.; Dadvar, A.; Dinh, D.; Khodabandehlou, K.; Liang, F.; Mishra, E.; Sidhu, M.; Brown, R.; et al. The Environmental Sustainability of Plant-Based Dietary Patterns: A Scoping Review. *J. Nutr.* **2023**, *153*, 857–869. [CrossRef]
9. Filippin, D.; Sarni, A.R.; Rizzo, G.; Baroni, L. Environmental Impact of Two Plant-Based, Isocaloric and Isoproteic Diets: The Vegan Diet vs. the Mediterranean Diet. *Int. J. Environ. Res. Public Health* **2023**, *20*, 3797. [CrossRef]
10. Storz, M.A. Will the Plant-Based Movement Redefine Physicians' Understanding of Chronic Disease? *New Bioeth.* **2020**, *26*, 141–157. [CrossRef]
11. Salehin, S.; Rasmussen, P.; Mai, S.; Mushtaq, M.; Agarwal, M.; Hasan, S.M.; Salehin, S.; Raja, M.; Gilani, S.; Khalife, W.I. Plant Based Diet and Its Effect on Cardiovascular Disease. *Int. J. Environ. Res. Public Health* **2023**, *20*, 3337. [CrossRef]
12. World Cancer Research Fund/American Institute for Cancer Research. Food, nutrition, physical activity, and the prevention of cancer: A global perspective. *Choice Rev. Online* **2008**, *45*, 5024.
13. ltd R and M. Global Plant Based Milk Market (Soy Milk, Almond Milk and Rice Milk): Insights, Trends and Forecast (2020–2024). Available online: https://www.researchandmarkets.com/reports/4992280/global-plant-based-milk-market-soy-milk-almond (accessed on 7 May 2023).
14. Munekata, P.E.S.; Domínguez, R.; Budaraju, S.; Roselló-Soto, E.; Barba, F.J.; Mallikarjunan, K.; Roohinejad, S.; Lorenzo, J.M. Effect of Innovative Food Processing Technologies on the Physicochemical and Nutritional Properties and Quality of Non-Dairy Plant-Based Beverages. *Foods* **2020**, *9*, 288. [CrossRef]
15. Paul, A.A.; Kumar, S.; Kumar, V.; Sharma, R. Milk Analog: Plant Based Alternatives to Conventional Milk, Production, Potential and Health Concerns. *Crit. Rev. Food Sci. Nutr.* **2020**, *60*, 3005–3023. [CrossRef]
16. Vanga, S.K.; Raghavan, V. How Well Do Plant Based Alternatives Fare Nutritionally Compared to Cow's Milk? *J. Food Sci. Technol.* **2018**, *55*, 10–20. [CrossRef]
17. CFR—Code of Federal Regulations Title 21. Available online: https://www.accessdata.fda.gov/scripts/cdrh/cfdocs/cfcfr/cfrsearch.cfm (accessed on 7 May 2023).

18. Verband Sozialer Wettbewerb eV v TofuTowncom GmbH [Internet]. 2017. Available online: https://eur-lex.europa.eu/legal-content/EN/TXT/?uri=CELEX%3A62016CJ0422 (accessed on 7 May 2023).
19. Nutrition C for FS and A. FDA Releases Draft Guidance on Labeling of Plant-Based Milk Alternatives. FDA. 22 February 2023. Available online: https://www.fda.gov/food/cfsan-constituent-updates/fda-releases-draft-guidance-labeling-plant-based-milk-alternatives (accessed on 7 May 2023).
20. Marangoni, F.; Pellegrino, L.; Verduci, E.; Ghiselli, A.; Bernabei, R.; Calvani, R.; Cetin, I.; Giampietro, M.; Perticone, F.; Piretta, L.; et al. Cow's Milk Consumption and Health: A Health Professional's Guide. *J. Am. Coll. Nutr.* **2019**, *38*, 197–208. [CrossRef]
21. Craig, W.J.; Fresán, U. International Analysis of the Nutritional Content and a Review of Health Benefits of Non-Dairy Plant-Based Beverages. *Nutrients* **2021**, *13*, 842. [CrossRef]
22. Rizzo, G.; Baroni, L. Soy, Soy Foods and Their Role in Vegetarian Diets. *Nutrients* **2018**, *10*, 43. [CrossRef]
23. Silva, A.R.A.; Silva, M.M.N.; Ribeiro, B.D. Health Issues and Technological Aspects of Plant-Based Alternative Milk. *Food Res. Int.* **2020**, *131*, 108972. [CrossRef]
24. Sousa, A.; Bolanz, K.A.K. Nutritional Implications of an Increasing Consumption of Non-Dairy Plant-Based Beverages Instead of Cow's Milk in Switzerland. *J. Adv. Dairy Res.* **2017**. Available online: https://www.omicsonline.org/open-access/nutritional-implications-of-an-increasing-consumption-of-nondairy-plantbased-beverages-instead-of-cow19516219483641948482s-milk-in-2329-888X-1000197-95593.html (accessed on 7 May 2023). [CrossRef]
25. Fructuoso, I.; Romão, B.; Han, H.; Raposo, A.; Ariza-Montes, A.; Araya-Castillo, L.; Zandonadi, R.P. An Overview on Nutritional Aspects of Plant-Based Beverages Used as Substitutes for Cow's Milk. *Nutrients* **2021**, *13*, 2650. [CrossRef] [PubMed]
26. Zuliani, G.; Galvani, M.; Leitersdorf, E.; Volpato, S.; Cavalieri, M.; Fellin, R. The Role of Polyunsaturated Fatty Acids (PUFA) in the Treatment of Dyslipidemias. *Curr. Pharm. Des.* **2009**, *15*, 4087–4093. [CrossRef] [PubMed]
27. Zielińska-Dawidziak, M. Plant Ferritin—A Source of Iron to Prevent Its Deficiency. *Nutrients* **2015**, *7*, 1184–1201. [CrossRef] [PubMed]
28. Romeiko, X.X.; Lee, E.K.; Sorunmu, Y.; Zhang, X. Spatially and Temporally Explicit Life Cycle Environmental Impacts of Soybean Production in the U.S. Midwest. *Environ. Sci. Technol.* **2020**, *54*, 4758–4768. [CrossRef] [PubMed]
29. Dreoni, I.; Matthews, Z.; Schaafsma, M. The Impacts of Soy Production on Multi-Dimensional Well-Being and Ecosystem Services: A Systematic Review. *J. Clean. Prod.* **2022**, *335*, 130182. [CrossRef]
30. USDA ERS-Soybeans and Oil Crops. Available online: https://www.ers.usda.gov/topics/crops/soybeans-and-oil-crops/ (accessed on 22 May 2023).
31. Messina, M. Perspective: Soybeans Can Help Address the Caloric and Protein Needs of a Growing Global Population. *Front. Nutr.* **2022**, *9*, 909464. [CrossRef]
32. Fraanje, W.; Garnett, T. *Soy: Food, Feed, and Land Use Change. (Foodsource: Building Blocks)*; Food Climate Research Network, University of Oxford: Oxford, UK, 2020. [CrossRef]
33. Coluccia, B.; Agnusdei, G.P.; De Leo, F.; Vecchio, Y.; La Fata, C.M.; Miglietta, P.P. Assessing the Carbon Footprint across the Supply Chain: Cow Milk vs Soy Drink. *Sci. Total Environ.* **2022**, *806*, 151200. [CrossRef]
34. Messina, M.; Mejia, S.B.; Cassidy, A.; Duncan, A.; Kurzer, M.; Nagato, C.; Ronis, M.; Rowland, I.; Sievenpiper, J.; Barnes, S. Neither Soyfoods nor Isoflavones Warrant Classification as Endocrine Disruptors: A Technical Review of the Observational and Clinical Data. *Crit. Rev. Food Sci. Nutr.* **2022**, *62*, 5824–5885. [CrossRef]
35. Rizzo, G.; Feraco, A.; Storz, M.A.; Lombardo, M. The Role of Soy and Soy Isoflavones on Women's Fertility and Related Outcomes: An Update. *J. Nutr. Sci.* **2022**, *11*, e17. [CrossRef]
36. Rizzo, G. The Antioxidant Role of Soy and Soy Foods in Human Health. *Antioxidants* **2020**, *9*, 635. [CrossRef]
37. Clark, B.E.; Pope, L.; Belarmino, E.H. Perspectives from Healthcare Professionals on the Nutritional Adequacy of Plant-Based Dairy Alternatives: Results of a Mixed Methods Inquiry. *BMC Nutr.* **2022**, *8*, 46. [CrossRef]
38. Pointke, M.; Ohlau, M.; Risius, A.; Pawelzik, E. Plant-Based Only: Investigating Consumers' Sensory Perception, Motivation, and Knowledge of Different Plant-Based Alternative Products on the Market. *Foods* **2022**, *11*, 2339. [CrossRef]
39. Home | Dietary Guidelines for Americans. Available online: https://www.dietaryguidelines.gov/ (accessed on 7 May 2023).
40. NHANES—About the National Health and Nutrition Examination Survey. 2022. Available online: https://www.cdc.gov/nchs/nhanes/about_nhanes.htm (accessed on 7 May 2023).
41. National Center for Health Statistics—National Health and Nutrition Examination Survey, 2013–2014. Overview. 2022. Available online: https://www.cdc.gov/nchs/data/nhanes/nhanes_13_14/2013-14_overview_brochure.pdf (accessed on 7 May 2023).
42. NHANES—NCHS Research Ethics Review Board Approval. 2022. Available online: https://www.cdc.gov/nchs/nhanes/irba98.htm. (accessed on 22 April 2023).
43. NHANES Questionnaires, Datasets, and Related Documentation. Available online: https://wwwn.cdc.gov/nchs/nhanes/continuousnhanes/default.aspx?BeginYear=2015 (accessed on 27 April 2023).
44. NHANES Questionnaires, Datasets, and Related Documentation. Available online: https://wwwn.cdc.gov/nchs/nhanes/continuousnhanes/default.aspx?cycle=2017-2020 (accessed on 27 April 2023).
45. Dan, M. Missing standard error because of stratum with single sampling unit. | Stata. Available online: https://www.stata.com/support/faqs/statistics/standard-error-because-of-stratum/ (accessed on 27 April 2023).
46. Heeringa, G.; West, B.T.; West, P.A. *Applied Survey Data Analysis*, 2nd ed.; Chapman and Hall/CRC: New York, NY, USA, 2017.

47. Parker, J.D.; Talih, M.; Malec, D.J.; Beresovsky, V.; Carroll, M.; Gonzalez, J.F.; Hamilton, B.E.; Ingram, D.D.; Kochanek, K.; McCarty, F.; et al. National Center for Health Statistics Data Presentation Standards for Proportions. *Vital Health Stat* **2017**, *2*, 1–22.
48. Ward, B.W. Kg_nchs: A Command for Korn-Graubard Confidence Intervals and National Center for Health Statistics' Data Presentation Standards for Proportions. *Stata J.* **2019**, *19*, 510–522. [CrossRef] [PubMed]
49. Dharmasena, S.; Capps, O. Unraveling Demand for Dairy-Alternative Beverages in the United States: The Case of Soymilk. *Agric. Resour. Econ. Rev.* **2014**, *43*, 140–157. [CrossRef]
50. Sethi, S.; Tyagi, S.K.; Anurag, R.K. Plant-Based Milk Alternatives an Emerging Segment of Functional Beverages: A Review. *J. Food Sci. Technol.* **2016**, *53*, 3408–3423. [CrossRef]
51. Basu, A. Plant-Based Milk Consumption in India: Motivators, Deterrents and Marketing Strategies in a Competitive Market. *J. Int. Food Agribus. Mark.* **2022**, 1–23. [CrossRef]
52. Laassal, M.; Kallas, Z. Consumers Preferences for Dairy-Alternative Beverage Using Home-Scan Data in Catalonia. *Beverages* **2019**, *5*, 55. [CrossRef]
53. Malekinejad, H.; Rezabakhsh, A. Hormones in Dairy Foods and Their Impact on Public Health—A Narrative Review Article. *Iran J. Public Health* **2015**, *44*, 742–758. [PubMed]
54. Kroenke, C.H.; Kwan, M.L.; Sweeney, C.; Castillo, A.; Caan, B.J. High- and Low-Fat Dairy Intake, Recurrence, and Mortality After Breast Cancer Diagnosis. *J. Natl. Cancer Inst.* **2013**, *105*, 616–623. [CrossRef]
55. Qin, L.-Q.; Xu, J.-Y.; Wang, P.-Y.; Tong, J.; Hoshi, K. Milk Consumption Is a Risk Factor for Prostate Cancer in Western Countries: Evidence from Cohort Studies. *Asia Pac. J. Clin. Nutr.* **2007**, *16*, 467–476.
56. Song, Y.; Chavarro, J.E.; Cao, Y.; Qiu, W.; Mucci, L.; Sesso, H.D.; Stampfer, M.J.; Giovannucci, E.; Pollak, M.; Liu, S.; et al. Whole Milk Intake Is Associated with Prostate Cancer-Specific Mortality among U.S. Male Physicians. *J. Nutr.* **2013**, *143*, 189–196. [CrossRef] [PubMed]
57. Zhang, X.; Chen, X.; Xu, Y.; Yang, J.; Du, L.; Li, K.; Zhou, Y. Milk Consumption and Multiple Health Outcomes: Umbrella Review of Systematic Reviews and Meta-Analyses in Humans. *Nutr. Metab.* **2021**, *18*, 7. [CrossRef] [PubMed]
58. Gil, Á.; Ortega, R.M. Introduction and Executive Summary of the Supplement, Role of Milk and Dairy Products in Health and Prevention of Noncommunicable Chronic Diseases: A Series of Systematic Reviews. *Adv. Nutr.* **2019**, *10*, S67–S73. [CrossRef] [PubMed]
59. Lu, L.J.; Anderson, K.E.; Grady, J.J.; Nagamani, M. Effects of Soya Consumption for One Month on Steroid Hormones in Premenopausal Women: Implications for Breast Cancer Risk Reduction. *Cancer Epidemiol. Biomark. Prev.* **1996**, *5*, 63–70.
60. Yan, L.; Spitznagel, E.L. Soy Consumption and Prostate Cancer Risk in Men: A Revisit of a Meta-Analysis. *Am. J. Clin. Nutr.* **2009**, *89*, 1155–1163. [CrossRef] [PubMed]
61. Teh, T.; Dougherty, M.P.; Camire, M.E. How Do Consumer Attitudes Influence Acceptance of a Novel Wild Blueberry–Soy Product? *J. Food Sci.* **2007**, *72*, S516–S521. [CrossRef]
62. Bosman, M.J.C.; Ellis, S.M.; Bouwer, S.C.; Jerling, J.C.; Erasmus, A.C.; Harmse, N.; Badham, J. South African Consumers' Opinions and Consumption of Soy and Soy Products. *Int. J. Consum. Stud.* **2009**, *33*, 425–435. [CrossRef]

*nutrients*

MDPI

*Article*

# Anti-Adipogenic Activity of *Rhaponticum carthamoides* and Its Secondary Metabolites

**Velislava Todorova [1], Martina S. Savova [2], Stanislava Ivanova [1,*], Kalin Ivanov [1] and Milen I. Georgiev [2]**

[1] Department of Pharmacognosy and Pharmaceutical Chemistry, Faculty of Pharmacy, Medical University-Plovdiv, 4002 Plovdiv, Bulgaria; velislava.todorova@mu-plovdiv.bg (V.T.); kalin.ivanov@mu-plovdiv.bg (K.I.)

[2] Laboratory of Metabolomics, Institute of Microbiology, Bulgarian Academy of Sciences, 4000 Plovdiv, Bulgaria; m.sav@abv.bg (M.S.S.); milengeorgiev@gbg.bg (M.I.G.)

* Correspondence: stanislava.ivanova@mu-plovdiv.bg

**Abstract:** Besides their common use as an adaptogen, *Rhaponticum carthamoides* (Willd.) Iljin. rhizome and its root extract (RCE) are also reported to beneficially affect lipid metabolism. The main characteristic secondary metabolites of RCE are phytoecdysteroids. In order to determine an RCE's phytoecdysteroid profile, a novel, sensitive, and robust high-performance thin-layer chromatography (HPTLC) method was developed and validated. Moreover, a comparative analysis was conducted to investigate the effects of RCE and its secondary metabolites on adipogenesis and adipolysis. The evaluation of the anti-adipogenic and lipolytic effects was performed using human Simpson–Golabi–Behmel syndrome cells, where lipid staining and measurement of released glycerol and free fatty acids were employed. The HPTLC method confirmed the presence of 20-hydroxyecdysone (20E), ponasterone A (PA), and turkesterone (TU) in RCE. The observed results revealed that RCE, 20E, and TU significantly reduced lipid accumulation in human adipocytes, demonstrating their anti-adipogenic activity. Moreover, RCE and 20E were found to effectively stimulate basal lipolysis. However, no significant effects were observed with PA and TU applications. Based on our findings, RCE and 20E affect both lipogenesis and lipolysis, while TU only restrains adipogenesis. These results are fundamental for further investigations.

**Keywords:** *Rhaponticum carthamoides* (Willd.) Iljin.; 20-hydroxyecdysone; ponasterone A; turkesterone; high-performance thin layer chromatography (HPTLC); obesity; adipocytes; adipogenesis; adipolysis

## 1. Introduction

Obesity and the state of being overweight are among the continuously growing public health concerns [1–4]. According to the World Health Organization (WHO), currently, almost 2 billion adults are considered overweight and 650 million of them are considered obese [5]. Common comorbidities attributed to obesity and the state of being overweight are hypertension, dyslipidemia, type 2 diabetes, sleep apnea, osteoarthritis, and cancer [2,6–8]. Current strategies for excess adiposity management include lifestyle modifications, pharmacotherapy, and bariatric surgery in the most severe cases [8–10]. However, the number of approved and safe drugs for the reduction of body weight is quite limited—orlistat, phentermine, topiramate, and semaglutide [11–13]. At present, plenty of studies are focused on the research of novel molecules with anti-obesity activity [14]. Many of these potential therapeutic molecules are plant secondary metabolites [15–17]. Numerous plants are reported to possess anti-obesity potential such as *Eleutherococcus senticosus*, *Bassia scoparia*, *Platycodon grandiflorum*, *Gypsophila oldhamiana*, *Momordica charantia*, *Rosmarinus officinalis*, *Citrus limon*, *Taraxacum officinale*, and *Ziziphus jujuba* [1,18,19]. The anti-obesity activity of plant species is related to their phytochemical content, especially: saponins (platycodin A, platycodin C, deapioplatycodin D, momordin Ic, escin Ia, escin IIa, escin Ib, etc.), polyphenols (caffeic acid, chlorogenic acid, resveratrol, curcumin, kaempferol, quercetin, cyanidin, naringenin, etc.), terpenoids (lycopene, lutein, and carotene), organosulfurs (allicin and alliin), and phytosterols (protodisoscin and diosgenin) [18,20]. These natural compounds may exert their anti-obesity effect through more than one of the following mechanisms: inhibition of pancreatic lipases, stimulation of lipolysis, inhibition of differentiation of preadipocytes, stimulation of adipose tissue browning, and induction apoptosis of existing hypertrophied adipocytes [18,20].

Although many bioactive compounds of plant origin possess anti-obesity potential, the specific role of phytoecdysteroids (PDs) remains incompletely understood. Noratto et al. reported that the intake of quinoa (a phytoecdysteroid-rich plant) is associated with positive effects on obesity in mice [21]. However, further research is needed to reveal the potential of PDs and phytoecdysteroid-containing plants on obesity. Among the phytoecdysteroid-rich plants is the endemic perennial plant *Rhaponticum carthamoides* (Willd.) Iljin. from the Asteraceae family, commonly known as maral root or Russian leuzea [22,23]. In traditional medicine, it has been used to improve physical strength [22]. In 1969, leuzea was systemized as one of the plant adaptogens by Brekman and Dardimov [22]. In recent decades, extracts from its rhizomes and roots have been used for physical weakness, to promote muscle growth, to treat impotency, etc. [22]. Various medicinal preparations from *R. carthamoides* rhizomes and roots have been reported to possess not only adaptogenic effects but also a broad spectrum of biological effects, such as antioxidant, immunomodulatory, anticancerogenic, antimicrobial, antiparasitic, and repellent activities [22–24]. The main isolated chemical classes from *R. carthamoides* rhizomes and roots are not only PDs but also phenolics (flavonoids and phenolic acids) [22]. Previous phytochemical reports regarding ecdysteroids of *R. carthamoides* from the underground parts of the plants revealed the isolation of 20-hydroxyecdysone, also known as ecdysterone (20E), ponasterone A (PA), and turkesterone (TU) [22,25,26]. Ecdysteroids are a group of polyhydroxylated sterols, structurally similar to androgens (Figure 1) [24,27,28].

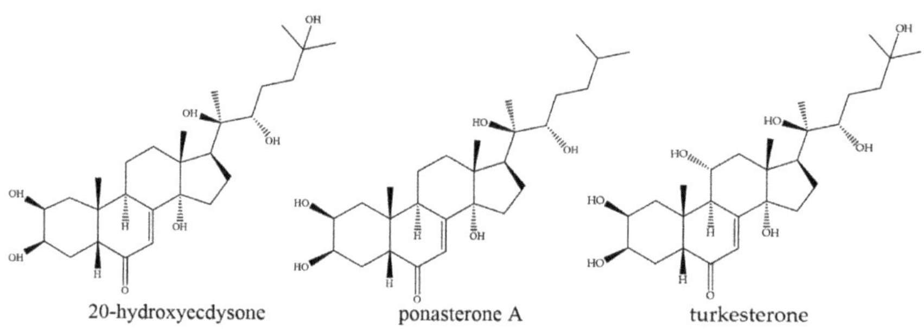


**Figure 1.** Chemical structures of the phytoecdysteroids–20-hydroxyecdysone, ponasterone A and turkesterone.

PDs possess a wide range of pharmacological properties, including antidiabetic and hepatoprotective properties [24,29]. Previous studies reported that 20E possesses anabolic, neuroprotective, and antitumor effects, restores renal dysfunction, and decreases triglycerides [28–34]. It has the potential to prevent adiposity, dyslipidemia, and hyperglycemia [35,36], while PA possesses anabolic activity [29]. Turkesterone has been associated with anabolic, antidiabetic, and hypoazotemic effects, as well as the ability to decrease cholesterol levels and restore renal function, according to previous investigations [29].

The current study aimed to evaluate the phytochemical profile of *R. carthamoides* rhizomes and roots extract (RCE) via an innovative high-performance thin layer chromatography (HPTLC) method. Moreover, the PDs in the extract—20E, PA, and TU—were quantified. Following the chemical analysis, the effect of RCE as well as its secondary metabolites on adipogenesis and adipolysis were investigated in an in vitro obesity model of human adipocytes.

## 2. Materials and Methods

### 2.1. Chemicals and Reagents

The reference standard of PA (molecular weight: 464.6 g·mol$^{-1}$; purity: HPLC $\geq$ 95%, #16,386) was purchased from Cayman Chemical, Ann Arbor, MI, USA. The reference standards of 20E (molecular weight 480.64 g·mol$^{-1}$; purity: HPLC $\geq$ 95%, #89,651) and TU (molecular weight: 496.6 g·mol$^{-1}$; purity: HPLC $\geq$ 95%, #85,781) were obtained from PhytoLab GmbH & Co. KG, Vestenbergsgreuth, Germany. Analytical grade dimethyl sulfoxide (DMSO), isopropanol, acetonitrile, methanol, cell culture medium Dulbecco's modified Eagle's medium/Nutrient F-12 Ham, Oil red O (ORO; 0.5% solution in isopropanol), fetal bovine serum, penicillin/streptomycin 10,000 IU/10 mg·mL$^{-1}$, d-biotin (purity > 99%), d-pantothenic acid (purity > 99%), human apo-transferrin (purity > 98%), rosiglitazone (purity: HPLC > 98%), human insulin, 3-isobutyl-1-methylxantine (purity: HPLC > 99%), dexamethasone (purity: HPLC > 98%), triiodothyronine (purity > 95%), cortisol (purity > 95%), and isoproterenol hydrochloride (purity: HPLC > 98%) were obtained from Merck KGaA (Darmstadt, Germany).

### 2.2. Plant Material and Extraction

The dried *R. carthamoides* rhizomes and roots were purchased from Russia. The plant material was characterized according to the Russian Pharmacopoeia by the Department of Pharmacognosy and pharmaceutical chemistry, Medical University of Plovdiv. The plant material was further frozen, freeze-dried, and ground before ultrasound-assisted extraction with 50% aqueous methanol at 20 °C for 30 min. The obtained RCE was filtered and concentrated via a rotary vacuum evaporator at 40 °C, further freeze-dried, and stored at −20 °C before use.

### 2.3. HPTLC Analyses

#### 2.3.1. Sample Preparation

The stock solutions for HPTLC analysis of 20E, PA, T, and the extract were prepared in acetonitrile in concentration 1 mg·mL$^{-1}$. Ultrasound was used for better dissolution. The prepared stock solutions were stored before use in brown vials, protected from light at 4 °C.

#### 2.3.2. Instrumentation

The method was developed using a CAMAG HPTLC system (CAMAG, Muttenz, Switzerland) in the following configuration: CAMAG Limomat 5, a software-controlled applicator of CAMAG, Muttenz, Switzerland); CAMAG Automatic Developing Chamber 2 (CAMAG, Muttenz, Switzerland), and CAMAG TLC Visualizer 2 (CAMAG, Muttenz, Switzerland). The software used was "VisionCATS" (version 3, CAMAG, Muttenz, Switzerland). An ultrasonic bath (Bandelin, Berlin, Germany) was used for better dissolution of the standard solutions.

#### 2.3.3. Method Development

The analyses were carried out using silica gel 60 F254 glass TLC plates of 10 × 20 cm size and with 200 µm layer thickness (E. Merck KGaA, Darmstadt, Germany). The mobile phase comprised methanol: acetonitrile at a ratio of 10:90 (*v*/*v*). The volume of the mobile phase was 10 mL. The application type was a band, and the front was 70 mm. The time for development was 10 min, followed by drying for 5 min. Detection was performed at 254 nm using CAMAG TLC Visualizer 2.

#### 2.3.4. Method Validation

The developed method was validated according to the International Council for Harmonization of Technical Requirements for Pharmaceuticals for Human Use (ICH) with the following validation parameters: linearity, range, precision, accuracy, and limits of detection (LD) and quantification (LQ) [37].

*2.4. Cell Culture and Treatment*

Human Simpson–Golabi–Behmel syndrome (SGBS) preadipocytes were kindly provided by Professor Martin Wabitsch (University of Ulm, Germany). The cells were cultured under optimal conditions [38,39]. The differentiation of near-confluent preadipocytes was carried out with the presence of RCE (5–50 μg·mL$^{-1}$), 20E (5–50 μM), PA (5–50 μM), TU (5–50 μM), or 0.02% DMSO as a vehicle. These concentrations were selected based on cell viability evaluation with the 3-(4,5-dimethylthiazol-2-yl)-2,5-diphenyltetrazolium bromide (MTT) assay. The experimental treatments were applied upon differentiation and on the fourth and eighth days with every culture media replacement process. Sample collection and subsequent analyses were performed 24 h after the last treatment. Each assay was performed at least in three independent experiments.

*2.5. Cell Viability Assay*

The preadipocytes were seeded in 96-well plates, grown to near confluence, and incubated for 48 h with increasing concentrations from 0.1 to 100 μM for the pure compounds and 0.1 to 100 μg·mL$^{-1}$ for the extract or 0.02% DMSO as a vehicle. The results are presented as the percentage of cell viability compared to the vehicle as the mean ± SEM and are representative of three independent experiments.

*2.6. Lipid Staining*

The procedure was performed as previously described [40]. Briefly, on day 9 of differentiation, the SGBS adipocytes were fixed with formalin and subsequently stained with freshly prepared ORO solution. Then, the representative microphotographs were taken using an Oxion Inverso OX.2053-PLPH inverted microscope, equipped with a DC.10,000-Pro CMEX camera (Euromex, Arnhem, The Netherlands). For the quantification of accumulated lipids for each group, the absorbance of the extracted lipid dye at 495 nm was measured using an Anthos Zenyth 340 multiplate reader from Biochrom Ltd. (Cambridge, United Kingdom). The results were represented as the percentage of accumulated lipids compared to the vehicle-treated group.

*2.7. Analysis of Basal and Stimulated Lipolysis*

The effect of increasing concentrations of RCE, 20E, PA, and TU, was evaluated through quantification of released glycerol and free fatty acids (FFAs) in the culture media, as products of lipid hydrolysis. Along with the last treatment, on day 8 of adipogenic differentiation, lipolysis was stimulated with 10 μM isoproterenol for 24 h [41]; then, culture media samples were collected from the tested treatments subjected to both basal and isoproterenol-stimulated conditions. Glycerol and FFA concentrations were determined using a glycerol assay kit (#MAK117) and a free fatty acid assay kit (#MAK044) from Merck KGaA according to the manufacturer's instructions.

*2.8. Statistical Analysis*

The resulting data were expressed as the mean ± SEM and statistical significance between groups was determined by one-way ANOVA, followed by Tukey's post hoc test, using SigmaPlot v11.0 software from Systat Software GmbH (Erkrath, Germany). Values of $p < 0.05$ were considered significant.

## 3. Results

*3.1. HPTLC Analysis*

3.1.1. Method Development

A rapid and sensitive HPTLC method was developed to quantify the PDs present in RCE. The method was effective for the estimation of 20E, PA, and TU.

The first step of the method development was to choose a suitable solvent system for the analyzed compounds. For the determination of a suitable phase, various proportions of acetonitrile and methanol were used. Proportions including acetonitrile/methanol

(85:15, *v/v*), acetonitrile/methanol (80:20, *v/v*), acetonitrile/methanol (10:90, *v/v*), acetonitrile/methanol (95:5, *v/v*), and acetonitrile/methanol (50:50, *v/v*) were investigated as the solvent systems for the development of a suitable band for quantitation. From the results, it was observed that the acetonitrile/methanol (85:15, *v/v*), acetonitrile/methanol (80:20, *v/v*), acetonitrile/methanol (10:90, *v/v*), acetonitrile/methanol (95:5, *v/v*), and acetonitrile/methanol (50:50, *v/v*) solvent systems presented a poor chromatogram of the examined PDs with a poor asymmetry factor. Among the tested solvent systems, acetonitrile/methanol (90:10, *v/v*) provided well-separated and compact chromatographic peaks of TU, 20E, and PA at Rf 0.2, 0.3, and 0.6, respectively. Hence, the acetonitrile/methanol (90:10, *v/v*) proportion was considered as a proper solvent system for the determination of 20E, PA, and TU in the HPTLC method. Figures 2 and 3 represent the HPTLC chromatogram and profiles of different concentration levels of the PDs and RCE, respectively.

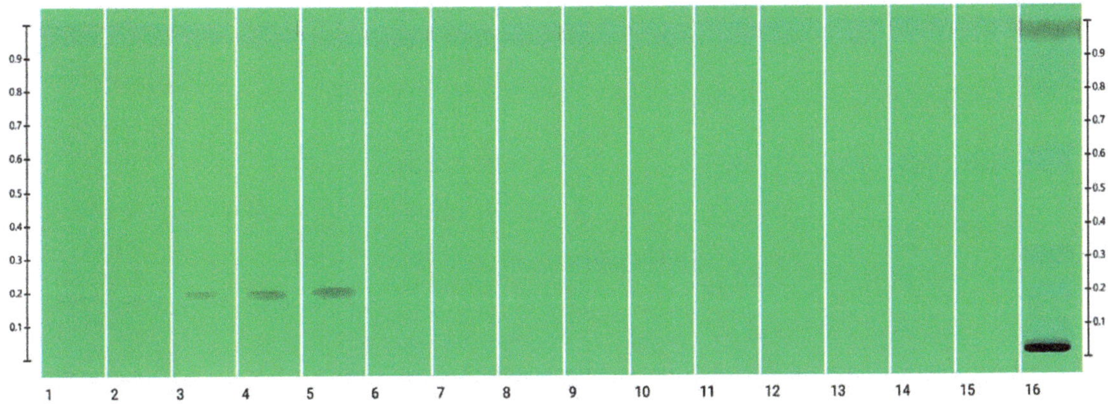


**Figure 2.** Comparison between different concentration levels of the standard solutions of PDs and RCE, where 1. TU 0.5 μg·band$^{-1}$; 2. TU 0.75 μg·band$^{-1}$; 3. TU 1 μg·band$^{-1}$; 4. TU 1.25 μg·band$^{-1}$; 5. TU 1.5 μg·band$^{-1}$; 6. 20E 0.5 μg·band$^{-1}$; 7. 20E 0.75 μg·band$^{-1}$; 8. 20E 1 μg·band$^{-1}$; 9. 20E 1.25 μg·band$^{-1}$; 10. 20E 1.5 μg·band$^{-1}$; 11. PA 0.5 μg.band$^{-1}$; 12. PA 0.75 μg·band$^{-1}$; 13. PA 1 μg·band$^{-1}$; 14. PA 1.25 μg·band$^{-1}$; 15. PA 1.5 μg·band$^{-1}$; 16. RCE.

#### 3.1.2. Method Validation

The method was validated according to ICH guidelines [37].

##### Linearity

To establish linearity, an external standard curve was employed. The calibration curves were plotted by concentrations and the peak area of each PD. To prepare the standard solution, 20E (0.5 to 1.5 μg·band$^{-1}$), PA (0.5 to 1.5 μg·band$^{-1}$), and TU (0.5 to 1.5 μg·band$^{-1}$) were dissolved in acetonitrile. The regression line was calculated with y = ax ± b, where x is the concentration and y is the peak area of each PD, b is the y-intercept, and a is the slope of the regression line. Moreover, the coefficient of determination ($R^2$) was established for the linearity.

The linearity of the method was determined in the 0.5–1.5 μg.band$^{-1}$ range for the tested substances. The regression line equation and the $R^2$ for 20E were y = 0.0027x + 0.0002 and $R^2$ = 0.9988, for PA, they were y = 0.0042x + 0.0003 and $R^2$ = 0.9986, and for TU, they were y = 0.004x + 0.0008 and $R^2$ = 0.997, respectively. These results showed a significant correlation and demonstrated the reliability of the method for estimating these PDs. Table 1 presents the results of the regression analysis, LD, and LQ.

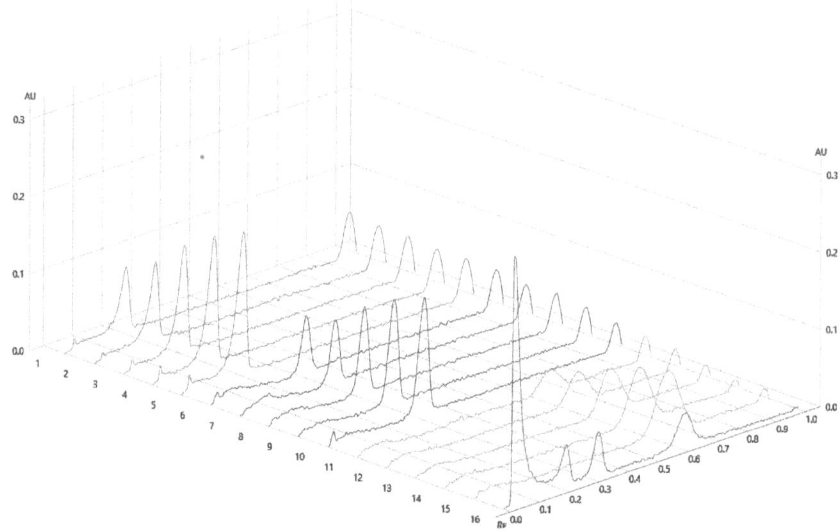


**Figure 3.** Profiles of different concentration levels of the standard solutions of PDs and RCE, where 1. TU 0.5 μg·band$^{-1}$; 2. TU 0.75 μg·band$^{-1}$; 3. TU 1 μg·band$^{-1}$; 4. TU 1.25 μg·band$^{-1}$; 5. TU 1.5 μg·band$^{-1}$; 6. 20E 0.5 μg·band$^{-1}$; 7. 20E 0.75 μg·band$^{-1}$; 8. 20E 1 μg·band$^{-1}$; 9. 20E 1.25 μg·band$^{-1}$; 10. 20E 1.5 μg·band$^{-1}$; 11. PA 0.5 μg·band$^{-1}$; 12. PA 0.75 μg·band$^{-1}$; 13. PA 1 μg·band$^{-1}$; 14. PA 1.25 μg·band$^{-1}$; 15. PA 1.5 μg·band$^{-1}$; 16. RCE.

**Table 1.** Linearity, LD, and LQ of the developed HPTLC method.

| Parameter | 20-Hydroxyecdysterone | Ponasterone A | Turkesterone |
|---|---|---|---|
| Range | 0.5–1.5 μg·band$^{-1}$ | 0.5–1.5 μg·band$^{-1}$ | 0.5–1.5 μg·band$^{-1}$ |
| Regression line | y = 0.0027x + 0.0002 | y = 0.0042x + 0.0003 | y = 0.004x + 0.0008 |
| $R^2$ | 0.9988 | 0.9986 | 0.997 |
| LD | 0.11 μg·band$^{-1}$ | 0.13 μg·band$^{-1}$ | 0.04 μg·band$^{-1}$ |
| LQ | 0.35 μg·band$^{-1}$ | 0.39 μg·band$^{-1}$ | 0.12 μg·band$^{-1}$ |

Accuracy

Accuracy was established across the specified range of the analytical procedure, which was determined to be from the 0.5 to 1.5 μg·band$^{-1}$ for 20E, PA, and TU.

The accuracy of the suggested HPTLC method was evaluated using the percentage of recovery of three concentration levels (low, medium, and high) with six replicates of each concentration. For the accuracy test, from each examined substance, three different quality control (QC) levels were used: lower QC (LQC: 0.75 μg·band$^{-1}$), middle QC (MQC: 1 μg·band$^{-1}$), and high QC (HQC: 1.25 μg·band$^{-1}$) with six replicates. Table 2 presents the results of the accuracy of the developed HPTLC method.

Precision

The precision of the proposed HPTLC method was evaluated for both intra-day and inter-day precision, with six replicates of the injection. Examining the intra-day variation for the examined substances involved quantifying fresh solutions at LQC, MQC, and HQC on the same day in six replicates ($n$ = 6). Inter-day variability for the examined substances was examined using the quantitation of freshly generated solutions at LQC, MQC, and HQC on three consecutive days in six replicates ($n$ =6). Table 3 presents the results for the precision of these PDs.

**Table 2.** Evaluating the accuracy of the developed HPTLC method.

| Concentration (μg·band$^{-1}$) | Mean (μg.band$^{-1}$) ± SD | Recovery % | CV% |
|---|---|---|---|
| | 20-hydroxyecdysone | | |
| 1.25 | 1.24 ± 0.010 | 99.06 | 0.82 |
| 1 | 0.99 ± 0.008 | 99.07 | 0.84 |
| 0.75 | 0.76 ± 0.008 | 100.90 | 1.10 |
| | Ponasterone A | | |
| 1.25 | 1.25 ± 0.006 | 99.62 | 0.49 |
| 1 | 0.99 ± 0.009 | 98.65 | 0.89 |
| 0.75 | 0.76 ± 0.007 | 100.95 | 0.93 |
| | Turkesterone | | |
| 1.25 | 1.26 ± 0.014 | 100.97 | 1.12 |
| 1 | 0.99 ± 0.010 | 99.21 | 1.01 |
| 0.75 | 0.74 ± 0.012 | 98.83 | 1.70 |

CV%—percent of coefficient of variation.

**Table 3.** The precision of the developed HPTLC method.

| Concentration (μg·band$^{-1}$) | Intraday Precision | | | Interday Precision | | |
|---|---|---|---|---|---|---|
| | Mean (μg·band$^{-1}$) ± SD | SE | CV% | Mean (μg·band$^{-1}$) ± SD | SE | CV% |
| | 20-hydroxyecdysone | | | | | |
| 1.25 | 1.24 ± 0.011 | 0.004 | 0.86 | 1.24 ± 0.011 | 0.003 | 0.95 |
| 1 | 1.00 ± 0.009 | 0.004 | 0.86 | 0.99 ± 0.009 | 0.004 | 0.96 |
| 0.75 | 0.75 ± 0.008 | 0.003 | 1.02 | 0.75 ± 0.010 | 0.004 | 1.27 |
| | Ponasterone A | | | | | |
| 1.25 | 1.25 ± 0.008 | 0.003 | 0.62 | 1.25 ± 0.007 | 0.003 | 0.53 |
| 1 | 0.99 ± 0.008 | 0.003 | 0.85 | 0.99 ± 0.008 | 0.003 | 0.77 |
| 0.75 | 0.75 ± 0.010 | 0.004 | 1.37 | 0.75 ± 0.009 | 0.004 | 1.16 |
| | Turkesterone | | | | | |
| 1.25 | 1.25 ± 0.010 | 0.004 | 0.79 | 1.24 ± 0.010 | 0.004 | 0.82 |
| 1 | 0.99 ± 0.017 | 0.007 | 1.66 | 0.99 ± 0.013 | 0.005 | 1.31 |
| 0.75 | 0.74 ± 0.008 | 0.003 | 1.06 | 0.74 ± 0.010 | 0.004 | 1.29 |

CV%—percent of coefficient of variation; SE—standard error.

Detection Limit (DL) and Quantitation Limit (QL)

The detection limit and quantification limit were expressed by the standard deviation of the slope (σ) and the slope of the calibration curve (S) using the following formulas: DL = 3.3 σ/S and QL = 10 σ/S, respectively.

The lowest concentrations for which a reliable spot was established were 0.11 μg·band$^{-1}$ for 20E, 0.13 μg·band$^{-1}$ for PA, and 0.04 μg·band$^{-1}$ for TU. The quantification limit for 20E was 0.35 μg·band$^{-1}$, for PA, it was 0.39 μg·band$^{-1}$, and for TU, it was 0.12 μg·band$^{-1}$, as shown in Table 1.

Robustness

The robustness of the proposed method was assessed by deliberately introducing variations in the mobile phase compositions and total run length. The solvents ratio of acetonitrile/methanol (90:10, $v/v$) was modified within a range of ±1%, and the HPTLC response was recorded for each set of conditions. The total solvent distance was altered to 72 mm and 68 mm from the initial 70 mm, and the HPTLC response was recorded. The observed changes in Rf values were within the range ± 0.02, which indicated that the method was robust.

In order to assess the stability of the standard solutions, they were stored at 2–8 °C for a week, visual inspection confirmed the clarity of the solutions, and subsequently, the obtained chromatograms from the freshly prepared solutions were compared with those derived from the stored solutions. The comparative analysis revealed that the samples maintained their stability throughout the entire duration of storage.

The close values of correlation factors to one, the high percentage of accuracy, and the low values of standard deviation suggested that the developed method is linear, accurate, precise, and reliable for the determination and quantification of 20E, PA, and TU. The developed and validated method was used for the quality determination of the three compounds in RCE. The amount of 20E was found to be 2.96 mg·g$^{-1}$, PA was found to be 1.75 mg·g$^{-1}$, and the amount of TU was found to be 1.65 mg·g$^{-1}$ crude dry extract. The obtained HPTLC results were confirmed through HPLC/UV analysis using the previously validated method [42].

### 3.2. *Effect of RCE, 20E, PA, and TU on Cell Viability*

The performed MTT assay revealed that the cell viability of the near-confluent preadipocytes was not affected upon incubation for 48 h with RCE µg·mL$^{-1}$ and 20E, PA, and TU in 0.1–100 µM, respectively (Figure 4). Consequently, the selected treatment concentrations are safe for application in the following experiments.

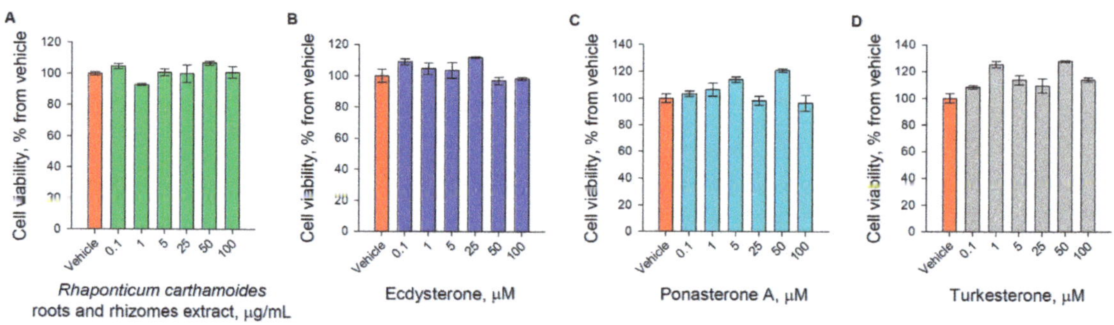


**Figure 4.** Cell viability was not affected upon RCE, 20E, PA, and TU treatment. Cell viability, expressed as the percentage of cell viability compared to the vehicle as the mean ± SEM upon treatment with (**A**) RCE, (**B**) 20E, (**C**) PA, and (**D**) TU.

### 3.3. *Effect of RCE, 20E, PA, and TU on Adipogenesis in Human Adipocytes*

The chemical profiling of RCE affirmed the presence of 20E, PA, and TU. To evaluate whether RCE and the identified PDs modulate adipogenesis, ORO lipid staining was performed. The observed tendency toward a reduction in accumulated lipids is represented through microscopic images of the treated groups (Figure 5A).

The results of total lipid quantification (Figure 5B) revealed a statistically significant reduction upon the administration of the following treatments—RCE (86.8, 87.1, 80.2, and 82.8% for 5, 10, 25 and 50 µg·mL$^{-1}$, respectively), 20E (97, 90.4, 90.2, and 88.3% for 5, 10, 25 and 50 µM, respectively), and TU (91.9, 82.3, 76, and 79.9% for 5, 10, 25 and 50 µM, respectively). Among the investigated treatments, the highest anti-adipogenic activity was observed for TU, followed by RCE and 20E. In the current experiment, PA did not affect adipogenic differentiation in human adipocytes.

Collectively, the screening, based on lipid staining, affirmed that RCE and the identified PDs—20E and TU—possess promising anti-adipogenic activity. Further experiments evaluated whether the modulation of adipolysis is involved in the observed decrease in total lipid content.

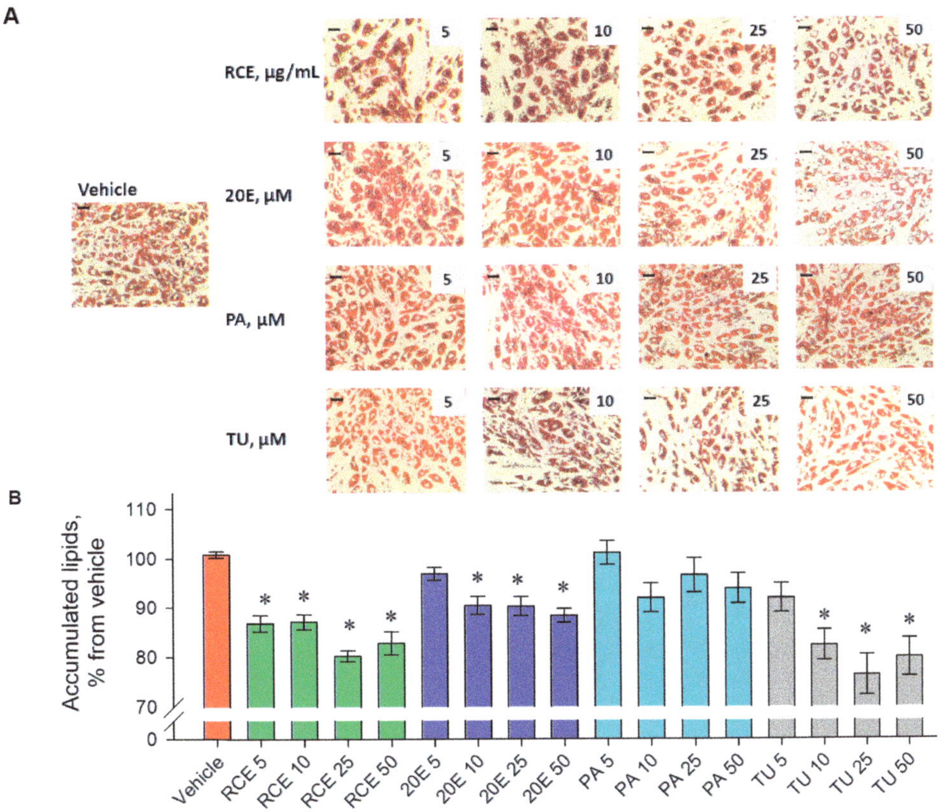


**Figure 5.** A significant decrease in adipogenic differentiation and lipid accumulation was observed upon RCE, 20E, and TU treatment. Representative microphotographs from the Oil red O staining of the experimental groups, 20x magnification (**A**). Quantification of accumulated lipids through spectrophotometric measures of the absorbance of the extracted Oil red O dye at 495 nm, represented as a percentage from vehicle (**B**). The data are expressed as the mean ± SEM. * $p < 0.05$ compared to the vehicle control group.

### *3.4. Effect of RCE, 20E, PA, and TU on Basal and Isoproterenol-Stimulated Lipolysis in Human Adipocytes*

To determine the effect of RCE, 20E, PA, and TU on basal and isoproterenol-stimulated lipolysis, quantification of glycerol and FFAs released in the culture media was performed.

Incubation with RCE (50 $\mu g \cdot mL^{-1}$) significantly increased the concentration of both glycerol (Figure 6A) and FFAs (Figure 6C) in the culture media under basal conditions. In a similar manner, in unstimulated adipocytes, 20E (50 µM) application only significantly increased the FFA concentration (Figure 6C). Treatment with PA and TU affected neither glycerol (Figure 6A) nor FFA (Figure 6C) concentrations. Therefore, we can suggest that both RCE and 20E significantly increased basal lipolysis, while such an effect was not observed upon PA or TU treatment (Figure 6A,C). Isoproterenol stimulation elevated the released glycerol and FFAs in comparison to the basal level. However, no significant effect on both glycerol (Figure 6B) and FFAs (Figure 6D) was detected upon all the treatments applied compared to the isoproterenol-stimulated vehicle.

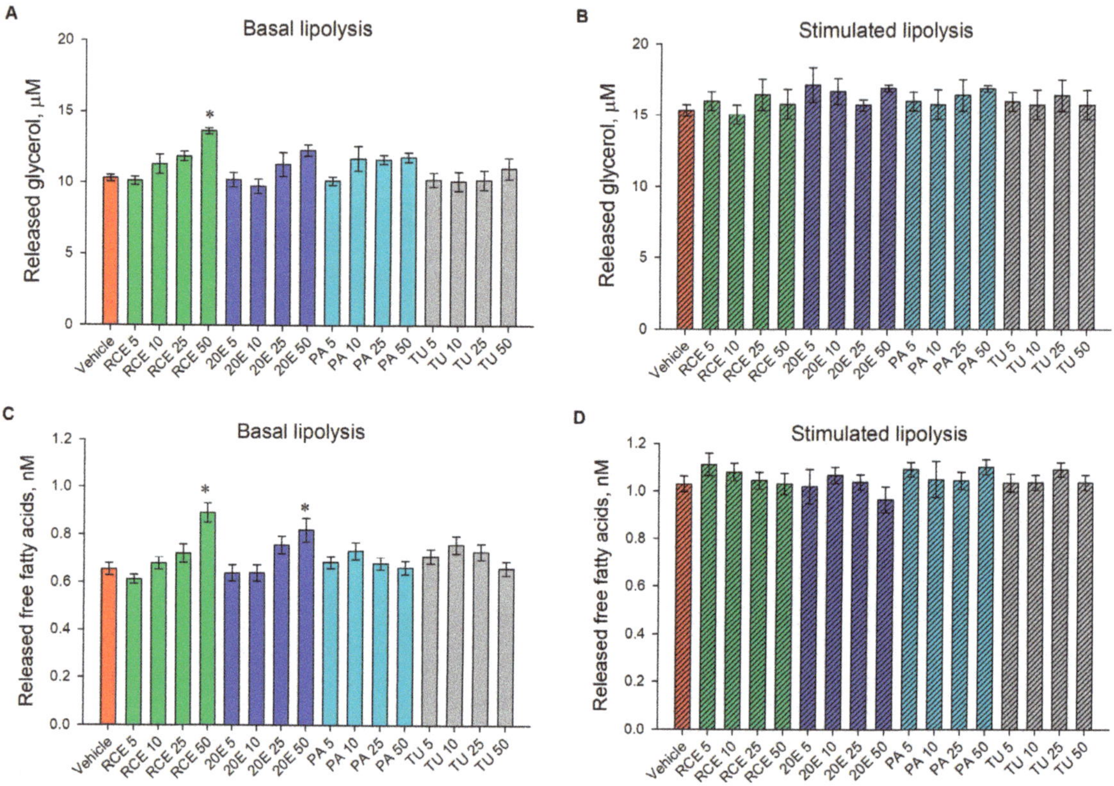


**Figure 6.** Only RCE and 20E stimulated basal lipolysis in human adipocytes. Glycerol concentration (µM) in cell culture media on day 9 of differentiation under basal conditions (**A**) and isoproterenol stimulation (10 µM for 24 h) (**B**). Free fatty acids concentration (nM) in cell culture media on day 9 of differentiation under basal conditions (**C**) and isoproterenol stimulation (**D**). The data are expressed as the mean ± SEM. * $p < 0.05$ compared to the vehicle control group.

Basal lipolysis was elevated only in the highest concentrations of RCE and 20E. However, none of the treatments affected isoproterenol-stimulated adipolysis.

## 4. Discussion

Considering the continuously increasing interest in plant products as food supplements due to the assumption of their safety [43], it is crucial to address the limited data regarding the control of their quality. Moreover, a lack of relevant scientific evidence confirming the biological activity and efficacy of some plant products [44] raises additional questions about the rationale of their use. Therefore, the development of fast, precise, and sensitive analytical methods is of great importance for the adequate control of plant products. RCE and PDs are widely used as adaptogens [22,45]. However, the available HPTLC methods for identifying and quantifying PDs, especially for PDs isolated from RCE, are currently quite limited, as evidenced by the data presented in Table 4 [46–50]. For that reason, a new HPTLC method that offers high sensitivity, efficiency, and reproducibility has been developed. The HPTLC technique has several advantages, including rapidity, cost-effectiveness, etc. [51,52], making it a highly suitable method for the future analysis of PDs.

**Table 4.** Comparison between chromatographic conditions of the HPTLC methods for PD determination.

| Purpose | Chromatographic Conditions | LD/LQ | Ref. |
|---|---|---|---|
| Ecdysteroids (20E, ponasterone A, and others) characterization of some *Silane* species | RP-HPTLC plates, mobile phase: chloroform: ethanol 4:1 (*v*/*v*), visualized under 254 nm. | - | [46] |
| Ecdysteroids (20E, ponasterone A, turkesterone, and others) characterization of some *Silane* species | RP-HPTLC plates, ethanol: water 3:2 (*v*/*v*) and acetone: water 3:2 (*v*/*v*), visualized under 254 nm. | - | [47] |
| Determination and quantitation of 20E in *Sida rhombifolia* L. and dietary supplements | HPTLC plates were prewashed with methanol and dried in an oven at 120 °C for three minutes, mobile phase: chloroform: methanol 8:2 (*v*/*v*), distance 60 mm, visualized under 250 nm. | LD 60 ng·spot$^{-1}$ LQ 200 ng·spot$^{-1}$ | [48] |
| Development and validation of an HPTLC method for the quantification of 20E | HPTLC plates, mobile phase: THF: toluene: 1 mM TFA in methanol: water 16:8:2:1 (*v*/*v*/*v*/*v*), a distance of 70 mm, visualized under 250 nm. | Lower limits of quantitation—70–100 μg·mL$^{-1}$ Upper limits of quantitation—815 μg·mL$^{-1}$ above 1000 μg·mL$^{-1}$. | [49] |
| Monitoring of ecdysteroids isolated from *Manduca sexta* pupae | HPTLC plates, mobile phase: chloroform: ethanol (65:35, *v*/*v*), chloroform: methanol: 10-N-ammonium hydroxide 28:20:2 (*v*/*v*/*v*) for ecdysteroid acids and 15:35:3.5 (*v*/*v*/*v*) for ecdysteroid conjugates, visualized under UV light and sprayed with 50% sulfuric acid solution. | - | [50] |

Except for the traditional adaptogenic activity of RCE, diverse biological activities are reported either for the extract or for the PDs investigated in this study. The extract has been evaluated for anti-neoplastic activity [53,54], cardioprotective effects [55], and the stimulation of muscle protein synthesis [56]. Moreover, an in vivo study indicates the beneficial effects of RCE on fat tissue expansion and hepatic triglyceride accumulation [57]. The reported biological activity of 20E includes anti-neoplastic activity [31,58], the modulation of mitochondrial bioenergetics [59], immunomodulatory effects [60], an increase in the muscle mass amelioration of the radiation-induced damage of oral mucosa [61], and neuroprotective [30,62,63], anti-fibrotic [64], wound-healing [65], and anti-inflammatory [66,67] activities. Several reports have proposed the potential of 20E to benefit metabolic disturbances such as obesity [36,68]; in addition, it has been reported to exert anti-diabetic [36,65,69,70] and anti-osteoporotic [71–73] effects. Moreover, as a food supplement in humans, 20E was found to increase strength performance with no effect on steroid profile [32]. Both PA and TU have not been investigated as natural compounds with anti-obesogenic effects.

The balance between adipogenesis and adipolysis determines the size of fat cells [74]. Thus, a decrease in lipid accumulation along with the stimulation of triglyceride mobilization are among the anti-obesogenic mechanisms of plant extracts and their constituents [75].

In order to affirm the available data for the potential of RCE and 20E in obesity management, as well as to evaluate the anti-adipogenic activity of PA and TU, the current investigation assessed the effect of RCE, 20E, PA, and TU on adipogenesis and lipolysis in vitro in human adipocytes. The applied cell-based platform provides fast and reliable screening of anti-adipogenic potential and accelerates the identification and selection of drugs which leads to their effects being subsequently evaluated in vivo.

The observed anti-adipogenic activity of RCE is in accordance with the previously reported decrease in the weight of epididymal fat tissue in rats [57]. Moreover, the obtained results suggested that among the identified PDs from the extract, only 20E and TU significantly decreased lipid accumulation during adipocyte differentiation. The detected effect upon 20E treatment is consistent with the literature data for reduced adipocyte size in diet-induced obesity in a murine model [68]. Interestingly, the current investigation suggested the notable anti-adipogenic activity of TU, which has not been previously reported.

Lipolysis is the process of triglyceride hydrolysis which is assumed to decrease the size of adipocytes [75] and can also be accepted as an indicator of energy expenditure [76]. Principally, there are two types of adipolysis—basal and stimulated (upon β3-adrenergic receptor activation by isoproterenol or catecholamines) [75]. Our findings suggest that RCE and 20E elevated basal lipolysis, which apparently contributes to the observed decrease in total lipid content.

In the current study, in comparison to 20E and TU, PA had no effect on adipogenesis and adipolysis, which have not been reported to our knowledge. Despite the common ecdysteroid structure in the investigated natural compounds, we could suggest that the observed difference in biological response is attributed to the lack of hydroxyl group on position 25 in PA, compared to 20E and TU.

The results of the present study demonstrated that RCE and 20E exhibit anti-obesity potential by reducing adipogenesis and promoting lipolysis in human adipocytes, while turkesterone promotes only adipogenesis. Further investigation is needed to fully understand the mechanism and affirm its potential therapeutic applications. Nevertheless, the findings highlight the importance of exploring the diversity of plant metabolites for drug discovery and development and suggest that *R. carthamoides* could be a promising source of natural anti-obesity agents or a combination of the most abundant secondary metabolites.

## 5. Conclusions

In summary, the developed and validated HPTLC method was demonstrated to be reliable for the estimation and quantification of the PDs 20E, PA, and TU. Using the developed HPTLC method, identification and quantification of these PDs in RCE were performed. Additionally, evaluation of anti-adipogenic activity revealed that RCE, 20E, and TU considerably decreased lipid accumulation in human adipocytes. Further experiments indicated that RCE and 20E significantly stimulated basal lipolysis, while no effect was observed upon PA and TU application. The obtained results from RCE, 20E, and TU are worth further mechanistic evaluation, which would provide a scientific rationale for subsequent in vivo experiments.

**Author Contributions:** Conceptualization, V.T., M.S.S., S.I., K.I. and M.I.G.; methodology, V.T., M.S.S., S.I. and K.I.; software, V.T. and M.S.S.; validation, V.T., S.I. and K.I.; formal analysis, V.T., M.S.S. and S.I.; investigation, V.T., M.S.S. and S.I.; resources, V.T.; data curation, V.T., S.I. and K.I.; writing—original draft preparation, V.T. and M.S.S.; writing—review and editing, S.I., K.I. and M.I.G.; visualization, V.T., M.S.S. and S.I.; supervision, S.I., K.I. and M.I.G. All authors have read and agreed to the published version of the manuscript.

**Funding:** This research received no external funding.

**Data Availability Statement:** Not applicable.

**Acknowledgments:** We gratefully acknowledge Martin Wabitsch (University of Ulm, Germany) for kindly providing SGBS preadipocyte cell line. The authors gratefully acknowledge the support of the Medical University of Plovdiv, project DPDP-06/2022.

**Conflicts of Interest:** The authors declare no conflict of interest.

## References

1. Gamboa-Gómez, C.I.; Rocha-Guzmán, N.E.; Gallegos-Infante, J.A.; Moreno-Jiménez, M.R.; Vázquez-Cabral, B.D.; González-Laredo, R.F. Plants with Potential Use on Obesity and Its Complications. *EXCLI J.* **2015**, *14*, 809–831. [CrossRef] [PubMed]
2. Dakanalis, A.; Mentzelou, M.; Papadopoulou, S.K.; Papandreou, D.; Spanoudaki, M.; Vasios, G.K.; Pavlidou, E.; Mantzorou, M.; Giaginis, C. The Association of Emotional Eating with Overweight/Obesity, Depression, Anxiety/Stress, and Dietary Patterns: A Review of the Current Clinical Evidence. *Nutrients* **2023**, *15*, 1173. [CrossRef] [PubMed]
3. Jakobsen, D.D.; Brader, L.; Bruun, J.M. Association between Food, Beverages and Overweight/Obesity in Children and Adolescents-A Systematic Review and Meta-Analysis of Observational Studies. *Nutrients* **2023**, *15*, 764. [CrossRef] [PubMed]
4. Tamel Selvan, K.; Goon, J.A.; Makpol, S.; Tan, J.K. Effects of Microalgae on Metabolic Syndrome. *Antioxidants* **2023**, *12*, 449. [CrossRef]
5. World Health Organisation. Obesity and Overweight. Available online: https://www.who.int/news-room/fact-sheets/detail/obesity-and-overweight (accessed on 12 March 2023).
6. Pronk, N.P.; Eneli, I.; Economos, C.D.; Bradley, D.; Fassbender, J.; Calancie, L.; Patawaran, W.; Hovmand, P.S. Using Systems Science for Strategic Planning of Obesity Prevention and Treatment: The Roundtable on Obesity Solutions Experience. *Curr. Prob. Cardiol.* **2022**, *48*, 101240. [CrossRef]
7. Ahn, J.; Suh, Y.; Lee, K. Chordin-like 1, a Novel Adipokine, Markedly Promotes Adipogenesis and Lipid Accumulation. *Cells* **2023**, *12*, 624. [CrossRef]
8. Ivanova, S.; Delattre, C.; Karcheva-Bahchevanska, D.; Benbasat, N.; Nalbantova, V.; Ivanov, K. Plant-Based Diet as a Strategy for Weight Control. *Foods* **2021**, *10*, 3052. [CrossRef]
9. Calcaterra, V.; Rossi, V.; Mari, A.; Casini, F.; Bergamaschi, F.; Zuccotti, G.V.; Fabiano, V. Medical Treatment of Weight Loss in Children and Adolescents with Obesity. *Pharmacol. Res.* **2022**, *185*, 106471. [CrossRef]
10. Kushner, R.F. Weight Loss Strategies for Treatment of Obesity. *Prog. Cardiovasc. Dis.* **2014**, *56*, 465–472. [CrossRef]
11. Rodgers, R.J.; Tschöp, M.H.; Wilding, J.P.H. Anti-Obesity Drugs: Past, Present and Future. *Dis. Model. Mech.* **2012**, *5*, 621–626. [CrossRef]
12. Derosa, G.; Maffioli, P. Anti-Obesity Drugs: A Review about Their Effects and Their Safety. *Expert Opin. Drug Saf.* **2012**, *11*, 459–471. [CrossRef]
13. Aaseth, J.; Ellefsen, S.; Alehagen, U.; Sundfør, T.M.; Alexander, J. Diets and Drugs for Weight Loss and Health in Obesity—An Update. *Biomed. Pharmacother.* **2021**, *140*, 111789. [CrossRef]
14. Hainer, V. Overview of New Antiobesity Drugs. *Expert Opin. Pharmacother.* **2014**, *15*, 1975–1978. [CrossRef]
15. Borah, A.K.; Sharma, P.; Singh, A.; Kalita, K.J.; Saha, S.; Chandra Borah, J. Adipose and Non-Adipose Perspectives of Plant Derived Natural Compounds for Mitigation of Obesity. *J. Ethnopharmacol.* **2021**, *280*, 114410. [CrossRef]
16. Wang, H.-N.; Xiang, J.-Z.; Qi, Z.; Du, M. Plant Extracts in Prevention of Obesity. *Crit. Rev. Food Sci. Nutr.* **2022**, *62*, 2221–2234. [CrossRef]
17. Shang, A.; Gan, R.-Y.; Xu, X.-Y.; Mao, Q.-Q.; Zhang, P.-Z.; Li, H.-B. Effects and Mechanisms of Edible and Medicinal Plants on Obesity: An Updated Review. *Crit. Rev. Food Sci. Nutr.* **2021**, *61*, 2061–2077. [CrossRef] [PubMed]
18. Marrelli, M.; Conforti, F.; Araniti, F.; Statti, G.A. Effects of Saponins on Lipid Metabolism: A Review of Potential Health Benefits in the Treatment of Obesity. *Molecules* **2016**, *21*, 1404. [CrossRef] [PubMed]
19. Savova, M.S.; Vasileva, L.V.; Mladenova, S.G.; Amirova, K.M.; Ferrante, C.; Orlando, G.; Wabitsch, M.; Georgiev, M.I. *Ziziphus Jujuba* Mill. Leaf Extract Restrains Adipogenesis by Targeting PI3K/AKT Signaling Pathway. *Biomed. Pharmacother.* **2021**, *141*, 111934. [CrossRef]
20. González-Castejón, M.; Rodriguez-Casado, A. Dietary Phytochemicals and Their Potential Effects on Obesity: A Review. *Pharmacol. Res.* **2011**, *64*, 438–455. [CrossRef]
21. Noratto, G.D.; Murphy, K.; Chew, B.P. Quinoa Intake Reduces Plasma and Liver Cholesterol, Lessens Obesity-Associated Inflammation, and Helps to Prevent Hepatic Steatosis in Obese Db/Db Mouse. *Food Chem.* **2019**, *287*, 107–114. [CrossRef] [PubMed]
22. Kokoska, L.; Janovska, D. Chemistry and Pharmacology of *Rhaponticum Carthamoides*: A Review. *Phytochemistry* **2009**, *70*, 842–855. [CrossRef] [PubMed]
23. Skała, E.; Sitarek, P.; Różalski, M.; Krajewska, U.; Szemraj, J.; Wysokińska, H.; Śliwiński, T. Antioxidant and DNA Repair Stimulating Effect of Extracts from Transformed and Normal Roots of *Rhaponticum Carthamoides* against Induced Oxidative Stress and DNA Damage in CHO Cells. *Oxid. Med. Cell Longev.* **2016**, *2016*, 5753139. [CrossRef]
24. Das, N.; Mishra, S.K.; Bishayee, A.; Ali, E.S.; Bishayee, A. The Phytochemical, Biological, and Medicinal Attributes of Phytoecdysteroids: An Updated Review. *Acta Pharm. Sin. B* **2021**, *11*, 1740–1766. [CrossRef] [PubMed]
25. Kosović, E.; Lino, K.; Kuchař, M. HPLC-MS Methodology for *R. Carthamoides* Extract Quality Evaluation: A Simultaneous Determination of Eight Bioactive Compounds. *Diversity* **2022**, *14*, 880. [CrossRef]
26. Buděšínský, M.; Vokáč, K.; Harmatha, J.; Cvačka, J. Additional Minor Ecdysteroid Components of *Leuzea Carthamoides*. *Steroids* **2008**, *73*, 502–514. [CrossRef] [PubMed]

27. Savchenko, R.G.; Veskina, N.A.; Odinokov, V.N.; Benkovskaya, G.V.; Parfenova, L.V. Ecdysteroids: Isolation, Chemical Transformations, and Biological Activity. *Phytochem. Rev.* **2022**, *21*, 1445–1486. [CrossRef]
28. Tóth, N.; Szabó, A.; Kacsala, P.; Héger, J.; Zádor, E. 20-Hydroxyecdysone Increases Fiber Size in a Muscle-Specific Fashion in Rat. *Phytomedicine* **2008**, *15*, 691–698. [CrossRef]
29. Bathori, M.; Toth, N.; Hunyadi, A.; Marki, A.; Zador, E. Phytoecdysteroids and Anabolic-Androgenic Steroids—Structure and Effects on Humans. *CMC* **2008**, *15*, 75–91. [CrossRef]
30. Xu, T.; Niu, C.; Zhang, X.; Dong, M. β-Ecdysterone Protects SH-SY5Y Cells against β-Amyloid-Induced Apoptosis via c-Jun N-Terminal Kinase- and Akt-Associated Complementary Pathways. *Lab. Investig.* **2018**, *98*, 489–499. [CrossRef]
31. Romaniuk-Drapała, A.; Lisiak, N.; Totoń, E.; Matysiak, A.; Nawrot, J.; Nowak, G.; Kaczmarek, M.; Rybczyńska, M.; Rubiś, B. Proapoptotic and Proautophagic Activity of 20-Hydroxyecdysone in Breast Cancer Cells in Vitro. *Chem. Biol. Interact.* **2021**, *342*, 109479. [CrossRef]
32. Isenmann, E.; Ambrosio, G.; Joseph, J.F.; Mazzarino, M.; de la Torre, X.; Zimmer, P.; Kazlauskas, R.; Goebel, C.; Botrè, F.; Diel, P.; et al. Ecdysteroids as Non-Conventional Anabolic Agent: Performance Enhancement by Ecdysterone Supplementation in Humans. *Arch. Toxicol.* **2019**, *93*, 1807–1816. [CrossRef] [PubMed]
33. Chen, L.; Zheng, S.; Huang, M.; Ma, X.; Yang, J.; Deng, S.; Huang, Y.; Wen, Y.; Yang, X. β-Ecdysterone from *Cyanotis Arachnoidea* Exerts Hypoglycemic Effects through Activating IRS-1/Akt/GLUT4 and IRS-1/Akt/GLUT2 Signal Pathways in KK-Ay Mice. *JFF* **2017**, *39*, 123–132. [CrossRef]
34. Catalán, R.E.; Martinez, A.M.; Aragones, M.D.; Miguel, B.G.; Robles, A.; Godoy, J.E. Alterations in Rat Lipid Metabolism Following Ecdysterone Treatment. *Comp. Biochem. Physiol. B Biochem. Mol. Biol.* **1985**, *81*, 771–775. [CrossRef] [PubMed]
35. Little, A.; Murphy, K.; Solverson, P. Quinoa's Potential to Enhance Dietary Management of Obesity and Type-2 Diabetes: A Review of the Current Evidence. *Diabetology* **2021**, *2*, 77–94. [CrossRef]
36. Kizelsztein, P.; Govorko, D.; Komarnytsky, S.; Evans, A.; Wang, Z.; Cefalu, W.T.; Raskin, I. 20-Hydroxyecdysone Decreases Weight and Hyperglycemia in a Diet-Induced Obesity Mice Model. *Am. J. Physiol. Endocrinol. Metab.* **2009**, *296*, E433–E439. [CrossRef] [PubMed]
37. EMA. ICH Q2(R2) Validation of Analytical Procedures—Scientific Guideline. Available online: https://www.ema.europa.eu/en/ich-q2r2-validation-analytical-procedures-scientific-guideline (accessed on 7 December 2022).
38. Vasileva, L.V.; Savova, M.S.; Amirova, K.M.; Balcheva-Sivenova, Z.; Ferrante, C.; Orlando, G.; Wabitsch, M.; Georgiev, M.I. Caffeic and Chlorogenic Acids Synergistically Activate Browning Program in Human Adipocytes: Implications of AMPK- and PPAR-Mediated Pathways. *Int. J. Mol. Sci.* **2020**, *21*, 9740. [CrossRef]
39. Wabitsch, M.; Brenner, R.E.; Melzner, I.; Braun, M.; Möller, P.; Heinze, E.; Debatin, K.-M.; Hauner, H. Characterization of a Human Preadipocyte Cell Strain with High Capacity for Adipose Differentiation. *Int. J. Obes.* **2001**, *25*, 8–15. [CrossRef]
40. Vasileva, L.V.; Savova, M.S.; Tews, D.; Wabitsch, M.; Georgiev, M.I. Rosmarinic Acid Attenuates Obesity and Obesity-Related Inflammation in Human Adipocytes. *FCT* **2021**, *149*, 112002. [CrossRef]
41. Lasa, A.; Schweiger, M.; Kotzbeck, P.; Churruca, I.; Simón, E.; Zechner, R.; Portillo, M.d.P. Resveratrol Regulates Lipolysis via Adipose Triglyceride Lipase. *J. Nutr. Biochem.* **2012**, *23*, 379–384. [CrossRef]
42. Todorova, V.; Ivanov, K.; Karcheva-Bahchevanska, D.; Ivanova, S. Development and Validation of High-Performance Liquid Chromatography for Identification and Quantification of Phytoecdysteroids Ecdysterone and Turkesterone in Dietary Supplements. *Processes* **2023**, *11*, 1786. [CrossRef]
43. Pasdaran, A.; Hamedi, A.; Shiehzadeh, S.; Hamedi, A. A Review of Citrus Plants as Functional Foods and Dietary Supplements for Human Health, with an Emphasis on Meta-Analyses, Clinical Trials, and Their Chemical Composition. *Clin. Nutr. ESPEN* **2023**, *54*, 311–336. [CrossRef] [PubMed]
44. Petroczi, A.; Taylor, G.; Naughton, D.P. Mission Impossible? Regulatory and Enforcement Issues to Ensure Safety of Dietary Supplements. *FCT* **2011**, *49*, 393–402. [CrossRef] [PubMed]
45. Sidorova, Y.S.; Shipelin, V.A.; Petrov, N.A.; Zorin, S.N.; Mazo, V.K. Adaptogenic Properties of a Phytoecdysteroid-Rich Extract from the Leaves of *Spinacia Oleracea* L. *Plants* **2021**, *10*, 2555. [CrossRef] [PubMed]
46. Claude, E.; Tower, M.; Lafont, R.; Wilson, I.D.; Plumb, R.S. High Performance Thin-Layer Chromatography of Plant Ecdysteroids Coupled with Desorption Electrospray Ionisation–Ion Mobility–Time of Flight High Resolution Mass Spectrometry (HPTLC/DESI/IM/ToFMS). *Chromatographia* **2020**, *83*, 1029–1035. [CrossRef]
47. Claude, E.; Lafont, R.; Plumb, R.S.; Wilson, I.D. High Performance Reversed-Phase Thin-Layer Chromatography-Desorption Electrospray Ionisation—Time of Flight High Resolution Mass Spectrometric Detection and Imaging (HPTLC/DESI/ToFMS) of Phytoecdysteroids. *J. Chromatogr. B* **2022**, *1200*, 123265. [CrossRef] [PubMed]
48. Jadhav, A.N.; Rumalla, C.S.; Avula, B.; Khan, I.A. HPTLC Method for Determination of 20-Hydroxyecdysone in *Sida Rhombifolia* L. and Dietary Supplements. *Chroma* **2007**, *66*, 797–800. [CrossRef]
49. Mamadalieva, N.Z.; Böhmdorfer, S.; Zengin, G.; Bacher, M.; Potthast, A.; Akramov, D.K.; Janibekov, A.; Rosenau, T. Phytochemical and Biological Activities of Silene Viridiflora Extractives. Development and Validation of a HPTLC Method for Quantification of 20-Hydroxyecdysone. *Ind. Crops Prod.* **2019**, *129*, 542–548. [CrossRef]
50. Lozano, R.; Thompson, M.J.; Svoboda, J.A.; Lusby, W.R. Isolation of Acidic and Conjugated Ecdysteroid Fractions from Manduca Sexta Pupae. *Insect Biochem.* **1988**, *18*, 163–168. [CrossRef]

51. Ivanova, S.; Todorova, V.; Dyankov, S.; Ivanov, K. High-Performance Thin-Layer Chromatography (HPTLC) Method for Identification of Meloxicam and Piroxicam. *Processes* **2022**, *10*, 394. [CrossRef]
52. Mukherjee, P.K. Chapter 9—High-Performance Thin-Layer Chromatography (HPTLC) for Analysis of Herbal Drugs. In *Quality Control and Evaluation of Herbal Drugs*; Mukherjee, P.K., Ed.; Elsevier: Amsterdam, The Netherlands, 2019; pp. 377–420; ISBN 978-0-12-813374-3.
53. Skała, E.; Sitarek, P.; Toma, M.; Szemraj, J.; Radek, M.; Nieborowska-Skorska, M.; Skorski, T.; Wysokińska, H.; Śliwiński, T. Inhibition of Human Glioma Cell Proliferation by Altered Bax/Bcl-2-P53 Expression and Apoptosis Induction by *Rhaponticum Carthamoides* Extracts from Transformed and Normal Roots. *J. Pharm. Pharmacol.* **2016**, *68*, 1454–1464. [CrossRef]
54. Gaube, F.; Wölfl, S.; Pusch, L.; Werner, U.; Kroll, T.C.; Schrenk, D.; Hartmann, R.W.; Hamburger, M. Effects of *Leuzea Carthamoides* on Human Breast Adenocarcinoma MCF-7 Cells Determined by Gene Expression Profiling and Functional Assays. *Planta Med.* **2008**, *74*, 1701–1708. [CrossRef] [PubMed]
55. Zheng, Z.; Xian, Y.; Jin, Z.; Yao, F.; Liu, Y.; Deng, Y.; Wang, B.; Chen, D.; Yang, J.; Ren, L.; et al. *Rhaponticum Carthamoides* Improved Energy Metabolism and Oxidative Stress through the SIRT6/Nrf2 Pathway to Ameliorate Myocardial Injury. *Phytomedicine* **2022**, *105*, 154197. [CrossRef] [PubMed]
56. Roumanille, R.; Vernus, B.; Brioche, T.; Descossy, V.; Van Ba, C.T.; Campredon, S.; Philippe, A.G.; Delobel, P.; Bertrand-Gaday, C.; Chopard, A.; et al. Acute and Chronic Effects of *Rhaponticum Carthamoides* and *Rhodiola Rosea* Extracts Supplementation Coupled to Resistance Exercise on Muscle Protein Synthesis and Mechanical Power in Rats. *J. Int. Soc. Sports Nutr.* **2020**, *17*, 58. [CrossRef]
57. Dushkin, M.; Khrapova, M.; Kovshik, G.; Chasovskikh, M.; Menshchikova, E.; Trufakin, V.; Shurlygina, A.; Vereschagin, E. Effects of *Rhaponticum Carthamoides* versus Glycyrrhiza Glabra and Punica Granatum Extracts on Metabolic Syndrome Signs in Rats. *BMC Complement. Altern. Med.* **2014**, *14*, 33. [CrossRef]
58. Shuvalov, O.; Fedorova, O.; Tananykina, E.; Gnennaya, Y.; Daks, A.; Petukhov, A.; Barlev, N.A. An Arthropod Hormone, Ecdysterone, Inhibits the Growth of Breast Cancer Cells via Different Mechanisms. *Front. Pharmacol.* **2020**, *11*, 561537. [CrossRef] [PubMed]
59. Baev, A.Y.; Charyshnikova, O.S.; Khasanov, F.A.; Nebesnaya, K.S.; Makhmudov, A.R.; Rahmedova, M.T.; Khushbaktova, Z.A.; Syrov, V.N.; Levitskaya, Y.V. Ecdysterone Prevents Negative Effect of Acute Immobilization Stress on Energy Metabolism of Rat Liver Mitochondria. *J. Steroid Biochem. Mol. Biol.* **2022**, *219*, 106066. [CrossRef]
60. Shakhmurova, G.A.; Syrov, V.N.; Khushbaktova, Z.A. Immunomodulating and Antistress Activity of Ecdysterone and Turkesterone Under Immobilization-Induced Stress Conditions in Mice. *Pharm. Chem. J.* **2010**, *44*, 7–9. [CrossRef]
61. Yang, L.; Pan, J. Therapeutic Effect of Ecdysterone Combine Paeonol Oral Cavity Direct Administered on Radiation-Induced Oral Mucositis in Rats. *IJMS* **2019**, *20*, 3800. [CrossRef]
62. Gholipour, P.; Komaki, A.; Ramezani, M.; Parsa, H. Effects of the Combination of High-Intensity Interval Training and Ecdysterone on Learning and Memory Abilities, Antioxidant Enzyme Activities, and Neuronal Population in an Amyloid-Beta-Induced Rat Model of Alzheimer's Disease. *Physiol. Behav.* **2022**, *251*, 113817. [CrossRef]
63. Wu, J.; Gao, L.; Shang, L.; Wang, G.; Wei, N.; Chu, T.; Chen, S.; Zhang, Y.; Huang, J.; Wang, J.; et al. Ecdysterones from *Rhaponticum Carthamoides* (Willd.) Iljin Reduce Hippocampal Excitotoxic Cell Loss and Upregulate MTOR Signaling in Rats. *Fitoterapia* **2017**, *119*, 158–167. [CrossRef]
64. Hung, T.-J.; Chen, W.-M.; Liu, S.-F.; Liao, T.-N.; Lee, T.-C.; Chuang, L.-Y.; Guh, J.-Y.; Hung, C.-Y.; Hung, Y.-J.; Chen, P.; et al. 20-Hydroxyecdysone Attenuates TGF-B1-Induced Renal Cellular Fibrosis in Proximal Tubule Cells. *JDC* **2012**, *26*, 463–469. [CrossRef] [PubMed]
65. Omanakuttan, A.; Bose, C.; Pandurangan, N.; Kumar, G.B.; Banerji, A.; Nair, B.G. Nitric Oxide and ERK Mediates Regulation of Cellular Processes by Ecdysterone. *Exp. Cell Res.* **2016**, *346*, 167–175. [CrossRef]
66. Jin, Z.; Wang, B.; Ren, L.; Yang, J.; Zheng, Z.; Yao, F.; Ding, R.; Wang, J.; He, J.; Wang, W.; et al. 20-Hydroxyecdysone Inhibits Inflammation via SIRT6-Mediated NF-KB Signaling in Endothelial Cells. *Biochim. Biophys. Acta Mol. Cell Res.* **2023**, *1870*, 119460. [CrossRef] [PubMed]
67. Zhang, X.; Xu, X.; Xu, T.; Qin, S. β-Ecdysterone Suppresses Interleukin-1β-Induced Apoptosis and Inflammation in Rat Chondrocytes via Inhibition of NF-KB Signaling Pathway. *Drug Dev. Res.* **2014**, *75*, 195–201. [CrossRef] [PubMed]
68. Foucault, A.-S.; Mathe, V.; Lafont, R.; Even, P.; Dioh, W.; Veillet, S.; Tome, D.; Huneau, J.-F.; Hermier, D.; Quignard-Boulange, A. Quinoa Extract Enriched in 20-Hydroxyecdysone Protects Mice From Diet-Induced Obesity and Modulates Adipokines Expression. *Obesity* **2012**, *20*, 270–277. [CrossRef]
69. Chen, Q.; Xia, Y.; Qiu, Z. Effect of Ecdysterone on Glucose Metabolism in Vitro. *Life Sci.* **2006**, *78*, 1108–1113. [CrossRef] [PubMed]
70. Xia, X.; Zhang, Q.; Liu, R.; Wang, Z.; Tang, N.; Liu, F.; Huang, G.; Jiang, X.; Gui, G.; Wang, L.; et al. Effects of 20-Hydroxyecdysone on Improving Memory Deficits in Streptozotocin-Induced Type 1 Diabetes Mellitus in Rat. *Eur. J. Pharmacol.* **2014**, *740*, 45–52. [CrossRef]
71. Kapur, P.; Wuttke, W.; Jarry, H.; Seidlova-Wuttke, D. Beneficial Effects of β-Ecdysone on the Joint, Epiphyseal Cartilage Tissue and Trabecular Bone in Ovariectomized Rats. *Phytomedicine* **2010**, *17*, 350–355. [CrossRef]
72. Tang, Y.-H.; Yue, Z.-S.; Li, G.-S.; Zeng, L.-R.; Xin, D.-W.; Hu, Z.-Q.; Xu, C.-D. Effect of Ḇ-ecdysterone on Glucocorticoid-induced Apoptosis and Autophagy in Osteoblasts. *Mol. Med. Rep.* **2018**, *17*, 158–164. [CrossRef]
73. You, W.-L.; Xu, Z.-L. β-Ecdysone Promotes Osteogenic Differentiation of Bone Marrow Mesenchymal Stem Cells. *J. Genet. Med.* **2020**, *22*, e3207. [CrossRef]

74. Bai, N.; Lu, X.; Jin, L.; Alimujiang, M.; Ma, J.; Hu, F.; Xu, Y.; Sun, J.; Xu, J.; Zhang, R.; et al. CLSTN3 Gene Variant Associates with Obesity Risk and Contributes to Dysfunction in White Adipose Tissue. *Mol. Metab.* **2022**, *63*, 101531. [CrossRef] [PubMed]
75. Kongthitilerd, P.; Suantawee, T.; Cheng, H.; Thilavech, T.; Marnpae, M.; Adisakwattana, S. Anthocyanin-Enriched Riceberry Rice Extract Inhibits Cell Proliferation and Adipogenesis in 3T3-L1 Preadipocytes by Downregulating Adipogenic Transcription Factors and Their Targeting Genes. *Nutrients* **2020**, *12*, 2480. [CrossRef] [PubMed]
76. Elmore, S.E.; Cano-Sancho, G.; La Merrill, M.A. Disruption of Normal Adipocyte Development and Function by Methyl- and Propyl- Paraben Exposure. *Toxicol. Lett.* **2020**, *334*, 27–35. [CrossRef] [PubMed]

nutrients

MDPI

*Article*

# Nitrogen Balance at the Recommended Dietary Allowance for Protein in Minimally Active Male Vegans

**Eric Bartholomae and Carol S. Johnston** *

College of Health Solutions, Arizona State University, Phoenix, AZ 85004, USA; ebartho2@asu.edu
* Correspondence: carol.johnston@asu.edu

**Abstract:** Vegan diets have gained popularity in recent years for reasons including health benefits and concerns for animal welfare. Although these diets are considered to be nutritionally adequate, questions remain over whether the current protein recommendation (0.8 g/kg/d) is sufficient. Protein status is determined through a nitrogen balance analysis when the protein content of the diet is known. A negative balance indicates a catabolic state, and a positive nitrogen balance indicates an anabolic state. In healthy adults, nitrogen equilibrium is the expectation reflecting the net synthesis and breakdown of proteins. Currently, there are no known studies measuring nitrogen balance in strict vegan men fed the protein requirement. Eighteen minimally active vegan men received a 5-day eucaloric diet (protein content: 0.8 g/kg/d). On day five, 24 h urine was collected for nitrogen analysis. Both the mean absolute nitrogen balance (−1.38 ± 1.22 g/d) and the mean relative nitrogen balance (−18.60 ± 16.96 mg/kg/d) were significantly lower than zero (equilibrium) ($p < 0.001$). There were no correlations seen between nitrogen balance and age, years as vegan, or fat-free mass. Consuming 0.8 g/kg/d of protein is not adequate to produce nitrogen balance in men adhering to typical strict vegan diets for at least one year.

**Keywords:** nitrogen balance; vegan; protein requirement

## 1. Introduction

In recent years, vegetarian diets have gained in popularity with 5% of United States (U.S.) adults aged 18–34 years old identifying as vegetarian, and half of those being vegan [1]. This amounts to 3.8 million vegetarians, nearly two million of whom are vegan. The popularity of vegetarian diets in the U.S. has been linked to ethical and environmental concerns, but the desire to have a healthier lifestyle was the most prominent reason for adopting vegetarianism [2]. Vegetarian diet adherence has been associated with reduced risk and mortality for several chronic conditions including cardiovascular disease and cancer [3,4]; however, vegetarian diet adherence is not consistently linked to reductions in all-cause mortality [5,6].

It is the position of the Academy of Nutrition and Dietetics that appropriately planned vegetarian diets are nutritionally adequate and appropriate for all stages of the life cycle [7]. Yet concern remains over the potential for inadequacies in several micronutrients, the omega-3 fatty acids, and protein [8–10]. Considering protein adequacy, the amino acid profile and the digestibility of dietary proteins differ between animal and plant sources. To support body protein synthesis, adequate amounts of indispensable amino acids must be ingested, e.g., those amino acids that cannot be synthesized in vivo. Many plant proteins have less optimal indispensable amino acid profiles in comparison with animal proteins [11]. Additionally, plant protein digestibility is reduced in comparison with animal proteins due to its structure and to the high levels of antinutritional factors present in many plants (e.g., protease inhibitors, insoluble fibers, and phytates) that interfere with the digestion and absorption of protein [12,13]. The digestible indispensable amino acid score [DIAAS] is the recommended manner for ranking the biological value of dietary proteins and is calculated using a protein's amino acid profile and ileal digestibility [14,15]. Animal proteins such as dairy have higher DIAAS values (>100) than plant proteins such as pea, soy, or wheat (62, 84, and 45, respectively) [16].

Due to the lower biological value of plant proteins in comparison with animal proteins, greater intakes of plant proteins are necessary to meet protein synthesis needs. Tang et al. demonstrated that whey protein ingestion (10 g) was superior to an equal dose of soy protein for stimulating muscle protein synthesis at rest as well as following resistance exercise in young, healthy men (+18% and +31%, respectively) [17]. Gorissen et al. showed that casein protein ingestion (35 g) produced a higher postprandial myofibrillar protein synthetic response versus the same amount of wheat protein in healthy older men (+56%) and that greater amounts of wheat protein (60 g) were required to increase myofibrillar protein synthetic rates to those observed for 35 g of casein protein [18]. Generally, the literature supports an adequate protein status in U.S. vegetarians [19]; however, less information is available specifically for vegan-diet adherence. Moreover, much of the available data are from cross-sectional trials, and protein and energy intakes are not controlled; hence, it is difficult to assess whether the current protein recommendations are adequate for individuals following a vegan diet exclusively.

The recommended dietary allowance (RDA) for protein is 0.80 g/kg/d for all adults over 18 years of age, including vegetarians and vegans. The RDA is based on the results of numerous nitrogen balance studies, which are considered the gold standard criteria for determining protein requirements [20]. Protein is the only macronutrient containing nitrogen; hence, protein status is determined by comparing the amount of nitrogen ingested to the amount of nitrogen which is excreted. A negative balance indicates net protein catabolism, and a positive nitrogen balance indicates a net anabolic state. In healthy adults, nitrogen equilibrium is the expectation reflecting the net synthesis and breakdown of proteins. Rand and colleagues analyzed data from twenty-nine nitrogen balance subtrials (twenty-three mixed diets and six vegetable diets; $n = 235$) and concluded that the estimated RDA was 0.83 g/kg/d for all healthy adults regardless of age, gender, or diet group [19]. The authors stated that there were no significant differences in dietary protein source (e.g., animal vs. plant sources) with regards to protein needs [19]; however, the 'plant-based diets' included in this meta-analysis were defined as diets with "vegetable sources providing > 90% of total protein", indicating that these diets could contain up to 10% animal protein. Furthermore, a close analysis of the data revealed an average nitrogen balance of $-2.21$ mg $N \cdot kg^{-1} \cdot d^{-1}$ and $+7.39$ mg $N \cdot kg^{-1} \cdot d^{-1}$ for the "vegetable diets" and mixed diets, respectively, and $+5.41$ mg $N \cdot kg^{-1} \cdot d^{-1}$ overall [19].

To date, a nitrogen balance trial in strict vegan participants has not been reported. The purpose of this study was to determine the nitrogen balance in minimally active, male vegans ingesting a controlled, eucaloric diet containing the protein RDA, 0.8 g/kg/d. It was hypothesized that participants would exhibit a negative nitrogen balance in response to this diet plan.

## 2. Materials and Methods

### *2.1. Participants and Study Design*

Minimally active, male adults (20–45 years) who adhered exclusively to a vegan diet for at least one year were recruited from the Phoenix metropolitan area between October 2020 and October 2021 using fliers, word of mouth, email listservs, and local social media groups. Participants were healthy by self-report and minimally active (<150 min of moderate to vigorous exercise per week). Further exclusion criteria included prescription medications, muscle-building supplements, such as protein or creatine powders, food allergies, an unwillingness to consume the trial foods exclusively, and/or those participating in or training for competitive sports in the past year. The stage of the menstrual cycle can impact nitrogen balance; hence, women were not recruited for this trial [21,22]. This study was approved by the Institutional Review Board at Arizona State University (STUDY00012662), and all participants provided written informed consent.

Following an initial screening via an internet questionnaire, potential participants took part in a separate, follow-up phone screening to explain to them the procedures and requirements of the study and ask any follow-up screening questions that may need clarification by the investigator. Upon agreement, qualifying participants were then scheduled to visit the lab where written informed consent was obtained. At the visit, anthropometric data (height, body mass, and waist circumference) were collected. Fat-free mass was assessed via bioelectrical impedance analysis following a 12 h fasting period in which no food, beverages, or water were consumed [23]. Participants received all foods for a complete 5-day menu plan personalized to provide maintenance energy for light activity (Harris–Benedict equation × 1.3) and 0.8 g/kg protein. Diets consisted of frozen meals, meal replacement shakes, and dried fruits with protein from mixed, complementary plant-based sources of varying degrees of protein quality based on DIAAS values, held constant at 0.8 g/kg/d (See Table 1). Participants were also allowed to eat selected foods from a list of fruits and vegetables, and logged all foods eaten in a daily food log (Table 2). Participants were scheduled to begin the 5-day feeding period immediately following the baseline visit.

**Table 1.** Example Meal Plans for Vegan Diets *.

| | Vegan Example Menu | | |
|---|---|---|---|
| | | **Protein (g)** | **Energy (kcal)** |
| Breakfast | Orgain Protein Shake | 20 | 150 |
| | Cinnamon Raisin Bagel | 9 | 280 |
| | Peanut Butter (2 T) | 8 | 180 |
| | Apple | 0 | 65 |
| Lunch | Amy's Indian Vegetable Korma | 9 | 330 |
| | Dried Pineapple (2 servings) | 0 | 280 |
| Dinner | Sweet Earth General Tso's Tofu | 10 | 330 |
| | Trader Joes Dried Mango (1/2 package) | 0 | 280 |
| | Peanut Butter (2 T) | 8 | 180 |
| | Fruit Snacks (2 packages) | 0 | 160 |
| Total | | 64 | 2235 |

* Example meal plan is for 80 kg male using the Harris–Benedict equation and a physical activity factor of 1.3 (seated work, no purposeful exercise). Meal plans provided 0.8 g protein/kg/d. Frozen entrees from Amy's Kitchen and Sweet Earth.

**Table 2.** List of Permitted Foods (≤3 servings/d) to Supplement Diet Plan.

| |
|---|
| 2 large celery stalks |
| 2 cups shredded romaine lettuce |
| ½ cucumber |
| 1 medium tomato |
| ½ cup sugar snap peas |
| 1 carrot |
| 1 cup jicama sticks |
| 1 peach |
| ½ grapefruit |
| 1 cup winter mix vegetables |
| 1 cup Tuscan-style vegetables |
| 1 cup mixed broccoli, cauliflower, and carrots |
| ¾ cup whole green beans |

Participants were provided instructions and a container for the 24 h urine collection on day 5, the final day of feeding. During the 5-day feeding period, participants were asked to refrain from any moderate–vigorous physical activity and limit all other activities in general. Participants tracked activity daily using the validated Godin leisure time physical activity questionnaire, and a score ≥24 METs × hours/week was the cutoff for 'active' [24]. Participants were instructed to record any uneaten food portions or additional foods eaten. For the 24 h urine collection, the first morning void was discarded, and all urine was collected throughout the day and overnight, including the first morning sample on day 6. No urine preservative was necessary and participants were asked to refrigerate the sample. The 24 h urine sample was delivered to the lab on the morning of day 6.

### *2.2. Diet and Urine Analysis*

Diet records were reviewed with the participants on their return to clarify any ambiguities and were analyzed by a trained investigator using the Food Processor software (version 7.71; ESHA Research, Salem, OR, USA). Urine samples were thoroughly mixed, total volume determined, and aliquots frozen at −80 °C for later analysis via photometric assay to determine nitrogen content by Sonora Quest Laboratories. Nitrogen balance was determined using the known protein content of the diet on the fifth day of consumption and the nitrogen content of the urine (as UUN) using the equation

$$\text{Nitrogen Balance (g/d)} = (\text{PRO intake (g/d)}/6.25) - \text{UUN (g/d)} - 4$$

where the coefficient of 6.25 is derived from the knowledge that protein is 16% nitrogen (e.g., there are 6.25 g of nitrogen per g of protein) [25]. A constant of 4 is used to account for obligatory nitrogen losses: 2 g urinary non-urea nitrogen excretion (e.g., ammonia, uric acid, creatinine, and amino acids) and 2 g gastrointestinal, integumentary (dermal), and sweat losses [26].

### *2.3. Statistical Analysis*

Data for this cross-sectional study are reported as the mean ± SD, and an a priori $\alpha$ of 0.05 used to determine significance. All outcome data were tested for normality and nonparametric statistics used when necessary. Statistical analyses were performed using SPSS version 27 (IBM, Armonk, NY, USA). To determine if calculated nitrogen balance values were different from zero (nitrogen equilibrium), a one-sample *t*-test was used. Simple regression analyses were used to understand whether nitrogen balance could be predicted based on diet duration, age, fat free mass, or physical activity (Spearman rank test). Sample size was determined using G*Power version 3.1 (Heinrich Heine Universität, Düsseldorf, Germany). Based on Rand et al. [19], given an expected change of 5 mg nitrogen/kg/d and an SD of 6.4 mg nitrogen/kg/d, this yields an effect size of 0.78 (e.g., 5/6.4 = 0.78). Using a predetermined $\alpha$ of 0.05, a sample size $N = 16$ yielded a power of 90%. Thus, allowing for an attrition rate of 20%, 20 participants was the enrollment goal.

## 3. Results

### *3.1. Participant Characteristics*

One hundred and twenty people responded to the online screening questionnaire, and thirty-five met the eligibility criteria for enrollment. Twelve of these qualifiers did not respond to emails, three declined to participate after a phone interview, and two withdrew from the study prior to any participation. Thus, 18 participants were enrolled and completed the study. Prior to analyses, age, years vegan, fat-free mass, physical activity, and nitrogen balance values were assessed for normality and potential outliers. A box plot analysis determined that only nitrogen balance had an outlier which was confirmed by Shapiro–Wilk normality testing ($W(18) = 0.89$, $p < 0.047$) (Figure 1). This participant was removed from all analyses, and data are presented for 17 participants.

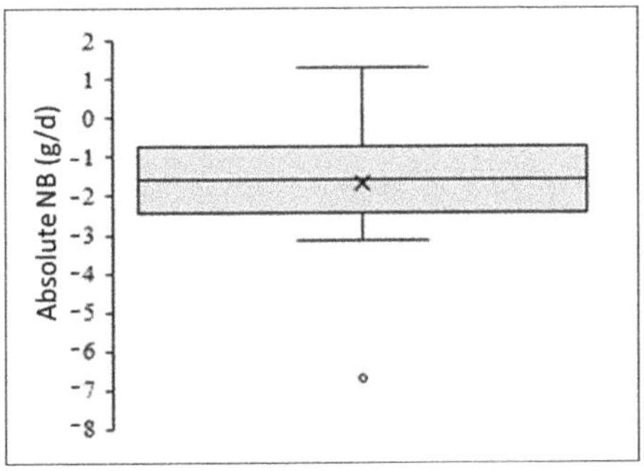


**Figure 1.** Nitrogen Balance (NB) (g/d) Box Plot Analysis displaying the median (×) and the outlier value (○).

Participants were young healthy male adults aged 31.6 ± 6.2 years (range: 25–43 years; body mass index: 24.2 ± 3.8 kg/m$^2$) (Table 3). Four participants were overweight (BMI 25.0–29.9 kg/m$^2$) and two were obese (BMI > 30.0 kg/m$^2$). Adherence to the vegan diet averaged 7.1 ± 6.5 years (range: 1–23 years). Maintenance energy was calculated using the Harris–Benedict equation, accounting for light activity (2377 ± 362 kcal) and protein needs (0.8 g/kg/d) averaged 60.9 ± 10.5 g/d (Table 3).

**Table 3.** Participant Characteristics [1].

| | *N* = 17 |
|---|---|
| Age (years) | 31.6 ± 6.2 |
| Years vegan (years) | 7.1 ± 6.5 |
| Height (cm) | 176.6 ± 8.1 |
| Weight (kg) | 75.5 ± 13.7 |
| Waist circumference (cm) | 85.9 ± 10.5 |
| Hip circumference (cm) | 101.3 ± 8.3 |
| Fat-free mass (kg) | 60.0 ± 7.5 |
| Fat mass (kg) | 15.1 ± 8.2 |
| Body fat (%) | 19.2 ± 7.2 |
| Body mass index (kg/m$^2$) | 24.2 ± 3.8 |
| Physical activity (METs × hours/week) | 18.1 ± 28.2 |
| Maintenance energy (kcal/d) | 2377 ± 362 |
| Protein requirement (g/d) | 60.9 ± 10.5 |
| Nitrogen balance (g/d) | −1.38 ± 1.22 * |
| Nitrogen balance (mg/kg/d) | −18.60 ± 16.96 * |

[1] Data are mean ± SD. Maintenance energy for light activity was calculated using the Harris–Benedict equation × 1.3. Protein requirement, 0.8 g/kg/d. Asterisk indicates significant difference from nitrogen equilibrium ($p < 0.05$; one sample $t$-test).

### 3.2. Nitrogen Balance

A one-sample $t$-test was performed to determine whether nitrogen balance values following the 5-day dietary protocol were statistically different than nitrogen equilibrium (a nitrogen balance value of zero). Nitrogen balance was analyzed as absolute nitrogen balance in grams per day (g/d) and, relative to body weight, as relative nitrogen balance in milligrams per kilogram per day (mg/kg/d). The mean absolute nitrogen balance (−1.38 ± 1.22 g/d) was statistically lower than the nitrogen equilibrium score of zero [(95% CI, −2.00 to −0.75), $t(16) = -4.643$, $p < 0.001$]. The mean relative nitrogen balance score (−18.60 ± 16.96 mg/kg/d) was statistically lower than the nitrogen equilibrium score of zero [(95% CI, −27.32 to −9.88), $t(16) = -4.522$, $p < 0.001$]. Individual participant nitrogen balance values are displayed in Figure 2A,B).

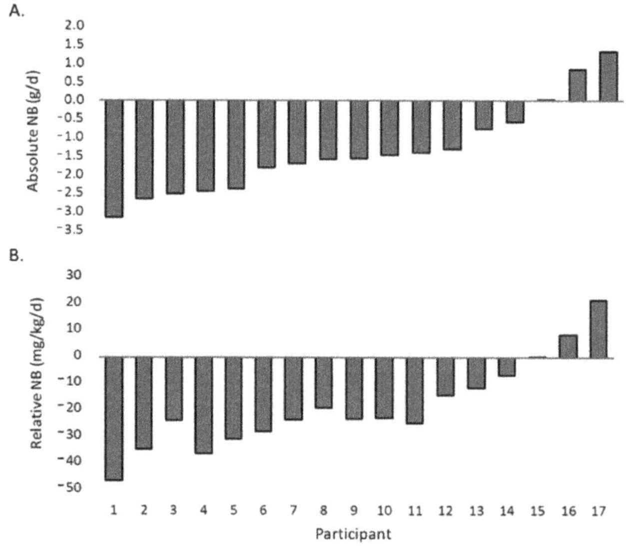


**Figure 2.** Individual participant nitrogen balance (NB) data: (**A**) Absolute NB (g/d) and (**B**) Relative NB (mg/kg/d).

There were no significant correlations between nitrogen balance and age, years vegan, fat-free mass, BMI, physical activity, or other descriptive variable ($p \geq 0.100$; Spearman rank correlation). A weak correlation was noted for age (r = −0.409; $p = 0.103$). The ages for the two participants displaying a positive nitrogen balance were 25 and 26 years. Daily energy intakes during the trial ranged from 1925 to 3231 kcals (average, 2338 ± 380 kcals/d; calculated average energy needs pre-trial, 2377 kcals/d), and the daily protein intake averaged 61 ± 9 g (calculated average protein need pre-trial, 60.9 g/d). Nitrogen balance was not related to energy or protein intakes.

## 4. Discussion

The U.S. protein RDA for adults (0.8 g/kg/d) is defined as the amount to achieve a 'zero nitrogen balance' [27]. The data presented herein suggest that 0.8 g/kg/d was not adequate to maintain nitrogen balance in men who have adhered to a strict vegan diet for at least one year. The U.S. protein requirement was informed by a series of nitrogen-balance studies systematically reviewed by Rand et al. [19], which incorporated trials focused mainly on animal proteins (trials = 23, participants = 247). Of the few trials that fed predominately plant-based proteins (trials = 6, participants = 73), animal proteins made up to 10% of the dietary protein in these trials, and participants were omnivores who only omitted animal foods for the purpose of these trials [19]. The present results, when compared with the plant-based protein data presented by Rand et al., showed a markedly decreased relative nitrogen balance (−18.60 ± 16.96 mg/kg/d versus −2.2 ± 7.75 mg/kg/d, respectively). Putting these results into perspective, a mean nitrogen balance of −1.38 g/d signifies a daily loss of 8.63 g body protein, or a loss of 3.1 kg body protein over one year.

Previous research that used 4-day diet recalls to calculate the protein digestibility corrected amino acid scores for the diet plans of 22 vegetarian women suggested that the protein requirement for vegetarians appeared to be 25% higher than that for omnivores [10]. In the present study, about 12 g of additional protein (incorporating a 74% digestibility factor for vegan diets [28]) is needed to counter the nitrogen losses, equating to a 20% increase in the protein requirement (e.g., 0.96 g/kg/d).

Nitrogen balance trials in vegetarian populations are scarce; however, several early studies support a protein requirement of 1 g/kg/d for individuals adhering to vegetarian diets. Yanez et al. [29] conducted a long-term nitrogen balance trial in eight Chilean men fed a controlled, eucaloric vegetarian diet for three months with protein at 1 g/kg/d. Body weight remained stable during the trial, and nitrogen balance averaged +6.7 mg/kg/d. Only one of the eight participants recorded a negative relative nitrogen balance (−2.3 mg/kg/d). Register et al. [30] also reported an overall positive nitrogen balance (+0.07 g/d) in six young adults fed a vegan, eucaloric diet for nine days with protein held at 1 g/kg/d; however, three of six participants reported a negative nitrogen balance (average: −3.4 g/d).

Negative nitrogen balance indicates a decline in body protein mass. For a healthy inactive adult consuming a eucaloric diet at the RDA of 0.8 g/kg/d, a negative nitrogen balance would suggest inferior protein quality and a lack of essential amino acids rather than an inadequate quantity of protein [31]. A chronic negative nitrogen balance would adversely impact the synthesis of new proteins and eventually reduce skeletal muscle mass and the synthesis of enzymes, hormones, and immune factors, and impede tissue maintenance and repair [32,33]. Negative nitrogen balances are noted in clinical cases including individuals with protein energy malnutrition and older adults suffering from sarcopenia [34,35]. Although muscle loss has not been studied over the long term in vegetarians, age-related muscle loss begins at about age 40, and up to 50% of muscle mass may be lost by age 80 [35,36]. The loss of muscle mass in older adults has been linked to lower protein intakes [37], and experts recommend a higher protein intake for older adults (1.0 to 1.5 g/kg/d) to combat muscle loss [38,39].

Vegan diet adherence has been linked to lower muscle mass in young adults in cross-sectional trials. Vanacore et al. [40] showed a nearly 5 kg difference in muscle mass between omnivore ($n$ = 10; 32.1 ± 0.81 kg) and long-term vegan ($n$ = 10; 27.3 ± 1.2 kg) cohorts, with no difference between vegetarians ($n$ = 10; 32.8 ± 1.4 kg) and omnivores. The study sample had a mean age of 29 ± 5 years and participants were age matched. Another study examined the relationship between protein intake from animal-based sources (1.05 g/kg/d) versus plant-based sources (0.98 g/kg/d) and muscle mass in healthy women [41]. They found that the vegetarian group ($n$ = 19, with only one strict vegan; mean age = 48 ± 12 years; mean years on diet = 12) had significantly lower muscle mass compared with the omnivore control group ($n$ = 21) (18.2 ± 3.9 kg vs. 22.6 ± 5.0 kg, respectively). There was also a significantly lower muscle mass index in vegetarians (6.7 ±1.2 kg/m$^2$) compared with omnivores (8.3 ± 1.5 kg/m$^2$). The data suggested that animal protein intake was an independent predictor of muscle mass index (adjusted $r^2$ = 0.42) [41]. Caso et al. demonstrated that albumin synthesis was lower in participants adhering to a vegetarian versus omnivore diet plan when protein intakes were held at 1 g/kg/d [42]. However, when supplementing 18 g soy protein to the vegetarian diet plan (raising protein intake to 1.25 g/kg/d), the albumin synthesis rate balanced between diet groups [42]. Monteyne et al. [43] randomized participants to two eucaloric-controlled diet groups (omnivore versus strict vegan) for 3 days (protein = 1.8 g/kg/d) and reported similar myofibrillar protein synthesis rates between diet groups for both rested and exercised muscle. Based on these results, as recommended for older adults to combat sarcopenia, vegetarian populations should be advised to consume protein at levels above the RDA (e.g., 1.2 to 1.8 g/kg/d).

The analyses of possible predictors of nitrogen balance in the present study (e.g., age, years vegan, FFM, or physical activity) yielded no significant relationships suggesting that minimum protein requirements are not influenced by these factors in healthy adult men, assuming overall energy intake is adequate and physical activity is minimal. Nitrogen balance is sensitive to variations in energy intake, and energy intakes were tightly controlled in the present trial. Basal metabolic rates were calculated for each participant and personalized menu plans were devised to provide energy to support light activity (basal metabolic rate $\times$ 1.3). All foods were provided during the 5-day feeding period, the minimum adaptation period recommended for protein equilibration [19]. Participants were mostly inactive prior to the study and were asked to remain sedentary during the study protocol to standardize physical activity.

Further strengths of this study include personalized menu planning to incorporate mixed, complementary proteins from various plant-based sources to reflect participants' normal diets, thus enhancing ecological validity (e.g., dietary protein was not limited to a single protein source). Importantly, this study was limited to long-term (>1 year), strict vegans, for which data in the literature was previously lacking. The current U.S. protein RDA was determined using nitrogen balance studies in omnivores and a few vegetarians—all of whom consume animal products, at least in part. The results of this study will serve as a starting point to better inform protein recommendations for those following a vegan lifestyle.

This study had several limitations. First, this was a short-term study, with an adaptation feeding period of five days. This is at the short end of what is considered adequate for nitrogen balance determination with standard protocol being between four days to several weeks adaptation to the experimental diet before the measurement of nitrogen balance [19]. Next, this was not an inpatient study, thus participants were free to live their daily lives during the study protocol. Because of this, dietary menu adherence was based on participants' trustworthiness in tracking their intake. Although all food was provided to participants at no cost, it is possible they may not have consumed all meals, added prohibited foods, or measured certain foods incorrectly, thus providing inaccurate information on total energy and protein intake. Like dietary intake, physical activity was based on participants' honesty of tracking outside of the laboratory as well. While participants were asked to keep all physical activity to a minimum, this definition may vary between individuals and can affect energy needs, thus nitrogen balance. Future studies of a similar design should better assess physical activity using body worn accelerometers to gather objective data. This study utilized a single protein intake for all individuals in order to test the adequacy of the U.S. protein RDA for a vegan population. While our data shows that the RDA was inadequate in achieving nitrogen balance, it is unknown at what intake this equilibrium could be achieved. Future studies could employ a crossover design, with participants consuming other protein amounts such as 1.0 g/kg/d, 1.2 g/kg/d, and so on in a randomized order to better determine protein adequacy. Lastly, this study used only a small sample of underactive males, thus these results are not generalizable to females or those engaging in physical activity or exercise. Further work is needed in these areas.

## 5. Conclusions

The results of this study suggest that the current U.S. RDA for protein, 0.8 g/kg/d, is not adequate to produce nitrogen equilibrium in underactive, vegan males consuming typical menu plans. This is important, given the increasing numbers of people who follow a vegan lifestyle, and the fact that high quality and quantity protein foods are less common in a vegan diet compared with an omnivore diet. Due to the inferior protein quality of most plant-based foods compared with animal-based foods, it is likely that the protein RDA should be amended with special recommendations for vegans, or at the very least highlight the importance of a diet with a higher protein intake to better guide and assure nutrient adequacy in vegans.

**Author Contributions:** Conceptualization, E.B. and C.S.J.; methodology, E.B. and C.S.J.; formal analysis, E.B. and C.S.J.; investigation, E.B.; resources, C.S.J.; data curation, E.B. and C.S.J.; writing—original draft preparation, E.B. and C.S.J.; writing—review and editing, E.B. and C.S.J.; supervision, C.S.J.; project administration, E.B. All authors have read and agreed to the published version of the manuscript.

**Funding:** This research received no external funding.

**Institutional Review Board Statement:** This study was conducted in accordance with the Declaration of Helsinki, and approved by the Institutional Review Board of Arizona State University [STUDY00012662; date approved: 10 February 2020].

**Informed Consent Statement:** Informed consent was obtained from all subjects involved in this study.

**Data Availability Statement:** Data will be shared upon request.

**Conflicts of Interest:** The authors declare no conflict of interest.

## References

1. Stahler, C. How Many People Are Vegan? How Many Eat Vegan When Eating Out? Asks the Vegetarian Resource Group. The Vegetarian Resource Group. Available online: https://www.vrg.org/nutshell/Polls/2019_adults_veg.htm (accessed on 23 June 2023).
2. Hopwood, C.J.; Bleidorn, W.; Schwaba, T.; Chen, S. Health, environmental, and animal rights motives for vegetarian eating. *PLoS ONE* **2020**, *15*, e0230609. [CrossRef] [PubMed]
3. Dinu, M.; Abbate, R.; Gensini, G.F.; Casini, A.; Sofi, F. Vegetarian, vegan diets and multiple health outcomes: A systematic review with meta-analysis of observational studies. *Crit. Rev. Food Sci. Nutr.* **2017**, *57*, 3640–3649. [CrossRef] [PubMed]
4. Oussalah, A.; Levy, J.; Berthezène, C.; Alpers, D.H.; Guéant, J.L. Health outcomes associated with vegetarian diets: An umbrella review of systematic reviews and meta-analyses. *Clin. Nutr.* **2020**, *39*, 3283–3307. [CrossRef] [PubMed]
5. Jabri, A.; Kumar, A.; Verghese, E.; Alameh, A.; Kumar, A.; Khan, M.S.; Khan, S.U.; Michos, E.D.; Kapadia, S.R.; Reed, G.W.; et al. Meta-analysis of effect of vegetarian diet on ischemic heart disease and all-cause mortality. *Am. J. Prev. Cardiol.* **2021**, *7*, 100182. [CrossRef]
6. Mihrshahi, S.; Ding, D.; Gale, J.; Allman-Farinelli, M.; Banks, E.; Bauman, A.E. Vegetarian diet and all-cause mortality: Evidence from a large population-based Australian cohort—The 45 and Up Study. *Prev. Med.* **2017**, *97*, 1–7. [CrossRef]
7. Melina, V.; Craig, W.; Levin, S. Position of the Academy of Nutrition and Dietetics: Vegetarian diets. *J. Acad. Nutr. Diet.* **2016**, *116*, 1970–1980. [CrossRef]
8. Key, T.J.; Appleby, P.N.; Rosell, M.S. Health effects of vegetarian and vegan diets. *Proc. Nutr. Soc.* **2006**, *65*, 35–41. [CrossRef]
9. Mariotti, F.; Gardner, C.D. Dietary Protein and Amino Acids in Vegetarian Diets-A Review. *Nutrients* **2019**, *11*, 2661. [CrossRef]
10. Kniskern, M.A.; Johnston, C.S. Protein dietary reference intakes may be inadequate for vegetarians if low amounts of animal protein are consumed. *Nutrition* **2011**, *27*, 727–730. [CrossRef]
11. Young, V.R.; Pellett, P.L. Plant proteins in relation to human protein and amino acid nutrition. *Am. J. Clin. Nutr.* **1994**, *59* (Suppl. S5), 1203S–1212S. [CrossRef]
12. Berrazaga, I.; Micard, V.; Gueugneau, M.; Walrand, S. The Role of the Anabolic Properties of Plant- versus Animal-Based Protein Sources in Supporting Muscle Mass Maintenance: A Critical Review. *Nutrients* **2019**, *1*, 1825. [CrossRef]
13. Gilani, S.G.; Xiao, C.W.; Cockell, K.A. Impact of antinutritional factors in food proteins on the digestibility of protein and the bioavailability of amino acids and on protein quality. *Br. J. Nutr.* **2012**, *108* (Suppl. S2), S315–S332. [CrossRef]
14. Dietary Protein Quality Evaluation in Human Nutrition. Food and Agriculture Organization of the United Nations. Available online: https://www.fao.org/ag/humannutrition/35978-02317b979a686a57aa4593304ffc17f06.pdf (accessed on 23 June 2023).
15. Wolfe, R.R.; Rutherfurd, S.M.; Kim, I.Y.; Moughan, P.J. Protein quality as determined by the Digestible Indispensable Amino Acid Score: Evaluation of factors underlying the calculation. *Nutr. Rev.* **2016**, *74*, 584–599. [CrossRef]
16. Mathai, J.K.; Liu, Y.; Stein, H.H. Values for digestible indispensable amino acid scores (DIAAS) for some dairy and plant proteins may better describe protein quality than values calculated using the concept for protein digestibility-corrected amino acid scores (PDCAAS). *Br. J. Nutr.* **2017**, *117*, 490–499. [CrossRef]
17. Tang, J.E.; Moore, D.R.; Kujbida, G.W.; Tarnopolsky, M.A.; Phillips, S.M. Ingestion of whey hydrolysate, casein, or soy protein isolate: Effects on mixed muscle protein synthesis at rest and following resistance exercise in young men. *J. Appl. Phys.* **2009**, *107*, 987–992. [CrossRef] [PubMed]
18. Gorissen, S.H.M.; Horstman, A.M.H.; Franssen, R.; Crombag, J.J.R.; Langer, H.; Bierau, J.; Respondek, F.; van Loon, L.J.C. Ingestion of wheat protein increases in vivo muscle protein synthesis rates in healthy older men in a randomized trial. *J. Nutr.* **2016**, *146*, 1651–1659. [CrossRef] [PubMed]
19. Rand, W.M.; Pellett, P.L.; Young, V.R. Meta-analysis of nitrogen balance studies for estimating protein requirements in healthy adults. *Am. J. Clin. Nutr.* **2003**, *77*, 109–127. [CrossRef]
20. Institute of Medicine. *Dietary Reference Intakes: The Essential Guide to Nutrient Requirements;* Otten, J.J., Hellwig, P., Meyers, L.D., Eds.; The National Academies Press: Washington, DC, USA, 2006. [CrossRef]
21. Calloway, D.H.; Kurzer, M.S. Menstrual cycle and protein requirements of women. *J. Nutr.* **1982**, *112*, 356–366. [CrossRef]
22. Draper, C.F.; Duisters, K.; Weger, B.; Chakrabarti, A.; Harms, A.C.; Brennan, L.; Hankemeier, T.; Goulet, L.; Konz Martin, F.P.; Moco, S.; et al. Menstrual cycle rhythmicity: Metabolic patterns in healthy women. *Sci. Rep.* **2018**, *8*, 14568. [CrossRef] [PubMed]
23. Walter-Kroker, A.; Kroker, A.; Mattiucci-Guehlke, M.; Glaab, T. A practical guide to bioelectrical impedance analysis using the example of chronic obstructive pulmonary disease. *Nutr. J.* **2011**, *10*, 35. [CrossRef] [PubMed]
24. Godin, G. The Godin-Shephard leisure-time physical activity questionnaire. *Health Fitness J. BC* **2011**, *4*, 18–22.

25. Richter, M.; Baerlocher, K.; Bauer, J.M.; Elmadfa, I.; Heseker, H.; Leschik-Bonnet, E.; Stangl, G.; Volkert, D.; Stehle, P. Revised reference values for the intake of protein. *Ann. Nutr. Metab.* **2019**, *74*, 242–250. [CrossRef] [PubMed]
26. Dickerson, R.N. Using nitrogen balance in clinical practice. *Hosp. Pharm.* **2005**, *40*, 1081–1087. [CrossRef]
27. Food and Nutrition Board; Institute of Medicine. *Dietary Reference Intakes for Energy, Carbohydrate, Fiber, Fat, Fatty Acids, Cholesterol, Protein, and Amino Acids*; The National Academies Press: Washington, DC, USA, 2005; p. 635.
28. Rojas Conzuelo, Z.; Bez, N.S.; Theobald, S.; Kopf-Bolanz, K.A. Protein Quality Changes of Vegan Day Menus with Different Plant Protein Source Compositions. *Nutrients* **2022**, *14*, 1088. [CrossRef] [PubMed]
29. Yáñez, E.; Uauy, R.; Zacarías, I.; Barrera, G. Long-term validation of 1 g of protein per kilogram body weight from a predominantly vegetable mixed diet to meet the requirements of young adult males. *J. Nutr.* **1986**, *116*, 865–872. [CrossRef]
30. Register, U.D.; Inano, M.; Thurston, C.E.; Vyhmeister, I.B.; Dysinger, P.W.; Blankenship, J.W.; Horning, M.C. Nitrogen-balance studies in human subjects on various diets. *Am. J. Clin. Nutr.* **1967**, *20*, 753–759. [CrossRef]
31. Kondrup, J. Basic concepts in nutrition: Energy and protein balance. *Clin. Nutr. ESPEN* **2008**, *3*, E117–E120. [CrossRef]
32. Wu, G. Dietary protein intake and human health. *Food Funct.* **2016**, *7*, 1251–1265. [CrossRef]
33. Nishimura, Y.; Højfeldt, G.; Breen, L.; Tetens, I.; Holm, L. Dietary protein requirements and recommendations for healthy older adults: A critical narrative review of the scientific evidence. *Nutr. Res. Rev.* **2023**, *36*, 69–85. [CrossRef]
34. Mathewson, S.L.; Azevedo, P.S.; Gordon, A.L.; Phillips, B.E.; Greig, C.A. Overcoming protein-energy malnutrition in older adults in the residential care setting: A narrative review of causes and interventions. *Ageing Res. Rev.* **2021**, *70*, 101401. [CrossRef]
35. Mitchell, W.K.; Williams, J.; Atherton, P.; Larvin, M.; Lund, J.; Narici, M. Sarcopenia, dynapenia, and the impact of advancing age on human skeletal muscle size and strength; a quantitative review. *Front. Phys.* **2012**, *3*, 260. [CrossRef] [PubMed]
36. Walston, J.D. Sarcopenia in older adults. *Curr. Opin. Rheumatol.* **2012**, *24*, 623–627. [CrossRef] [PubMed]
37. Huang, R.Y.; Yang, K.C.; Chang, H.H.; Lee, L.T.; Lu, C.W.; Huang, K.C. The Association between Total Protein and Vegetable Protein Intake and Low Muscle Mass among the Community-Dwelling Elderly Population in Northern Taiwan. *Nutrients* **2016**, *8*, 373. [CrossRef] [PubMed]
38. Bauer, J.; Biolo, G.; Cederholm, T.; Cesari, M.; Cruz-Jentoft, A.J.; Morley, J.E.; Phillips, S.; Sieber, C.; Stehle, P.; Teta, D.; et al. Evidence-based recommendations for optimal dietary protein intake in older people: A position paper from the PROT-AGE Study Group. *J. Am. Med. Dir. Assoc.* **2013**, *14*, 542–559. [CrossRef]
39. Morley, J.E.; Argiles, J.M.; Evans, W.J.; Bhasin, S.; Cella, D.; Deutz, N.E.; Doehner, W.; Fearon, K.C.; Ferrucci, L.; Hellerstein, M.K.; et al. Nutritional recommendations for the management of sarcopenia. *J. Am. Med. Dir. Assoc.* **2010**, *11*, 391–396. [CrossRef]
40. Vanacore, D.; Messina, G.; Lama, S.; Bitti, G.; Ambrosio, P.; Tenore, G.; Messina, A.; Monda, V.; Zappavigna, S.; Boccellino, M.; et al. Effect of restriction vegan diet's on muscle mass, oxidative status, and myocytes differentiation: A pilot study. *J. Cell Physiol.* **2018**, *233*, 9345–9353. [CrossRef]
41. Aubertin-Leheudre, M.; Adlercreutz, H. Relationship between animal protein intake and muscle mass index in healthy women. *Br. J. Nutr.* **2009**, *102*, 1803–1810. [CrossRef]
42. Caso, G.; Scalfi, L.; Marra, M.; Covino, A.; Muscaritoli, M.; McNurlan, M.A.; Garlick, P.J.; Contaldo, F. Albumin synthesis is diminished in men consuming a predominantly vegetarian diet. *J. Nutr.* **2000**, *130*, 528–533. [CrossRef]
43. Monteyne, A.J.; Dunlop, M.V.; Machin, D.J.; Coelho, M.O.C.; Pavis, G.F.; Porter, C.; Murton, A.J.; Abdelrahman, D.R.; Dirks, M.L.; Stephens, F.B.; et al. A mycoprotein-based high-protein vegan diet supports equivalent daily myofibrillar protein synthesis rates compared with an isonitrogenous omnivorous diet in older adults: A randomised controlled trial. *Br. J. Nutr.* **2021**, *126*, 674–684. [CrossRef]

*nutrients*

MDPI

*Article*

# The Role of a Plant-Only (Vegan) Diet in Gastroesophageal Reflux Disease: Online Survey of the Italian General Population

**Gianluca Rizzo [1], Luciana Baroni [2,*], Chiara Bonetto [3], Pierfrancesco Visaggi [4], Mattia Orazzini [4], Irene Solinas [4], Giada Guidi [4], Jessica Pugliese [4], Giulia Scaramuzza [4], Filippo Ovidi [4], Irene Buselli [4], Massimo Bellini [4], Edoardo V. Savarino [5] and Nicola de Bortoli [4,6]**

1 Independent Researcher, 98121 Messina, Italy; drgianlucarizzo@gmail.com
2 Scientific Society for Vegetarian Nutrition, 30171 Venice, Italy
3 Section of Psychiatry, Department of Neurosciences, Biomedicine and Movement Sciences, University of Verona, 37134 Verona, Italy; chiara.bonetto@univr.it
4 Division of Gastroenterology, Department of Translational Research and New Technologies in Medicine and Surgery, University of Pisa, 56126 Pisa, Italy; pierfrancesco.visaggi@phd.unipi.it (P.V.); m.orazzini4@studenti.unipi.it (M.O.); i.solinas1@studenti.unipi.it (I.S.); 27627122@studenti.unipi.it (G.G.); j.pugliese1@studenti.unipi.it (J.P.); g.scaramuzza@studenti.unipi.it (G.S.); f.ovidi2@studenti.unipi.it (F.O.); i.buselli2@studenti.unipi.it (I.B.); massimo.bellini@unipi.it (M.B.); nicola.debortoli@unipi.it (N.d.B.)
5 Division of Gastroenterology, Department of Surgery, Oncology and Gastroenterology, University of Padua, 35124 Padua, Italy; edoardo.savarino@unipd.it
6 NUTRAFOOD, Interdepartmental Center for Nutraceutical Research and Nutrition for Health, University of Pisa, 56124 Pisa, Italy
* Correspondence: luciana.baroni@scienzavegetariana.it

**Abstract:** The relationship between food and the pathophysiological mechanisms of gastroesophageal reflux disease (GERD) is unclear. There are few data on the impact of dietary habits on GERD symptoms and on the incidence of GERD in subjects undergoing plant-based diets. In this study, we investigated the association between diet and GERD, using data collected through an online survey of the Italian general population. In total, 1077 subjects participated in the study. GERD was defined according to the Montreal Consensus. For all subjects age, gender, body mass index (BMI), marital status, education, occupation, alcohol consumption, and smoking habits were recorded. All participants also completed the SF-36 questionnaire on Quality of Life. A total of 402 subjects (37.3%) were vegans and 675 (62.7%) non-vegans. The prevalence of GERD in the total population was 9%. Subjects with GERD-related symptoms recorded a worse quality of life according to SF-36 analysis ($p < 0.05$ for all dimensions). In multivariate analysis, after adjusting for confounders, participants undergoing a vegan diet had a significantly lower risk of GERD (OR = 0.47, 95% CI 0.28–0.81, $p = 0.006$). These findings should be taken into account to inform the lifestyle management of GERD.

**Keywords:** gastroesophageal reflux disease; GERD; plant-based diet; plant-only diet; vegan diet; heartburn; regurgitation; non-cardiac chest pain; lifestyle habits; Quality of Life; QoL; SF-36

## 1. Introduction

Gastroesophageal reflux disease (GERD) occurs when the passage of gastric contents back into the esophagus causes either mucosal damage or symptoms [1]. When GERD is defined as heartburn and/or acid regurgitation occurring at least weekly, its prevalence is less than 5% in Asia, and ranges from 10% to 20% in Western countries [2–4]. There is evidence that the prevalence of GERD has increased over the past two decades [4–6].

The main pathological mechanism is the passage of gastric contents into the esophagus and the dysfunction of the esophageal anti-reflux barrier. The former is primarily brought about by delayed stomach emptying and the creation of gastric acid pockets. The latter is mostly brought on by the lower esophageal sphincter's (LES) malfunction. Among other things, there is an increase in the frequency of transient lower esophageal sphincter relaxation (TLESR) and a reduction in esophageal clearing mechanisms [7,8].

However, the reason for the increase in GERD and its complications is not yet clear. It is likely that the general change in dietary habits plays an important role: diets in Western countries are now mainly characterized by the consumption of sugars, fats, and animal foods instead of plant foods [9]. Many studies have indicated a relationship between the increasing prevalence of obesity and GERD [10,11]. Accordingly, it has been shown that a diet planned to induce weight loss decreases symptoms and PPI consumption in overweight/obese GERD subjects [10]. Few studies have investigated the role of different dietary patterns in the development of reflux symptoms, often leading to conflicting results [12,13]. The American College of Gastroenterology recommends that subjects with GERD reduce their intake of total fat, chocolate, alcohol, citrus fruits, tomato products, coffee, tea, and large meals, and make lifestyle changes, including quitting smoking and loosing body weight. It has been suggested that there is a potential difference in dietary style among patients with erosive and non-erosive GERD [14]. More recently, a potential role of functional foods seems playing some role in GERD management [15]. However, due to the paucity of evidence, routine global elimination of foods that may trigger reflux is not recommended for the treatment of all subjects with GERD [16–18]. To date, there are few data on the role of different dietary patterns on GERD symptoms, which affect the quality of daily life, interfering with physical activity, social life, sleep, and productivity at work [19–21]. According to previous guidelines, a negative impact on quality of life is a criterion for the diagnosis of GERD in subjects with frequent heartburn [22,23].

In this study, we investigated the association between a plant-only (vegan) diet and GERD-related symptoms after adjusting for socio-demographic characteristics, life habits, and health-related quality of life by using data collected through an online survey.

## 2. Materials and Methods

### 2.1. Data Collection

The INVITA study (INVestigation on ITAlians' habits and health) uses an online survey launched on 26 July 2022, with the aim of cross-sectionally collecting data on the lifestyle, health status, and diet of the Italian general population. Participants were voluntarily recruited online by advertising the access link of the study through social media and newsletters. The exclusion criteria were age < 18 years, pregnancy or breastfeeding, and plant-based dietary restrictions (macrobiotic, fruit-based, raw-food, hygienist diets). The survey ensured anonymity and informed consent was obtained from all the participants. The online questionnaire was hosted by the Scientific Society for Vegetarian Nutrition (an Italian non-profit organization) in a dedicated application on the domain www.studioinvita.it (accessed on 26 July 2022) and could be accessed from computers, tablets, and smartphones. The data collected were downloaded and managed by data management personnel who had no possibility to identify study participants. This study was approved by the Bioethics Committee of the University of Pisa, Italy (Prot. N. 0116339/2021, approval date 29 September 2021).

### 2.2. Assessments

The dietary pattern ('vegan' or 'non-vegan') classification was established by categorizing participants who consumed at least one food item among meat, fish, poultry, dairy, or eggs as 'non-vegan,' and those who did not consume any food among meat, fish, poultry, dairy, or eggs as 'vegan.' GERD was diagnosed according to the Montreal consensus [23] by evaluating the presence of chest pain, regurgitation, and heartburn. Subjects were diagnosed as either having (GERD+) or not having (GERD−). To be considered as GERD-related, symptoms were required to have occurred two or more times per week over the previous 30 days. An ad hoc question about medications was used to classify those subjects who were controlling GERD symptoms with antiacids, histamine-2 blockers and/or proton pump inhibitors as GERD+.

The health-related quality of life was assessed by the self-reported Medical Outcomes Study 36-item Short Form Survey (SF-36; Italian version) [24]. The scale comprises 36 items. Item 1 asks participants to judge their health condition in general as excellent, very good, good, fair, or poor. Item 2 asks to rate their health in general compared to one year ago (from 1 'Much better now than one year ago' to 5 'Much worse now than one year ago'). Items 3–12 describe how their health status could limit a series of activities usually performed during a typical day (vigorous activities such as running, lifting heavy objects etc.; moderate activities such as moving a table, pushing a vacuum cleaner, etc.; lifting or carrying groceries; climbing several flights of stairs; climbing one flight of stairs; bending, kneeling, or stooping; walking more than a mile; walking several blocks; walking one block; bathing or dressing yourself). Items 13–16 list (with an option of 'Yes' or 'No') some problems with work or other daily activities as a result of physical health in the past 4 weeks (cut down the amount of time spent on work or other activities; accomplished less than a subject would like; limited in the kind of work or other activities; difficulty performing the work or other activities). Items 17–19 ask (with an option of 'Yes' or 'No') about problems with work or other regular activities as a result of emotional problems in the past 4 weeks (cut down the amount of time spent on work or other activities; accomplished less than a subject would like; did not work or do other activities as carefully as usual). Item 20 'During the past 4 weeks, to what extent has your physical health or emotional problems interfered with your normal social activities with family, friends, neighbors, or groups?' was scored from 1 'Not at all' to 5 'Extremely'. Item 21 explores how much bodily pain was experienced during the past 4 weeks (from 1 'None' to 6 'Very severe'), while item 22 asks how much pain interfered with the normal work (from 1 'Not at all' to 5 'Extremely). Items 23–31 assess how participants felt during the past 4 weeks (very nervous, down in the dumps, calm and peaceful, with a lot of energy, etc.) by scoring from 1 'All of the time' to 6 'None of the time'. Item 32 'During the past 4 weeks, how much of the time has your physical health or emotional problems interfered with your social activities?' was scored from 1 'All of the time' to 5 'None of the time'. Finally, items 33–36 ask participants to judge as true or false statements about their health (to become sick a little easier than other people; healthy as anybody I know; to expect health becoming worse; to have excellent health). All items were recorded so that a high score defined a more favorable health status. In addition, each item was scored on a range from 0 to 100 to represent the percentage of total possible score achieved. After that, items were averaged together to create 8 dimensions: general health (5 items), physical functioning (10 items), role limitations due to emotional problems (3 items), bodily pain (2 items), emotional well-being (5 items), role limitations due to physical health (4 items), energy/fatigue (4 items), and social functioning (2 items).

Moreover, ad hoc forms were used to collect sociodemographic characteristics and lifestyle habits: gender, age, marital status, education level, occupation, self-reported height and weight (BMI was computed by dividing weight in kilograms by height in meters squared), smoking history (yes/no), and alcohol consumption per month (1 alcohol unit, AU = 12 gr of pure alcohol, which corresponds to an average 330 cc of beer or 125 cc of wine or 80 cc of vermouth or 40 cc of liquor. 'At risk' consumption was defined as >60 AUs for males and >30 AUs for females [25,26]).

### 2.3. Statistical Analyses

Categorical variables were described as absolute numbers and percentages; continuous variables were summarized as means and standard deviations (SDs). Comparisons between groups were performed by Fisher's exact test (4 cells) or Chi-square test (more than 4 cells) in the case of categorical variables, and by $t$ test in the case of continuous variables. Subsequently, univariate logistic regression models with GERD+ as the dependent variable and each characteristic (dietary pattern and a set of possible confounding factors such as gender, age, marital status, education, occupation, BMI, alcohol consumption, smoking, and the 8 quality of life dimensions) as the independent variable were estimated to calculate unadjusted ORs. The characteristics that were found to be associated (at $p < 0.05$) with GERD+ entered the multivariate logistic regression model, returning adjusted ORs. All tests were two-tailed, with a significance level of 0.05. Analyses were performed by Stata 17 for Windows.

## 3. Results

At the time data were extracted (16 May 2023), 4352 subjects completed socio-demographics and life habits questionnaires. Of these, 1077 (24.7%) completed both the GERD survey and the SF-36 assessment and were included in the study (Figure 1).

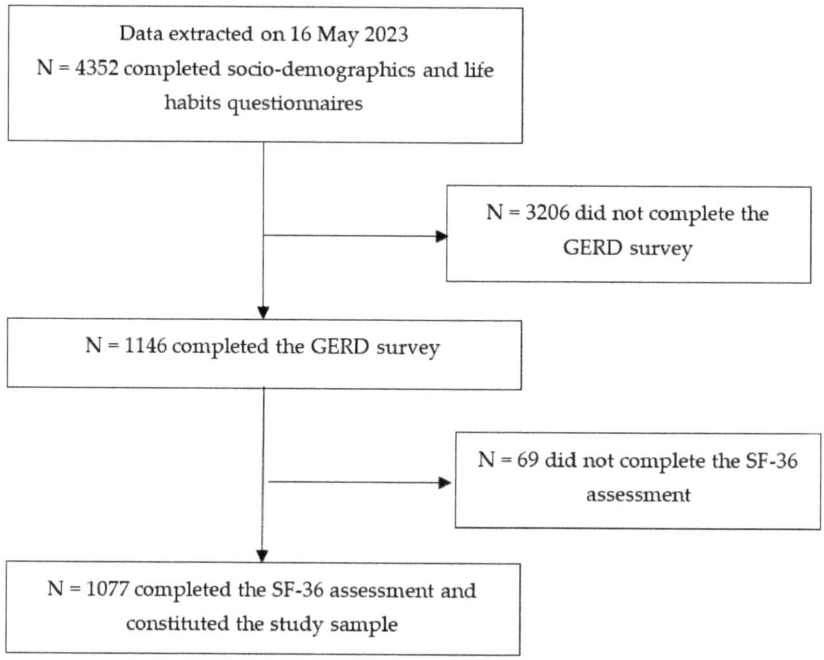


**Figure 1.** Flowchart of participants throughout the study.

A percentage of about 9% were found to have GERD symptoms and were categorized as GERD+. The number of participants in the sample giving information about medications were 929. In this sub-sample, the number of subjects taking antiacids, histamine 2 blockers, and/or proton pump inhibitors (PPI) were 16. Furthermore, 93% of participants were female, the mean age of the overall population was 37 $\pm$ 12 years, more than 60% were married, about 65% had a high education level (a degree or a post-degree), and more than 70% were employed. The mean BMI was 22.2 (SD 3.8) (Table 1, part a). By considering life habits (Table 1, part b), 4.9% declared a monthly alcohol consumption at risk, 9% were smokers, and 37.3% were vegans. By comparing socio-demographic characteristics and life habits between the study sample (n = 1077) and the subjects who did not complete the GERD survey or the SF-36 (n = 3275), age (37.1, SD 12.0 vs. 35.2, SD 11.8; $p < 0.001$ *t* test), vegan dietary pattern (37.3% vs. 31.7%; $p < 0.001$ Fisher's test), and monthly alcohol consumption (no consumption 21.4% vs. 1.1%, low/moderate 73.7% vs. 90.8%, at risk 4.9% vs. 8.2%; $p < 0.001$ Chi-square test) were the only variables reaching a statistical significance. By considering the health-related quality of life (Table 1, part c), the mean scores for the eight dimensions ranged from 53.8 (SD 18.4) for Energy/fatigue to 94.6 (SD 9.9) for Physical functioning.

**Table 1.** Socio-demographic characteristics of (a) life habits, (b) health-related quality of life (SF-36), and (c) of the overall sample, and of GERD+ and GERD− participants (n = 1077).

| **a. Socio-Demographic Characteristics** | **Overall Sample n = 1077** | **GERD− n = 982 (91.2%)** | **GERD+ n = 95 (8.8%)** | ***p*-Value** |
|---|---|---|---|---|
| Gender, n (%)<br>Male<br>Female | <br>75 (7.0%)<br>1002 (93.0%) | <br>70 (7.1%)<br>912 (92.9%) | <br>5 (5.3%)<br>90 (94.7%) | 0.672<br>Fisher |
| Age, mean (SD) | 37.1 (12.0) | 37.0 (11.9) | 37.7 (12.9) | 0.583<br>*t* test |
| BMI, mean (SD) | 22.2 (3.8) | 22.0 (3.5) | 24.1 (5.4) | <0.001<br>*t* test |
| Marital status, n (%)<br>Married<br>Not married | <br>664 (61.7%)<br>413 (38.3%) | <br>602 (61.3%)<br>380 (38.7%) | <br>62 (65.3%)<br>33 (34.7%) | 0.508<br>Fisher |
| Education, n (%)<br>Professional qualification/Diploma<br>Degree/Post-degree | <br>362 (33.6%)<br>715 (66.4%) | <br>321 (32.7%)<br>661 (67.3%) | <br>41 (43.2%)<br>54 (56.8%) | 0.027<br>Fisher |
| Occupation, n (%)<br>Employed<br>Not employed | <br>765 (71.0%)<br>312 (29.0%) | <br>705 (71.8%)<br>277 (28.2%) | <br>60 (63.2%)<br>35 (36.8%) | 0.097<br>Fisher |
| **b. Life habits** | **Overall Sample n = 1077** | **GERD− n = 982 (91.2%)** | **GERD+ n = 95 (8.8%)** | ***p*-value** |
| Dietary pattern, n (%)<br>Vegan<br>Non-vegan | <br>402 (37.3%)<br>675 (62.7%) | <br>379 (38.6%)<br>603 (61.4%) | <br>23 (24.2%)<br>72 (75.8%) | 0.005<br>Fisher |
| Monthly alcohol consumption, n (%)<br>No consumption<br>Low/Moderate [1]<br>At risk [2] | 32 missing<br>224 (21.4%)<br>770 (73.7%)<br>51 (4.9%) | 30 missing<br>206 (21.6%)<br>700 (73.5%)<br>46 (4.8%) | 2 missing<br>18 (19.4%)<br>70 (75.3%)<br>5 (5.4%) | 0.864<br>Chi-square |
| Currently smoking, n (%)<br>No<br>Yes | 5 missing<br>975 (91.0%)<br>97 (9.0%) | 4 missing<br>896 (91.6%)<br>82 (8.4%) | 1 missing<br>79 (84.0%)<br>15 (16.0%) | 0.022<br>Fisher |
| **c. Health-related quality of life (SF-36), mean (SD)** | **Overall Sample n = 1077** | **GERD− n = 982 (91.2%)** | **GERD+ n = 95 (8.8%)** | ***p*-value *t* test** |
| General health | 68.4 (17.2) | 69.7 (16.0) | 54.3 (22.5) | <0.001 |
| Physical functioning | 94.6 (9.9) | 95.2 (8.7) | 88.3 (17.4) | <0.001 |
| Role limitations due to emotional problems | 58.9 (40.9) | 60.0 (40.7) | 48.2 (41.5) | 0.007 |
| Bodily pain | 82.7 (20.3) | 84.0 (19.4) | 68.4 (23.4) | <0.001 |
| Emotional well-being | 65.8 (17.1) | 66.6 (16.7) | 57.9 (18.7) | <0.001 |
| Role limitations due to physical health | 84.6 (28.8) | 86.0 (27.2) | 70.0 (39.4) | <0.001 |
| Energy/fatigue | 53.8 (18.4) | 54.8 (17.9) | 43.9 (20.8) | <0.001 |
| Social functioning | 74.3 (22.7) | 75.4 (22.0) | 63.0 (25.8) | <0.001 |

[1] ≤60 alcohol units for males; ≤30 alcohol units for females [26]. [2] >60 alcohol units for males; >30 alcohol units for females [26].

GERD+ subjects had a higher BMI (24.1, SD 5.4 vs. 22.0, SD 3.5; $p < 0.001$ *t* test), a lower education level (degree/post-degree 56.8% vs. 67.3%; $p = 0.027$ Fisher's test), a lower percentage of vegan dietary pattern (24.2% vs. 38.6%; $p = 0.005$ Fisher's test), and a higher percentage of smoking habit (16.0% vs. 8.4%; $p = 0.022$ Fisher's test). All the health-related quality of life dimensions showed that the GERD+ group had mean scores lower than the GERD− group.

The unadjusted ORs estimated by univariate logistic regression models confirmed the association between GERD+ and BMI, education, dietary pattern, current smoking, and all the health-related quality of life dimensions ($p < 0.05$ for all) (Table 2).

**Table 2.** Univariate logistic models for GERD+ participants: unadjusted ORs (n = 1077).

| Independent Variable | OR (Unadjusted) | 95% CI | *p*-Value |
|---|---|---|---|
| Gender | | | |
| Male | Ref. | - | - |
| Female | 1.38 | 0.54–3.51 | 0.497 |
| Age | 1.01 | 0.99–1.02 | 0.345 |
| BMI | 1.12 | 1.07–1.17 | <0.001 |
| Marital status | | | |
| Married | Ref. | - | - |
| Not married | 0.84 | 0.54–1.31 | 0.449 |
| Education | | | |
| Professional qualification/Diploma | Ref. | - | - |
| Degree/Post-degree | 0.64 | 0.42–0.98 | 0.040 |
| Occupation | | | |
| Employed | Ref. | - | - |
| Not employed | 1.48 | 0.96–2.30 | 0.078 |
| Dietary pattern | | | |
| Non-vegan | Ref. | - | - |
| Vegan | 0.51 | 0.31–0.83 | 0.006 |
| Monthly alcohol consumption | | | |
| No consumption | Ref. | - | - |
| Low/Moderate [1] | 1.14 | 0.67–1.96 | 0.625 |
| At risk [2] | 1.24 | 0.44–3.52 | 0.681 |
| Currently smoking | | | |
| No | Ref. | - | - |
| Yes | 2.07 | 1.14–3.77 | 0.016 |
| General health | 0.96 | 0.95–0.97 | <0.001 |
| Physical functioning | 0.98 | 0.98–0.99 | <0.001 |
| Role limitations due to emotional problems | 0.99 | 0.98–0.99 | 0.008 |
| Bodily pain | 0.97 | 0.96–0.98 | <0.001 |
| Emotional well-being | 0.97 | 0.96–0.98 | <0.001 |
| Role limitations due to physical health | 0.96 | 0.94–0.97 | <0.001 |
| Energy/fatigue | 0.97 | 0.96–0.98 | <0.001 |
| Social functioning | 0.98 | 0.97–0.99 | <0.001 |

[1] ≤60 alcohol units for males; ≤30 alcohol units for females [26]. [2] >60 alcohol units for males; >30 alcohol units for females [26].

These characteristics entered the multivariate logistic regression model ultimately providing adjusted ORs (adj-ORs) (Table 3). A higher BMI (adj-OR = 1.07, $p = 0.007$), smoking (adj-OR = 1.97, $p = 0.039$), a worse General health (adj-OR = 0.97, $p = 0.001$), and a worse Bodily pain (adj-OR = 0.98, $p = 0.005$) were significantly associated with GERD+ condition, while a vegan dietary pattern was inversely associated with GERD+ status (adj-OR = 0.47, $p = 0.006$).

**Table 3.** Multivariate logistic model for GERD+ participants: adjusted ORs (only independent variables significantly associated at $p < 0.05$ in univariate logistic regression models entered the multivariate logistic regression model).

| Independent Variable | OR (Adjusted) | 95% CI | *p*-Value |
|---|---|---|---|
| BMI | 1.07 | 1.02–1.13 | 0.007 |
| Education | | | |
| Professional qualification/Diploma | Ref. | - | - |
| Degree/Post-degree | 0.74 | 0.46–1.19 | 0.219 |
| Dietary pattern | | | |
| Non-vegan | Ref. | - | - |
| Vegan | 0.47 | 0.28–0.81 | 0.006 |
| Currently smoking | | | |
| No | Ref. | - | - |
| Yes | 1.97 | 1.03–3.74 | 0.039 |
| General health | 0.97 | 0.96–0.99 | 0.001 |
| Physical functioning | 1.00 | 0.99–1.01 | 0.721 |
| Role limitations due to emotional problems | 1.00 | 0.99–1.01 | 0.317 |
| Bodily pain | 0.98 | 0.97–0.99 | 0.005 |
| Emotional well-being | 0.99 | 0.97–1.01 | 0.544 |
| Role limitations due to physical health | 1.00 | 0.98–1.02 | 0.921 |
| Energy/fatigue | 0.99 | 0.97–1.01 | 0.547 |
| Social functioning | 1.00 | 0.98–1.01 | 0.583 |
| Number of observations | | 1077 | |
| LR test, *p*-value | | Chi2(12) = 94.45, $p < 0.001$ | |
| Hosmer—Lemeshow goodness-of-fit (10 groups) | | | |
| Chi2(df), *p*-value | | Chi2(8) = 7.55, $p = 0.479$ | |
| Pearson goodness-of-fit | | | |
| Number of covariate patterns | | 1072 | |
| Chi2(df), *p*-value | | Chi2(1059) = 1060.64, $p = 0.480$ | |
| Area under ROC curve | | 0.78 | |

## 4. Discussion

GERD is a very common disease, affecting about 1 billion people worldwide with some degree of variability according to the geographical location. In Europe, the prevalence of GERD is about 14.12% [3,27]. Typically reported risk factors are represented by sex, age, BMI, use of non-steroidal anti-inflammatory drugs, and smoking [3,27,28]. Additionally, diet is a potential risk factor for GERD symptoms; however, there is currently limited research on the impact of dietary choices on reflux symptoms [16,29]. The clinical diagnosis of GERD is based on the frequency of troublesome symptoms such as heartburn, regurgitation, and chest pain [23,30]. The recently updated version of the Lyon Consensus 2.0 suggests that only patients with typical symptoms (without clinical red signs) should be approached with a short empiric trial of proton pump inhibitors (PPIs) because the likelihood of GERD is quite high compared to atypical or extraesophageal presentations [31].

Our results showed a very strong association between some dietary choices and GERD: a plant-only (vegan) diet was inversely associated with the GERD+ condition (about halving the risk, compared to any other animal-based dietary patterns (OR = 0.47, 95% CI 0.28–0.81, $p = 0.006$)).

Moreover, we confirmed other established GERD risk factors, including smoking cigarettes (OR 1.97) and increased BMI (OR 1.07). In addition, the Quality-of-Life (SF-36) perception resulted lower in GERD+ subjects.

The American College of Gastroenterology guidelines [17] suggest, in the statement regarding lifestyle modifications for GERD treatment, avoiding trigger foods (indicated individually), reducing body weight for overweight and obese subjects, avoiding tobacco smoking, and head of bed elevation for subjects with nighttime symptoms. Despite the low level of evidence, the American College of Gastroenterology suggests cessation of foods that potentially aggravate reflux symptoms such as coffee, chocolate, carbonated beverages, spicy foods, and acidic foods such as citrus and tomatoes [11,17].

Only a few studies have evaluated the role of food components in the genesis of reflux symptoms, with conflicting results [9,12,18]. Moreover, eating animal food has been associated with a worsening of GERD symptoms. Similarly, a high-fat diet, including mainly animal fats, is considered a risk factor for the development of GERD complications such as Barrett esophagus [9,32,33].

Zalvan et al. suggested that a plant-based Mediterranean diet should be considered in the treatment of laryngopharyngeal reflux. A Mediterranean diet includes plant foods such as vegetables, bread and other grains, potatoes, beans, nuts and seeds, fresh fruit as the typical daily dessert, olive oil as the principal source of fat, dairy products (principally cheese and yoghurt), and fish and poultry consumed in low to moderate amounts, zero to four eggs consumed weekly, red meat consumed in low amounts, and wine consumed in low to moderate amounts, normally at mealtime [34].

Another study by Jung J.G. et al. suggested that a vegetarian diet may offer a protective effect for reflux esophagitis [35]. Similarly, Martinucci I. et al. [9] have shown that plant foods are associated with a lower number of reflux episodes, particularly acid refluxes, and with a reduced number of symptoms during the first postprandial hour. Unfortunately, these studies included a relatively small sample of individuals, and their findings warrant further investigation. Vegetarians may experience fewer symptoms of gastroesophageal reflux due to a typically healthier lifestyle [36], and some research has indicated that a vegetarian diet may be associated with improved mood and reduced stress [37]; these factors could potentially reduce reflux symptoms [38]. Nevertheless, it is yet to be determined whether subjects with GERD symptoms and related issues can benefit from adopting a vegetarian diet. In support of the potential anti-reflux effect of fiber, it was shown that fiber food improved heartburn symptoms in a randomized controlled trial [39]. The vegetarian diet is also rich in antioxidants and maintains a higher antioxidant vitamin status (vitamin C, vitamin E, ß-carotene) [40]. a chronic oxidative stress has been shown to contribute to the development of GERD [41,42], and diets high in vitamin C content were associated with a lower risk of GERD [43].

The determinant role of vegetables and fibers in the diet has been underlined in many different studies. A very elegant study provided from Houston team (US) discovered that a daily intake of more than 1.58 cups of vegetables and 0.18 cups of dark green vegetables per 1000 calories was associated with a lower risk of intestinal metaplasia in the esophagus (Barrett Esophagus, BE) [44].

Kubo et al., in a population-based case–control study conducted in the United States, observed that the consumption of veggies was associated with a lower risk of BE [45]. Similarly, a nice research study, conducted in Washington State with 170 hospitalized cases and 182 controls from the general population, showed that a global vegetable intake was linked to a 60–70% risk decrease for BE [46].

Anderson and colleagues found an inverse correlation between fruit and vegetable intake and the risk of complicated GERD [47]. However, consumption of leafy or dark green vegetables has consistently been linked to a lower risk of cancer [48–50]. Different reports have shown that dietary fibers are known to play a determinant role in the prevention of different gastrointestinal diseases such as constipation, hemorrhoids, colon cancer, gastroesophageal reflux disease, duodenal ulcer, and diverticulitis, as well in serious and systemic diseases such as obesity, diabetes, stroke, hypertension, and cardiovascular diseases [51–53].

A reduction in Quality-of-Life in GERD subjects has been reported in previous studies [54–57]. The QoL in patients with GERD-related symptoms was lower than that associated with untreated duodenal ulcer, angina, mild heart failure, diabetes, and hypertension [58,59]. Importantly, when compared with population normal values, the decrements QoL in GERD patients were independent of whether patients have erosive or nonerosive disease [60].

Some literature reports have highlighted that the presence of mucosal injury has little impact on how reflux symptoms affect individual quality of life. This result is in line with the observation that patients with symptomatic GERD (without any mucosal lesion) experience symptoms that are comparable to those of patients with erosive GERD [61]. Numerous studies have also revealed that the impact on the QoL is often proportional to symptom improvement, and that improvements in QoL in response to treatment are independent of whether esophagitis is present or not [62]. According to our results, we may speculate that the different QoL perception is not only related to the prevalence of GERD-related symptoms. Some reports describe a reduced QoL in subjects with dietary habits based on a Western diet. Moreover, a healthy Mediterranean diet-lifestyle was associated with a lower risk of depression onset [63,64], especially when it was compared with a Western dietary style including processed foods, meat, and dairy, which seems to be associated with an increased risk of depression [65,66]. Accordingly, some randomized control trials described an improvement in depression-related symptom scores when subjects changed from an unhealthy diet (Western) to a healthy diet based on plant foods [63,67,68].

The main strength of this study is the large sample: 1077 questionnaires on GERD-related symptoms and SF-36 were received, in addition to questionnaires about food choices; almost 40% of those who took part in the study declared to follow a vegan diet. Such a large sample, with 402 participants following a diet based exclusively on plant foods, is larger than that of other studies, and provides results with a higher strength of evidence.

Some limitations are also present in this study: data collection relied on self-reported data, thus resulting in possible recall bias and a biased interpretation of the questions. In addition, the design of the study was cross-sectional, which does not allow for the identification of causal relationships. The study was conducted in Italy, hampering the generalizability of the findings to other countries. Moreover, despite the large sample size of participants in the INVITA study (n = 4352), the percentage of those who completed the GERD survey and the SF-36 assessment was relatively low (24.7%). The comparison between those who completed GERDQ and SF-36 (n = 1077) and those who did not complete them (n = 3275) showed that completers were slightly older, more often vegans, and had a lower alcohol consumption. The comparison between the whole INVITA sample (n = 4352) and the Italian general population ($\geq$18 years) showed that there are differences in some characteristics: gender (females 92.2% vs. 51.2%), BMI (>25 kg/m$^2$ 17.5% vs. 43%), age (<50 56.3% vs. 85.2%), education (university degree: 52.7% vs. 22.4%), smoking habit (10.1% vs. 24.2%), and 'at risk' alcohol consumption (7.0% vs. 17.3%). The vegan dietary pattern, as mentioned above, was over-represented (33.1% vs. 2.4%) [69,70]. All in all, in our study, GERD was defined based on the presence of typical symptoms according to the Montreal Consensus [23] and cannot be considered an objective diagnosis of GERD. Anyway, both versions of the Lyon Consensus [31,71] suggest that typical symptoms are associated with a high likelihood of having objective GERD, corroborating the use of a short course of PPIs in primary care. Finally, the dietary pattern classification in 'vegan' vs. 'non-vegan' did not permit an evaluation of the quality of the diet.

## 5. Conclusions

In conclusion, this study confirmed that a plant-only (vegan) diet is associated with a lower risk of GERD-related symptoms and could therefore prevent the onset of GERD. The results about quality of life (SF-36 questionnaire, QoL) have shown how the GERD+ participants had a lower score on the SF-36 questionnaire in comparison to GERD− participants. These findings suggest that GERD subjects have a lower perception of their health status, stressing the impact of this disease on the QoL. Considering the low level of evidence of guidelines in suggesting the avoidance of some type of food as a first-line therapy of this disease, the possibility of following a vegan diet, or at least of decreasing the consumption of animal foods, is worthy of consideration as a first-line therapy approach.

**Author Contributions:** Conceptualization, L.B., G.R. and N.d.B.; methodology, C.B.; software, C.B.; validation, I.S., P.V. and F.O.; formal analysis, M.O. and C.B.; investigation, L.B. and G.S.; data curation, M.O. and M.B.; writing—original draft preparation, L.B., C.B. and N.d.B.; writing—review and editing, G.G., G.R., P.V., I.B. and J.P.; supervision, L.B., E.V.S., G.R. and G.G. All authors have read and agreed to the published version of the manuscript.

**Funding:** This research received no external funding.

**Institutional Review Board Statement:** The study was conducted in accordance with the Declaration of Helsinki and approved by the Bioethical Committee of the University of Pisa, (Prot. N. 0116339/2021, approval date 29 September 2021).

**Informed Consent Statement:** Informed consent was obtained from all subjects involved in the study.

**Data Availability Statement:** The data presented in this study are available on the request from the corresponding author. The data are not publicly available due to privacy law.

**Acknowledgments:** Authors wish to thank all the participants to the INVITA study, and the Scientific Society for Vegetarian Nutrition of Italy for providing the technical support to the survey.

**Conflicts of Interest:** The authors declare no conflict of interest.

## References

1. Savarino, E.; Bredenoord, A.J.; Fox, M.; Pandolfino, J.E.; Roman, S.; Gyawali, C.P.; International Working Group for Disorders of Gastrointestinal Motility and Function. Advances in the Physiological Assessment and Diagnosis of GERD. *Nat. Rev. Gastroenterol. Hepatol.* **2018**, *15*, 323. [CrossRef] [PubMed]
2. Gyawali, C.P.; Azagury, D.E.; Chan, W.W.; Chandramohan, S.M.; Clarke, J.O.; de Bortoli, N.; Figueredo, E.; Fox, M.; Jodorkovsky, D.; Lazarescu, A.; et al. Nonerosive Reflux Disease: Clinical Concepts. *Ann. N. Y. Acad. Sci.* **2018**, *1434*, 290–303. [CrossRef] [PubMed]
3. Savarino, E.; Marabotto, E.; Bodini, G.; Pellegatta, G.; Coppo, C.; Giambruno, E.; Brunacci, M.; Zentilin, P.; Savarino, V. Epidemiology and Natural History of Gastroesophageal Reflux Disease. *Minerva Gastroenterol. Dietol.* **2017**, *63*, 175–183. [CrossRef] [PubMed]
4. Savarino, E.; de Bortoli, N.; De Cassan, C.; Della Coletta, M.; Bartolo, O.; Furnari, M.; Ottonello, A.; Marabotto, E.; Bodini, G.; Savarino, V. The Natural History of Gastro-Esophageal Reflux Disease: A Comprehensive Review. *Dis. Esophagus* **2017**, *30*, 1–9. [CrossRef] [PubMed]
5. Navarro Silvera, S.A.; Mayne, S.T.; Gammon, M.D.; Vaughan, T.L.; Chow, W.-H.; Dubin, J.A.; Dubrow, R.; Stanford, J.L.; West, A.B.; Rotterdam, H.; et al. Diet and Lifestyle Factors and Risk of Subtypes of Esophageal and Gastric Cancers: Classification Tree Analysis. *Ann. Epidemiol.* **2014**, *24*, 50–57. [CrossRef] [PubMed]
6. Akiyama, J.; Kuribayashi, S.; Baeg, M.K.; de Bortoli, N.; Valitova, E.; Savarino, E.V.; Kusano, M.; Triadafilopoulos, G. Current and Future Perspectives in the Management of Gastroesophageal Reflux Disease. *Ann. N. Y. Acad. Sci.* **2018**, *1434*, 70–83. [CrossRef]
7. Tack, J.; Pandolfino, J.E. Pathophysiology of Gastroesophageal Reflux Disease. *Gastroenterology* **2018**, *154*, 277–288. [CrossRef]
8. Lacy, B.E.; Weiser, K.; Chertoff, J.; Fass, R.; Pandolfino, J.E.; Richter, J.E.; Rothstein, R.I.; Spangler, C.; Vaezi, M.F. The Diagnosis of Gastroesophageal Reflux Disease. *Am. J. Med.* **2010**, *123*, 583–592. [CrossRef] [PubMed]
9. Martinucci, I.; Guidi, G.; Savarino, E.V.; Frazzoni, M.; Tolone, S.; Frazzoni, L.; Fuccio, L.; Bertani, L.; Bodini, G.; Ceccarelli, L.; et al. Vegetal and Animal Food Proteins Have a Different Impact in the First Postprandial Hour of Impedance-pH Analysis in Patients with Heartburn. *Gastroenterol. Res. Pract.* **2018**, *2018*, 7572430. [CrossRef] [PubMed]
10. de Bortoli, N.; Guidi, G.; Martinucci, I.; Savarino, E.; Imam, H.; Bertani, L.; Russo, S.; Franchi, R.; Macchia, L.; Furnari, M.; et al. Voluntary and Controlled Weight Loss Can Reduce Symptoms and Proton Pump Inhibitor Use and Dosage in Patients with Gastroesophageal Reflux Disease: A Comparative Study. *Dis. Esophagus* **2016**, *29*, 197–204. [CrossRef] [PubMed]
11. Fox, M.; Gyawali, C.P. Dietary Factors Involved in GERD Management. *Best Pract. Res. Clin. Gastroenterol.* **2023**, *62–63*, 101826. [CrossRef]
12. Nilsson, M.; Johnsen, R.; Ye, W.; Hveem, K.; Lagergren, J. Lifestyle Related Risk Factors in the Aetiology of Gastro-Oesophageal Reflux. *Gut* **2004**, *53*, 1730–1735. [CrossRef] [PubMed]

13. Murao, T.; Sakurai, K.; Mihara, S.; Marubayashi, T.; Murakami, Y.; Sasaki, Y. Lifestyle Change Influences on GERD in Japan: A Study of Participants in a Health Examination Program. *Dig. Dis. Sci.* **2011**, *56*, 2857–2864. [CrossRef] [PubMed]
14. Chen, Y.; Sun, X.; Fan, W.; Yu, J.; Wang, P.; Liu, D.; Song, M.; Liu, S.; Zuo, X.; Zhang, R.; et al. Differences in Dietary and Lifestyle Triggers between Non-Erosive Reflux Disease and Reflux Esophagitis-A Multicenter Cross-Sectional Survey in China. *Nutrients* **2023**, *15*, 3400. [CrossRef]
15. Herdiana, Y. Functional Food in Relation to Gastroesophageal Reflux Disease (GERD). *Nutrients* **2023**, *15*, 3583. [CrossRef]
16. Martinucci, I.; de Bortoli, N.; Savarino, E.; Nacci, A.; Romeo, S.O.; Bellini, M.; Savarino, V.; Fattori, B.; Marchi, S. Optimal Treatment of Laryngopharyngeal Reflux Disease. *Ther. Adv. Chronic Dis.* **2013**, *4*, 287–301. [CrossRef] [PubMed]
17. Katz, P.O.; Dunbar, K.B.; Schnoll-Sussman, F.H.; Greer, K.B.; Yadlapati, R.; Spechler, S.J. ACG Clinical Guideline for the Diagnosis and Management of Gastroesophageal Reflux Disease. *Am. J. Gastroenterol.* **2022**, *117*, 27–56. [CrossRef]
18. Zheng, Z.; Nordenstedt, H.; Pedersen, N.L.; Lagergren, J.; Ye, W. Lifestyle Factors and Risk for Symptomatic Gastroesophageal Reflux in Monozygotic Twins. *Gastroenterology* **2007**, *132*, 87–95. [CrossRef] [PubMed]
19. Lee, S.-W.; Chang, C.-M.; Chang, C.-S.; Kao, A.-W.; Chou, M.-C. Comparison of Presentation and Impact on Quality of Life of Gastroesophageal Reflux Disease between Young and Old Adults in a Chinese Population. *World J. Gastroenterol.* **2011**, *17*, 4614–4618. [CrossRef] [PubMed]
20. Wahlqvist, P.; Karlsson, M.; Johnson, D.; Carlsson, J.; Bolge, S.C.; Wallander, M.-A. Relationship between Symptom Load of Gastro-Oesophageal Reflux Disease and Health-Related Quality of Life, Work Productivity, Resource Utilization and Concomitant Diseases: Survey of a US Cohort. *Aliment. Pharmacol. Ther.* **2008**, *27*, 960–970. [CrossRef]
21. Wiklund, I. Review of the Quality of Life and Burden of Illness in Gastroesophageal Reflux Disease. *Dig. Dis.* **2004**, *22*, 108–114. [CrossRef] [PubMed]
22. Dent, J.; Brun, J.; Fendrick, A.; Fennerty, M.; Janssens, J.; Kahrilas, P.; Lauritsen, K.; Reynolds, J.; Shaw, M.; Talley, N. An Evidence-Based Appraisal of Reflux Disease Management--the Genval Workshop Report. *Gut* **1999**, *44* (Suppl. S2), S1–S16. [CrossRef]
23. Vakil, N.; van Zanten, S.V.; Kahrilas, P.; Dent, J.; Jones, R.; Global Consensus Group. The Montreal Definition and Classification of Gastroesophageal Reflux Disease: A Global Evidence-Based Consensus. *Am. J. Gastroenterol.* **2006**, *101*, 1900–1920; quiz 1943. [CrossRef]
24. Apolone, G.; Mosconi, P. The Italian SF-36 Health Survey: Translation, Validation and Norming. *J. Clin. Epidemiol.* **1998**, *51*, 1025–1036. [CrossRef] [PubMed]
25. Ministero Della Salute, Italia. Alcol, Zero o Il Meno Possibile. Available online: https://www.salute.gov.it/portale/alcol/dettaglioContenutiAlcol.jsp?lingua=italiano&id=5526&area=alcol&menu=vuoto (accessed on 14 September 2023).
26. Istituto Superiore di Sanità. Indicatori Passi: Consumo Di Bevande Alcoliche. Available online: https://www.epicentro.iss.it/passi/indicatori/alcol (accessed on 14 September 2023).
27. Nirwan, J.S.; Hasan, S.S.; Babar, Z.-U.-D.; Conway, B.R.; Ghori, M.U. Global Prevalence and Risk Factors of Gastro-Oesophageal Reflux Disease (GORD): Systematic Review with Meta-Analysis. *Sci. Rep.* **2020**, *10*, 5814. [CrossRef] [PubMed]
28. Martinucci, I.; Natilli, M.; Lorenzoni, V.; Pappalardo, L.; Monreale, A.; Turchetti, G.; Pedreschi, D.; Marchi, S.; Barale, R.; de Bortoli, N. Gastroesophageal Reflux Symptoms among Italian University Students: Epidemiology and Dietary Correlates Using Automatically Recorded Transactions. *BMC Gastroenterol.* **2018**, *18*, 116. [CrossRef] [PubMed]
29. Tosetti, C.; Savarino, E.; Benedetto, E.; De Bastiani, R.; Study Group for the Evaluation of GERD Triggering Foods. Elimination of Dietary Triggers Is Successful in Treating Symptoms of Gastroesophageal Reflux Disease. *Dig. Dis. Sci.* **2021**, *66*, 1565–1571. [CrossRef]
30. Savarino, V.; Marabotto, E.; Zentilin, P.; Furnari, M.; Bodini, G.; De Maria, C.; Tolone, S.; De Bortoli, N.; Frazzoni, M.; Savarino, E. Pathophysiology, Diagnosis, and Pharmacological Treatment of Gastro-Esophageal Reflux Disease. *Expert Rev. Clin. Pharmacol.* **2020**, *13*, 437–449. [CrossRef] [PubMed]
31. Gyawali, C.P.; Yadlapati, R.; Fass, R.; Katzka, D.; Pandolfino, J.; Savarino, E.; Sifrim, D.; Spechler, S.; Zerbib, F.; Fox, M.R.; et al. Updates to the Modern Diagnosis of GERD: Lyon Consensus 2.0. *Gut* **2023**, 1–11. [CrossRef] [PubMed]
32. Ledeboer, M.; Masclee, A.A.; Batstra, M.R.; Jansen, J.B.; Lamers, C.B. Effect of Cholecystokinin on Lower Oesophageal Sphincter Pressure and Transient Lower Oesophageal Sphincter Relaxations in Humans. *Gut* **1995**, *36*, 39–44. [CrossRef]
33. Chirila, I.; Morariu, I.D.; Barboi, O.B.; Drug, V.L. The Role of Diet in the Overlap between Gastroesophageal Reflux Disease and Functional Dyspepsia. *Turk. J. Gastroenterol.* **2016**, *27*, 73–80. [CrossRef] [PubMed]
34. Zalvan, C.H.; Hu, S.; Greenberg, B.; Geliebter, J. A Comparison of Alkaline Water and Mediterranean Diet vs Proton Pump Inhibition for Treatment of Laryngopharyngeal Reflux. *JAMA Otolaryngol. Head Neck Surg.* **2017**, *143*, 1023–1029. [CrossRef] [PubMed]
35. Jung, J.G.; Kang, H.W.; Hahn, S.J.; Kim, J.H.; Lee, J.K.; Lim, Y.J.; Koh, M.-S.; Lee, J.H. Vegetarianism as a Protective Factor for Reflux Esophagitis: A Retrospective, Cross-Sectional Study between Buddhist Priests and General Population. *Dig. Dis. Sci.* **2013**, *58*, 2244–2252. [CrossRef] [PubMed]
36. McEvoy, C.T.; Temple, N.; Woodside, J.V. Vegetarian Diets, Low-Meat Diets and Health: A Review. *Public Health Nutr.* **2012**, *15*, 2287–2294. [CrossRef] [PubMed]
37. Beezhold, B.L.; Johnston, C.S.; Daigle, D.R. Vegetarian Diets Are Associated with Healthy Mood States: A Cross-Sectional Study in Seventh Day Adventist Adults. *Nutr. J.* **2010**, *9*, 26. [CrossRef]

38. Okuyama, M.; Takaishi, O.; Nakahara, K.; Iwakura, N.; Hasegawa, T.; Oyama, M.; Inoue, A.; Ishizu, H.; Satoh, H.; Fujiwara, Y. Associations among Gastroesophageal Reflux Disease, Psychological Stress, and Sleep Disturbances in Japanese Adults. *Scand. J. Gastroenterol.* **2017**, *52*, 44–49. [CrossRef] [PubMed]
39. DiSilvestro, R.A.; Verbruggen, M.A.; Offutt, E.J. Anti-Heartburn Effects of a Fenugreek Fiber Product. *Phytother. Res.* **2011**, *25*, 88–91. [CrossRef]
40. Rauma, A.L.; Mykkänen, H. Antioxidant Status in Vegetarians versus Omnivores. *Nutrition* **2000**, *16*, 111–119. [CrossRef]
41. Olyaee, M.; Sontag, S.; Salman, W.; Schnell, T.; Mobarhan, S.; Eiznhamer, D.; Keshavarzian, A. Mucosal Reactive Oxygen Species Production in Oesophagitis and Barrett's Oesophagus. *Gut* **1995**, *37*, 168–173. [CrossRef]
42. Peng, D.; Zaika, A.; Que, J.; El-Rifai, W. The Antioxidant Response in Barrett's Tumorigenesis: A Double-Edged Sword. *Redox Biol.* **2021**, *41*, 101894. [CrossRef]
43. Veugelers, P.J.; Porter, G.A.; Guernsey, D.L.; Casson, A.G. Obesity and Lifestyle Risk Factors for Gastroesophageal Reflux Disease, Barrett Esophagus and Esophageal Adenocarcinoma. *Dis. Esophagus* **2006**, *19*, 321–328. [CrossRef]
44. Jiao, L.; Kramer, J.R.; Rugge, M.; Parente, P.; Verstovsek, G.; Alsarraj, A.; El-Serag, H.B. Dietary Intake of Vegetables, Folate, and Antioxidants and the Risk of Barrett's Esophagus. *Cancer Causes Control* **2013**, *24*, 1005–1014. [CrossRef] [PubMed]
45. Kubo, A.; Levin, T.R.; Block, G.; Rumore, G.J.; Quesenberry, C.P.; Buffler, P.; Corley, D.A. Dietary Antioxidants, Fruits, and Vegetables and the Risk of Barrett's Esophagus. *Am. J. Gastroenterol.* **2008**, *103*, 1614–1623; quiz 1624. [CrossRef] [PubMed]
46. Thompson, O.M.; Beresford, S.A.A.; Kirk, E.A.; Vaughan, T.L. Vegetable and Fruit Intakes and Risk of Barrett's Esophagus in Men and Women. *Am. J. Clin. Nutr.* **2009**, *89*, 890–896. [CrossRef] [PubMed]
47. Anderson, L.A.; Watson, R.G.P.; Murphy, S.J.; Johnston, B.T.; Comber, H.; Mc Guigan, J.; Reynolds, J.V.; Murray, L.J. Risk Factors for Barrett's Oesophagus and Oesophageal Adenocarcinoma: Results from the FINBAR Study. *World J. Gastroenterol.* **2007**, *13*, 1585–1594. [CrossRef] [PubMed]
48. Hughes, M.C.B.; Antonsson, A.; Rodriguez-Acevedo, A.J.; Liyanage, U.E.; Green, A.C.; van der Pols, J.C. Dark Green Leafy Vegetable Intake, MTHFR Genotype, and Risk of Cutaneous Squamous Cell Carcinoma. *Dermatology* **2022**, *238*, 657–661. [CrossRef]
49. Kubo, A.; Corley, D.A.; Jensen, C.D.; Kaur, R. Dietary Factors and the Risks of Oesophageal Adenocarcinoma and Barrett's Oesophagus. *Nutr. Res. Rev.* **2010**, *23*, 230–246. [CrossRef]
50. Hajizadeh, B.; Jessri, M.; Moasheri, S.M.; Rad, A.H.; Rashidkhani, B. Fruits and Vegetables Consumption and Esophageal Squamous Cell Carcinoma: A Case-Control Study. *Nutr. Cancer* **2011**, *63*, 707–713. [CrossRef] [PubMed]
51. Otles, S.; Ozgoz, S. Health Effects of Dietary Fiber. *Acta Sci. Pol. Technol. Aliment.* **2014**, *13*, 191–202. [CrossRef]
52. Lattimer, J.M.; Haub, M.D. Effects of Dietary Fiber and Its Components on Metabolic Health. *Nutrients* **2010**, *2*, 1266–1289. [CrossRef] [PubMed]
53. Birt, D.F.; Boylston, T.; Hendrich, S.; Jane, J.-L.; Hollis, J.; Li, L.; McClelland, J.; Moore, S.; Phillips, G.J.; Rowling, M.; et al. Resistant Starch: Promise for Improving Human Health. *Adv. Nutr.* **2013**, *4*, 587–601. [CrossRef] [PubMed]
54. Velanovich, V. Comparison of Generic (SF-36) vs. Disease-Specific (GERD-HRQL) Quality-of-Life Scales for Gastroesophageal Reflux Disease. *J. Gastrointest. Surg.* **1998**, *2*, 141–145. [CrossRef] [PubMed]
55. Eloubeidi, M.A.; Provenzale, D. Health-Related Quality of Life and Severity of Symptoms in Patients with Barrett's Esophagus and Gastroesophageal Reflux Disease Patients without Barrett's Esophagus. *Am. J. Gastroenterol.* **2000**, *95*, 1881–1887. [CrossRef] [PubMed]
56. Maleki, I.; Masoudzadeh, A.; Khalilian, A.; Daheshpour, E. Quality of Life in Patients with Gastroesophageal Reflux Disease in an Iranian Population. *Gastroenterol. Hepatol. Bed Bench* **2013**, *6*, 96–100. [PubMed]
57. Cheung, T.K.; Lam, P.K.Y.; Wei, W.I.; Wong, W.M.; Ng, M.L.; Gu, Q.; Hung, I.F.; Wong, B.C.Y. Quality of Life in Patients with Laryngopharyngeal Reflux. *Digestion* **2009**, *79*, 52–57. [CrossRef] [PubMed]
58. Dimenäs, E.; Glise, H.; Hallerbäck, B.; Hernqvist, H.; Svedlund, J.; Wiklund, I. Quality of Life in Patients with Upper Gastrointestinal Symptoms. An Improved Evaluation of Treatment Regimens? *Scand. J. Gastroenterol.* **1993**, *28*, 681–687. [CrossRef]
59. Revicki, D.A.; Wood, M.; Maton, P.N.; Sorensen, S. The Impact of Gastroesophageal Reflux Disease on Health-Related Quality of Life. *Am. J. Med.* **1998**, *104*, 252–258. [CrossRef]
60. Wiklund, I.; Bardhan, K.D.; Müller-Lissner, S.; Bigard, M.A.; Bianchi Porro, G.; Ponce, J.; Hosie, J.; Scott, M.; Weir, D.; Fulton, C.; et al. Quality of Life during Acute and Intermittent Treatment of Gastro-Oesophageal Reflux Disease with Omeprazole Compared with Ranitidine. Results from a Multicentre Clinical Trial. The European Study Group. *Ital. J. Gastroenterol. Hepatol.* **1998**, *30*, 19–27.
61. Mathias, S.D.; Colwell, H.H.; Miller, D.P.; Pasta, D.J.; Henning, J.M.; Ofman, J.J. Health-Related Quality-of-Life and Quality-Days Incrementally Gained in Symptomatic Nonerosive GERD Patients Treated with Lansoprazole or Ranitidine. *Dig. Dis. Sci.* **2001**, *46*, 2416–2423. [CrossRef] [PubMed]
62. Ofman, J.J. The Economic and Quality-of-Life Impact of Symptomatic Gastroesophageal Reflux Disease. *Am. J. Gastroenterol.* **2003**, *98*, S8–S14. [CrossRef]
63. Jacka, F.N.; O'Neil, A.; Opie, R.; Itsiopoulos, C.; Cotton, S.; Mohebbi, M.; Castle, D.; Dash, S.; Mihalopoulos, C.; Chatterton, M.L.; et al. A Randomised Controlled Trial of Dietary Improvement for Adults with Major Depression (the "SMILES" Trial). *BMC Med.* **2017**, *15*, 23. [CrossRef]

64. Yin, W.; Löf, M.; Chen, R.; Hultman, C.M.; Fang, F.; Sandin, S. Mediterranean Diet and Depression: A Population-Based Cohort Study. *Int. J. Behav. Nutr. Phys. Act.* **2021**, *18*, 153. [CrossRef] [PubMed]
65. Jacka, F.N.; Pasco, J.A.; Mykletun, A.; Williams, L.J.; Hodge, A.M.; O'Reilly, S.L.; Nicholson, G.C.; Kotowicz, M.A.; Berk, M. Association of Western and Traditional Diets with Depression and Anxiety in Women. *Am. J. Psychiatry* **2010**, *167*, 305–311. [CrossRef] [PubMed]
66. Matison, A.P.; Mather, K.A.; Flood, V.M.; Reppermund, S. Associations between Nutrition and the Incidence of Depression in Middle-Aged and Older Adults: A Systematic Review and Meta-Analysis of Prospective Observational Population-Based Studies. *Ageing Res. Rev.* **2021**, *70*, 101403. [CrossRef] [PubMed]
67. Parletta, N.; Zarnowiecki, D.; Cho, J.; Wilson, A.; Bogomolova, S.; Villani, A.; Itsiopoulos, C.; Niyonsenga, T.; Blunden, S.; Meyer, B.; et al. A Mediterranean-Style Dietary Intervention Supplemented with Fish Oil Improves Diet Quality and Mental Health in People with Depression: A Randomized Controlled Trial (HELFIMED). *Nutr. Neurosci.* **2019**, *22*, 474–487. [CrossRef]
68. Francis, H.M.; Stevenson, R.J.; Chambers, J.R.; Gupta, D.; Newey, B.; Lim, C.K. A Brief Diet Intervention Can Reduce Symptoms of Depression in Young Adults—A Randomised Controlled Trial. *PLoS ONE* **2019**, *14*, e0222768. [CrossRef] [PubMed]
69. Istituto Superiore di Sanità. Sorveglianza PASSI 2021–2022. Available online: https://www.epicentro.iss.it/passi/dati/socio (accessed on 28 August 2023).
70. Eurispes. Rapporto Italia 2023. Available online: https://eurispes.eu/news/risultati-del-rapporto-italia-2023/ (accessed on 28 August 2023).
71. Gyawali, C.P.; Kahrilas, P.J.; Savarino, E.; Zerbib, F.; Mion, F.; Smout, A.J.P.M.; Vaezi, M.; Sifrim, D.; Fox, M.R.; Vela, M.F.; et al. Modern Diagnosis of GERD: The Lyon Consensus. *Gut* **2018**, *67*, 1351–1362. [CrossRef] [PubMed]

*nutrients*

MDPI

*Article*

# Plant-Based Diet Indices and Their Association with Frailty in Older Adults: A CLHLS-Based Cohort Study

**Ran Qi, Yun Yang, Baihe Sheng, Huiping Li and Xinyu Zhang ***

School of Public Health, Tianjin Medical University, Tianjin 300070, China; qiran@tmu.edu.cn (R.Q.); yunyang@tmu.edu.cn (Y.Y.); shengbaihe@tmu.edu.cn (B.S.); lihuiping1222@163.com (H.L.)
* Correspondence: zhangxinyu@tmu.edu.cn; Tel.: +86-15122431228

**Abstract:** Within the realm of aging, the nexus between diet and health has garnered considerable attention. However, only select studies have amalgamated insights into the correlation between plant and animal food consumption and frailty. Our aim was to appraise the connections between the overall plant-based diet index (PDI), healthful plant-based diet index (hPDI), and unhealthful plant-based diet index (uPDI) and frailty in the elderly, utilizing data from the Chinese Longitudinal Healthy Longevity Survey (CLHLS). This cohort study drew upon CLHLS data spanning from 2008 to 2018. The PDI, hPDI, and uPDI were gauged using a simplified food frequency questionnaire (FFQ). A frailty index, encompassing 35 variables across major health domains, was formulated. Cox proportional hazard models were employed to scrutinize the associations between the three plant-based dietary indices and frailty in older adults, including an exploration of gender disparities in these associations. A cohort of 2883 study participants was encompassed, with 1987 (68.9%) observed to be either frail or in the pre-frail stage. The Cox model with penalized spline exhibited linear associations of PDI, hPDI, and uPDI with the frailty index. Following covariate adjustments, it was discerned that older adults situated in the highest quartiles of PDI (HR = 0.86, 95% CI: 0.77–0.95) and hPDI (HR = 0.83, 95% CI: 0.74–0.93) experienced a 14% and 17% diminished risk of frailty compared to those in the lowest quartiles of PDI and hPDI, respectively. Conversely, when contrasted with those in the lowest quartile of uPDI, older adults adhering to the highest tertile of uPDI exhibited a 21% elevated risk of frailty (HR = 1.21, 95% CI: 1.08–1.36), with both associations achieving statistical significance ($p < 0.01$). Moreover, additional subgroup analyses revealed that the protective effects of PDI and hPDI against frailty and the deleterious effects of uPDI were more conspicuous in men compared to women. To forestall or decelerate the progression of frailty in the elderly, tailored dietary interventions are imperative, particularly targeting male seniors.

**Keywords:** Chinese longitudinal healthy longevity survey; older adults; plant-based diet indices; frailty

## 1. Introduction

Frailty, defined as a state of vulnerability marked by cumulative decline in physiological systems and a diminished resistance to stressors [1], constitutes an escalating global health concern, notably prevalent among the elderly. Previous data have indicated that the prevalence of frailty and pre-frailty in the elderly reached 24% and 49%, respectively [2]. Projections suggest that the prevalence of frailty will continue to escalate in the context of the ongoing global ageing trend [3]. Frailty typically manifests as a general decline in various systems and organs, characterized by compromised resistance and responsiveness to stressors [4]. This condition not only gives rise to heightened clinical symptoms and adverse outcomes, including mobility disability, falls, cardiovascular diseases, and cognitive decline, but also elevates the risk of hospitalization and mortality in the elderly [5–8]. The public health implications associated with frailty exert substantial pressure on healthcare systems worldwide, and the health of older individuals is increasingly under scrutiny. While frailty is dynamic and preventable, effective interventions become challenging when it progresses to an advanced stage before death [9]. Therefore, adopting proactive strategies to prevent frailty or identify and delay its onset in the early stages is pivotal for enhancing the quality of life and well-being of the elderly in their later years.

The etiology of frailty in the elderly is multifactorial, influenced by environmental, behavioural, and nutritional factors [10–13]. As a modifiable aspect of lifestyle, diet has garnered increasing attention for its role in promoting human health. It has been demonstrated that habitual tea consumption and a high intake of fruits and vegetables are efficacious in preventing frailty development [14–16], whereas habitual red meat intake is associated with an elevated risk of frailty [17]. However, assessing only individual foods and the relative limitations of nutrients can be mitigated by the plant-based diet index, which incorporates multiple food groups and comprehensively considers their health benefits [18–20]. By encompassing common food groups in the population and categorizing them into healthful plant-based foods, unhealthful plant-based foods, and animal-based foods based on their health benefits, the plant-based diet index offers greater flexibility and enhanced population promotion compared to the conventional "Mediterranean diet" and "Western diet" [21–23].

Only three studies have investigated the correlation between a plant-based dietary index and frailty. Two of these studies were conducted among female nurses [24] and community-dwelling older adults [25], resulting in limitations related to the generalization of findings to broader populations. Another study, exclusive to Chinese elderly participants, solely examined the association between the Plant-based diet index (PDI) and frailty [26]. Furthermore, all these studies employed the physical frailty phenotype as the basis for defining frailty, a categorization that does not directly correlate with a specific disease or significant disability. This phenotype overlooks cognitive and emotional aspects and proves inadequate for characterizing frailty linked to known comorbidities [27]. Divergent from the frailty phenotype, the deficit accumulation model incorporates numerous candidate factors, encompassing all major health domains (e.g., cognition, emotion, chronic disease, and cognitive function), and its multidimensional advantage facilitates the understanding of frailty across various pathogenic pathways. The frailty index employed in this study is grounded in the deficit accumulation model, offering a pragmatic measure of frailty. This study sought to investigate the associations between three plant-based dietary indices and frailty in individuals aged 65 and above in China, utilizing nationally representative cohort data. Additionally, the study aimed to explore gender-specific differences in these associations, providing a scientific reference for older individuals to adapt their dietary habits and forestall frailty.

## 2. Objects and Methods

### 2.1. Study Population

The Chinese Longitudinal Healthy Longevity Survey (CLHLS) commenced in 1998 with the aim of conducting a nationally representative survey of Chinese individuals aged 65 years and above. The primary objective of the CLHLS is to scrutinize the correlation between common health-related factors and health outcomes in the elderly, providing a valuable reference for promoting healthy ageing. The survey encompassed 23 provinces, municipalities, and autonomous regions, covering approximately 85% of China's population. Information gathered by the project included fundamental characteristics, socioeconomic features, behavioural habits, dietary status, and physical health status of the elderly. More detailed descriptions of the CLHLS project can be found elsewhere [28–30]. The CLHLS received ethical approval from the Biomedical Ethics Committee of Peking University, China (IRB00001052–13074).

This study utilised data extracted from the 2008–2018 CLHLS. A total of 16,954 participants aged 65 years and older were enrolled for this follow-up analysis. Exclusions were applied to those with missing dietary information, frailty details, and covariates at baseline and during follow up. Additionally, older adults presenting with frailty at baseline or in the pre-frailty stage were excluded, retaining only those without predisposition to frailty at baseline. Furthermore, individuals who experienced mortality or were lost to follow up without an outcome of interest during the follow-up period were also excluded. The analysis ultimately included a final cohort of 2883 participants. A comprehensive depiction of participant enrolment and exclusion processes is presented in Figure 1.

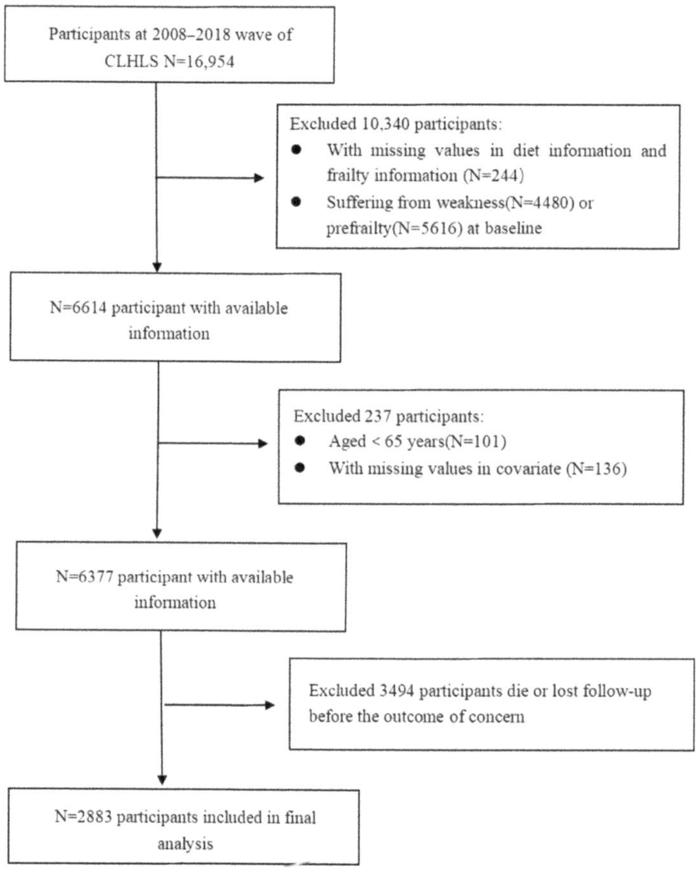


**Figure 1.** Flowchart of Participant Screening Flowchart.

## 2.2. Calculation of Plant-Based Diet Indices

The dietary information of the subjects was acquired through a simplified food frequency questionnaire (FFQ). A total of 16 common food groups in the daily Chinese diet were encompassed, categorised into three groups based on the nature of the food: healthful plant-based foods (whole grains, vegetable oils, fruits, vegetables, soy products, garlic, nuts, and tea), unhealthful plant-based foods (refined grains, preserved vegetables, and sugar), and animal-based foods (animal fats, meat, fish and other aquatic products, eggs, and dairy products). From the self-reported dietary frequency, we computed three plant-based diet indices: an overall plant-based diet index (PDI), a healthful plant-based diet index (hPDI), and an unhealthful plant-based diet index (uPDI). The consumption of each food was taken into account in the calculation of the three plant-based diet indices. Drawing from prior research [18,31–33], each food item was assigned a score between 1 and 5, with subtle variations in emphasis for the three plant-based diet indices. Among them, PDI focuses on the high consumption of plant food and the low consumption of animal food in the study population. hPDI highlights the high consumption of healthy plant foods and the low consumption of unhealthy plant foods; uPDI, in contrast to hPDI, focuses on high consumption of unhealthy plant foods and low consumption of healthy plant foods. For the PDI, scores were allocated based on the frequency of consumption, favouring healthful plant-based diets over unhealthful ones (5 points for the most frequent consumption, and 1 point for rarely or never consumption). In the case of hPDI, a higher frequency of consumption of healthful plant-based diets garnered a higher score (5 points for the most frequent consumption, and 1 point for rarely or never consumption), while unhealthful plant-based and animal-based diets were inversely scored (1 point for the most frequent consumption, and 5 points for rarely or never consumption). The uPDI assigned a higher score for a more frequent consumption of an unhealthful plant-based diet (5 points for the most frequent consumption, and 1 point for rarely or never consumption), with an inverse scoring for healthful plant-based diets and animal-based diets (1 point for the most frequent consumption, and 5 points for rarely or never consumption). For animal foods, 1 point is given for most frequent consumption and 5 points for rarely or never consumption. Detailed information regarding food grouping and assignment can be found in Table S1. In this study, PDI, hPDI, and uPDI were further stratified into three groups (T1, T2, and T3) based on the tertiles of the subjects' scores.

### 2.3. Assessment of Frailty

In adherence to the frailty index (FI) construction standard [34], this study employed 35 health-related variables to formulate the FI. These variables encompassed self-rated health, psychological status, activities of daily living, sensory status, physical limitations, and chronic diseases (Table S2). Health status was assigned a score ranging from 0 to 1, contingent on the participant's response to the respective variable. For instance, self-rated health status was categorised as healthy, moderately healthy, fair, unhealthy, and very unhealthy, with scores of 0, 0.25, 0.5, 0.75, and 1, respectively. Notably, 2 points were assigned if the subject had experienced two or more severe illnesses in the preceding two years. The FI was computed by dividing the aggregate health score by the total number of variables. In instances where study subjects had missing information on certain variables, deductions were applied in both the numerator and denominator. However, if the count of missing variables exceeded 30%, it was categorised as missing FI. In line with established literature [9,34,35], the FI was categorised into three scales: non-frail (FI $\leq$ 0.10), pre-frail (0.10 $<$ FI $\leq$ 0.21), and frail (FI $>$ 0.21). For our study, either prefrailty or frailty at the conclusion of the follow-up period was considered as the outcome of interest.

### 2.4. Assessment of Covariates

In consideration of factors identified in prior studies as potential influences on frailty, the covariates encompassed age (years), sex (male and female), type of residence (urban and rural), economic status (wealthy or not wealthy), living arrangement (solitary or not living alone), marital status (married and cohabiting or other), smoking status (current, former, or never), alcohol consumption (current, former, or never), exercise status (current, former, or never), and body-mass index (BMI; underweight, normal, overweight, or obese). The subjects' height and weight were measured using standard methods and employed to calculate BMI = weight (kg)/height (m)$^2$.

### 2.5. Statistical Analysis

Descriptive statistics were employed to calculate baseline characteristics. Cox proportional hazard models were constructed to scrutinize the association between the three plant-based diet indices and frailty in older adults, utilizing Schoenfeld residuals to assess the proportional risk hypothesis. Participant follow up was computed from baseline until the initial occurrence of the outcome of interest, death, loss to follow up, or the conclusion of the follow-up period, whichever transpired first. Restricted cubic spline curves, with 4 nodes chosen at the 5th, 35th, 65th, and 95th percentiles, were employed to explore potential nonlinear associations of baseline PDI, hPDI and uPDI with the frailty index. The models integrated multiple covariates to adjust for potential confounding factors affecting study outcomes. Model 1 incorporated adjustments for age and sex, while Model 2 additionally adjusted for type of residence, economic situation, residence status, marital status, smoking status, alcohol consumption, exercise status, and body mass index (BMI) based on Model 1. Subgroup analyses were conducted based on Model 2 to investigate whether the associations between plant-based diet indices and frailty exhibited variations by gender. The statistical analysis of this study was conducted using IBM SPSS version 20.0 and R version 4.2.1. GraphPad version 8.3 was utilised for visualising the results of subgroup analyses. A two-sided test with $p < 0.05$ was deemed statistically significant.

## 3. Results

### *3.1. Basic Information*

A total of 2883 subjects, with an average age of 81 years, were included in this study, comprising 1331 females (46.2%) and 1552 males (53.8%). At the conclusion of the follow-up period, 1987 participants (68.9%) were either frail or pre-frail. The results indicated differences in PDI, hPDI, and uPDI scores at baseline among older adults by age, genders, marital statuses, smoking statuses, and BMI. There were differences in PDI and uPDI scores among individuals residing in different locations. Nevertheless, in different economic situations, residence statuses, alcohol consumption, and exercise statuses of the elderly, uPDI significant differences in scores. ($p < 0.05$) (Table 1). In addition, we compared the basic characteristics of participants of different genders, and there were statistically significant differences between males and females in age, residential status, marital status, smoking status, alcohol consumption status, exercise status, and BMI among older adults ($p < 0.001$) (Table S3).

### *3.2. Association between Baseline Plant-Based Diet Index and Frailty Index*

The outcomes of the restricted cubic spline curves demonstrated statistically significant correlations ($p < 0.05$) of PDI, hPDI, and uPDI with the frailty index among older participants. Moreover, the correlations of PDI, hPDI, and uPDI with the frailty index exhibited linear tendencies (Figure 2). Upon stratifying the three plant-based diet indices into three groups based on participants' scores' tertiles, the highest tertile of PDI scores correlated with a 14% lower risk of frailty compared to participants in the lowest tertile of PDI in the fully adjusted model (HR = 0.86, 95% CI: 0.77–0.95, $p < 0.01$). Likewise, participants with the highest hPDI scores exhibited a 17% lower risk of frailty compared to those in the lowest hPDI tertile (HR = 0.83, 95% CI: 0.74–0.93, $p < 0.01$). Conversely, the highest quartile of uPDI scores correlated with a 21% increased risk of frailty compared to participants in the lowest quartile of uPDI scores (HR = 1.21, 95% CI: 1.08–1.36, $p < 0.01$) (Table 2).

**Table 1.** Baseline characteristics of participants.

| Characteristics | N(%) | PDI | | | p-Value | hPDI | | | p-Value | uPDI | | | p-Value |
|---|---|---|---|---|---|---|---|---|---|---|---|---|---|
| | | T1 | T2 | T3 | | T1 | T2 | T3 | | T1 | T2 | T3 | |
| Age (years) | 2883 (100) | 82 (11) | 81 (11) | 79 (10) | <0.001 | 83 (11) | 80 (11) | 80 (10) | <0.001 | 80 (11) | 81 (11) | 82 (11) | <0.001 |
| Sex | | | | | <0.05 | | | | <0.001 | | | | <0.001 |
| Male | 1552 (53.8) | 562 (36.2) | 469 (30.2) | 521 (33.6) | | 479 (30.9) | 567 (37.1) | 497 (32.0) | | 622 (40.1) | 525 (33.8) | 405 (26.1) | |
| Female | 1331 (46.2) | 506 (38.0) | 439 (33.0) | 386 (29.0) | | 486 (36.5) | 508 (38.2) | 337 (25.3) | | 403 (30.3) | 497 (37.3) | 431 (32.4) | |
| Resdic | | | | | <0.01 | | | | 0.09 | | | | <0.001 |
| Urban | 361 (12.5) | 122 (33.8) | 142 (39.3) | 97 (26.9) | | 103 (28.5) | 142 (39.3) | 116 (32.1) | | 235 (65.1) | 78 (21.6) | 48 (13.3) | |
| Town | 2522 (87.5) | 946 (37.5) | 766 (30.4) | 810 (32.1) | | 862 (34.2) | 942 (37.4) | 718 (28.5) | | 790 (31.3) | 944 (37.4) | 788 (31.2) | |
| Economic situation | | | | | 0.23 | | | | 0.31 | | | | <0.001 |
| Wealthy | 483 (16.8) | 189 (39.1) | 158 (32.7) | 136 (28.2) | | 162 (33.5) | 169 (35.0) | 152 (31.5) | | 257 (53.2) | 145 (30.0) | 81 (16.8) | |
| Not wealthy | 2400 (83.2) | 879 (36.6) | 750 (31.2) | 771 (32.1) | | 803 (33.5) | 915 (38.1) | 682 (28.4) | | 768 (32.0) | 877 (36.5) | 755 (31.5) | |
| Cohabitation status | | | | | 0.15 | | | | 0.62 | | | | <0.001 |
| Solitude | 544 (18.9) | 220 (40.4) | 168 (30.9) | 156 (28.7) | | 190 (34.9) | 205 (37.7) | 149 (27.4) | | 140 (25.7) | 189 (34.7) | 215 (39.5) | |
| Not living alone | 2339 (81.1) | 848 (36.3) | 740 (31.6) | 751 (32.1) | | 775 (33.1) | 879 (37.6) | 685 (29.3) | | 885 (37.8) | 833 (35.6) | 621 (26.5) | |
| Marital status | | | | | <0.001 | | | | <0.001 | | | | <0.001 |
| Married/cohabitating | 1306 (45.3) | 415 (31.8) | 400 (30.6) | 491 (37.6) | | 363 (27.8) | 508 (38.9) | 435 (33.3) | | 539 (41.3) | 451 (34.5) | 316 (24.2) | |
| Others | 1577 (54.7) | 653 (41.4) | 508 (32.2) | 416 (26.4) | | 602 (38.2) | 576 (36.5) | 399 (25.3) | | 486 (30.8) | 571 (36.2) | 520 (33.0) | |
| Smoking status | | | | | <0.01 | | | | <0.01 | | | | <0.01 |
| never | 1718 (59.6) | 675 (39.3) | 542 (31.5) | 501 (29.2) | | 613 (35.7) | 630 (36.7) | 475 (27.6) | | 576 (33.5) | 608 (35.4) | 534 (31.1) | |
| former | 429 (14.9) | 153 (35.7) | 134 (31.2) | 142 (33.1) | | 132 (30.8) | 180 (42.0) | 117 (27.3) | | 177 (71.3) | 151 (35.2) | 101 (23.5) | |
| now | 736 (25.5) | 240 (32.6) | 232 (31.5) | 264 (35.9) | | 220 (29.9) | 274 (37.2) | 242 (32.9) | | 272 (37.0) | 263 (35.7) | 201 (27.3) | |
| Alcohol consumption | | | | | 0.53 | | | | 0.12 | | | | <0.001 |
| never | 1813 (62.9) | 687 (37.9) | 573 (31.6) | 553 (30.5) | | 619 (34.1) | 694 (38.3) | 500 (27.6) | | 598 (33.0) | 646 (35.6) | 569 (31.4) | |
| former | 357 (12.4) | 124 (34.7) | 118 (33.1) | 115 (32.2) | | 126 (35.3) | 118 (33.1) | 113 (31.7) | | 134 (37.5) | 122 (34.2) | 101 (28.3) | |
| now | 713 (24.7) | 257 (36.0) | 217 (30.4) | 239 (33.5) | | 220 (30.9) | 272 (38.1) | 221 (31.0) | | 293 (41.1) | 254 (35.6) | 166 (23.3) | |
| Physical exercise | | | | | 0.18 | | | | 0.09 | | | | <0.001 |
| never | 1611 (55.9) | 622 (38.6) | 494 (30.7) | 495 (30.7) | | 569 (35.3) | 602 (37.4) | 440 (27.3) | | 470 (29.2) | 618 (38.4) | 523 (32.5) | |
| former | 255 (8.8) | 97 (38.0) | 73 (28.6) | 85 (33.3) | | 73 (28.6) | 99 (38.8) | 83 (32.5) | | 90 (35.3) | 92 (36.1) | 73 (28.6) | |
| now | 1017 (35.3) | 349 (34.3) | 341 (333.5) | 327 (32.2) | | 323 (31.8) | 383 (37.7) | 311 (30.6) | | 465 (45.7) | 312 (30.7) | 240 (23.6) | |
| BMI (kg/m$^2$) | | | | | <0.001 | | | | <0.001 | | | | |
| low | 696 (24.1) | 317 (45.5) | 214 (30.7) | 165 (23.7) | | 283 (40.7) | 238 (34.2) | 175 (25.1) | | 212 (30.5) | 258 (37.1) | 226 (32.5) | <0.001 |
| nomal | 1749 (60.7) | 619 (35.4) | 549 (31.4) | 581 (33.2) | | 575 (32.9) | 664 (38.0) | 510 (29.2) | | 610 (34.9) | 624 (35.7) | 515 (29.4) | |
| overweight | 355 (12.3) | 112 (31.5) | 116 (32.7) | 127 (35.8) | | 89 (25.1) | 146 (41.1) | 120 (33.8) | | 157 (44.2) | 120 (33.8) | 78 (22.0) | |
| Obesity | 83 (2.9) | 20 (24.1) | 29 (34.9) | 34 (41.0) | | 18 (21.7) | 36 (43.4) | 29 (34.9) | | 46 (55.4) | 20 (24.1) | 17 (20.5) | |

PDI—overall plant-based diet index; hPDI—healthful plant-based diet index; uPDI—unhealthful plant-based diet index; BMI—body-mass index.

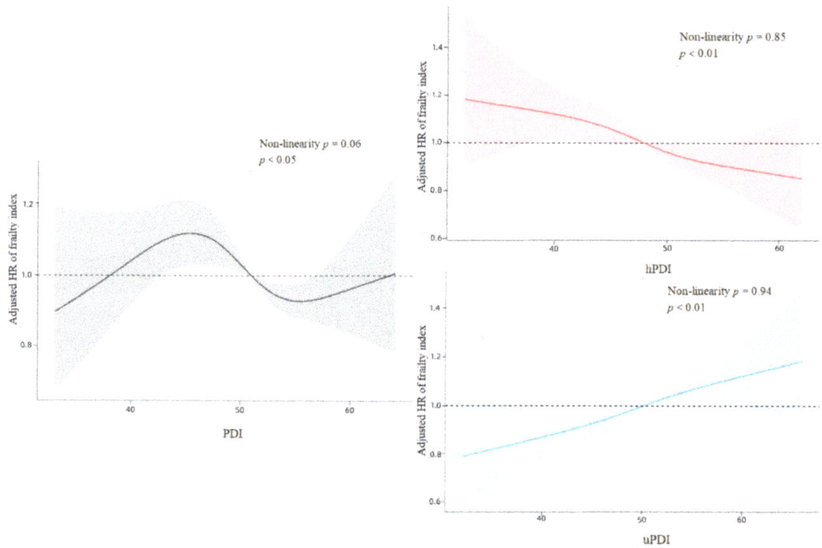


**Figure 2.** Cubic Spline Curves for PDI, hPDI, and uPDI Versus Association with Frailty.

**Table 2.** Association of Baseline PDI, hPDI and uPDI with Incidence of Frailty Risk.

| | T1 | T2 | | T3 | |
|---|---|---|---|---|---|
| | | HR (95% CI) | $p$-Value | HR (95% CI) | $p$-Value |
| PDI | | | | | |
| Model 1 | 1 | 0.93 (0.84–1.04) | 0.21 | 0.85 (0.77–0.95) | <0.01 |
| Model 2 | 1 | 0.93 (0.83–1.04) | 0.19 | 0.86 (0.77–0.95) | <0.01 |
| hPDI | | | | | |
| Model 1 | 1 | 0.87 (0.79–0.97) | <0.05 | 0.82 (0.73–0.92) | <0.001 |
| Model 2 | 1 | 0.87 (0.79–0.97) | <0.05 | 0.83 (0.74–0.93) | <0.001 |
| uPDI | | | | | |
| Model 1 | 1 | 1.07 (0.96–1.19) | 0.21 | 1.23 (1.10–1.38) | <0.001 |
| Model 2 | 1 | 1.05 (0.94–1.18) | 0.37 | 1.21 (1.08–1.36) | <0.01 |

Note: OR—odds ratio; CI—confidence interval. Grouping basis of three plant-based diet indices: PDI (T1 ≤ 48, 49 ≤ T2 ≤ 53, T3 ≥ 54); hPDI (T1 ≤ 45, 46 ≤ T2 ≤ 50, T3 ≥ 51); uPDI (T1 ≤ 47, 48 ≤ T2 ≤ 53, T3 ≥ 54). Model 1 adjusted for age and gender; Model 2 adjusted for type of residence, economic situation, residence status, marital status, smoking status, alcohol consumption, exercise status, and BMI based on Model 1.

### 3.3. *Gender Differences in the Association between Plant-Based Diet Index and Frailty Index*

To further investigate potential gender differences in the association between PDI, hPDI, uPDI and the onset of frailty in older adults, subgroup analyses were conducted based on gender subgroups. The results (Figure 3) demonstrated that the association between the highest tertile of PDI (HR = 0.77, 95% CI: 0.66–0.89, $p < 0.001$) and hPDI (HR = 0.79, 95% CI: 0.68–0.93, $p < 0.01$) scores and a reduced risk of frailty in males, compared to study participants in the lowest tertile of PDI and hPDI, was statistically significant. However, this association was not significant in females. Conversely, the association between the highest quartile of uPDI scores and an increased risk of developing frailty was statistically significant in both men (HR = 1.26, 95% CI: 1.07–1.48, $p < 0.01$) and women (HR = 1.19, 95% CI: 1.01–1.41) when compared to study participants in the lowest quartile of uPDI scores. Nevertheless, the detrimental effect was more pronounced in the male population than in the female population.

| | | HR(95% CI) | *p*–value |
|---|---|---|---|
| PDI | Male | 0.77(0.66–0.89) | < 0.001 |
| | | 0.90(0.77–1.05) | 0.18 |
| | | 1 | |
| | Famale | 0.97(0.82–1.14) | 0.69 |
| | | 0.97(0.83–1.14) | 0.74 |
| | | 1 | |
| hPDI | Male | 0.79(0.68–0.93) | < 0.01 |
| | | 0.89(0.77–1.04) | 0.15 |
| | | 1 | |
| | Famale | 0.88(0.74–1.04) | 0.14 |
| | | 0.84(0.72–0.98) | < 0.05 |
| | | 1 | |
| uPDI | Male | 1.26(1.07–1.48) | < 0.01 |
| | | 1.07(0.92–1.24) | 0.39 |
| | | 1 | |
| | Famale | 1.19(1.01–1.41) | < 0.05 |
| | | 1.08(0.91–1.27) | 0.39 |
| | | 1 | |

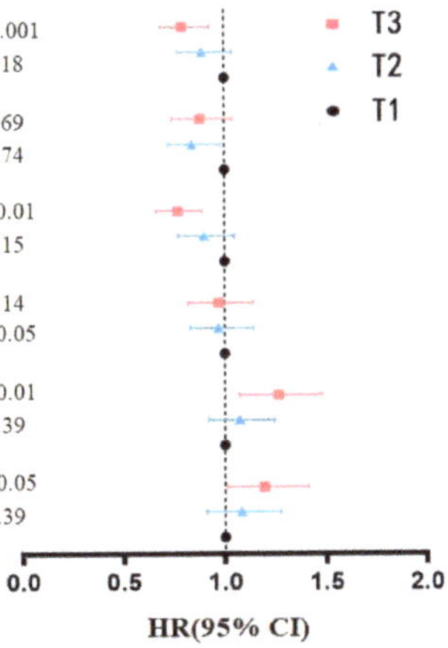


**Figure 3.** Association of baseline PDI, hPDI and uPDI with incidence of frailty risk.

## 4. Discussion

The outcomes of the investigation revealed a correlation between overall plant-based diet index, healthful plant-based diet index (hPDI), and unhealthful plant-based diet index (uPDI) with the propensity for developing frailty. The outcomes from the restricted cubic spline analysis indicated that the consumption of a diet rich in plant-based constituents and low in animal-derived components exhibited an inversely proportional relationship with the likelihood of frailty onset in the elderly. Conversely, an increased risk of frailty was evident with elevated consumption of animal-based foods and diminished intake of plant-based foods in the geriatric population. Notably, PDI and hPDI exhibited a negative correlation with the susceptibility to frailty in the elderly, while uPDI demonstrated a positive association with frailty risk in this demographic. Furthermore, heightened adherence to PDI and hPDI exerted a more pronounced protective effect against frailty in males compared to females. Conversely, greater adherence to uPDI was notably linked to an increased risk of frailty in males. These findings suggest that the rationalization of dietary habits may function as a mitigating factor against frailty in the elderly.

Our findings indicate that higher PDI and hPDI are associated with a decreased risk of frailty in older adults. The role of a balanced diet in safeguarding the physical and mental health of a population has been extensively discussed [36–39]. Nonetheless, few studies have specifically evaluated the connection between the quality of a plant-based diet and the risk of frailty. Unlike specific diseases, frailty is often accompanied by a decline in the functioning of multiple physiological systems. Despite its prevalence increasing with age, frailty is an extreme consequence of normal aging. A previous cohort study with female nurses demonstrated that a higher adherence to a healthful plant-based diet was linked to a lower risk of frailty, while an unhealthful plant-based diet was associated with an increased risk [24]. Additionally, a study focused on older Brazilian and Italian women observed that older Brazilian women with a higher plant protein intake exhibited better physical functioning [40]. Similarly, a study based on a Chinese cohort found a significant negative association between high PDI and the risk of frailty in older adults [26]. However, contrasting findings exist. Another Chinese cohort study suggested that a dietary pattern including eggs, fish, and meat might reduce the incidence of frailty in older adults [41]. A cross-sectional study from Brazil indicated that relatively low meat consumption was linked to a high prevalence of frailty in edentulous individuals [42]. Hence, exploring the association between specific food groups and frailty warrants further investigation.

Our study also revealed that a higher adherence to uPDI was associated with an increased risk of frailty in older adults. A U.S.-based cohort study noted that habitual consumption of unprocessed or processed red meat was associated with a higher risk of frailty [17]. Similarly, a study among community-dwelling older adults in Spain found that uPDI was associated with a higher risk of frailty, while the opposite was true for hPDI [25]. Some findings suggest that the consumption of ultra-processed foods, including dairy and meat products, strongly correlates with the risk of frailty in older adults. These findings emphasize the critical role of consuming unprocessed or minimally processed foods, such as vegetables and fruits, in preventing age-related frailty [43]. Interestingly, our results suggest that the protective effect of hPDI against frailty appears to be more pronounced in older adults compared to PDI. This implies that a reduced intake of refined grains, preserved vegetables, and sugar may be associated with a further reduction in the risk of frailty. However, the cause of this discrepancy, particularly whether it is related to the low intake of unhealthful plant-based foods, warrants further discussion. In future clinical practice, controlled clinical interventions around the role of specific food types in frailty related health disorders can be appropriately conducted.

Several pathophysiological mechanisms may help elucidate our findings. Firstly, inflammation and oxidative stress may contribute to frailty by inducing dysregulation in the organism. Plant-based foods, rich in flavonoids and antioxidants with anti-inflammatory and antioxidant properties, may mitigate the risk of frailty [44]. Secondly, imbalances in gut ecology can lead to immune responses and low-grade inflammation. Plant-based foods have been associated with greater gut microbiota diversity in older adults, potentially reducing inflammation and oxidative stress [45]. Additionally, insulin resistance (IR) increases as an individual ages [46]. Insulin resistance can cause frailty related health deficits by causing problems such as altered lipid metabolism, increased inflammatory status, impaired endothelial function, pro-thrombotic status, and atherosclerosis [47–49]. Moreover, deficiencies in macronutrients, such as protein, and micronutrients, such as vitamins, zinc and magnesium, negatively affect anabolic responses, levels of oxidative stress and levels of inflammation in the body in the elderly, leading to loss of individual muscle mass and tissue damage, thereby increasing the risk of frailty in the elderly [50–54]. Vegetable, fruit and other plant foods are often rich in macronutrients and micronutrients. Finally, a high consumption of animal diets, including meat, sugar, and dairy products, is often associated with unfavourable levels of low-grade inflammation and glucose metabolic biomarkers, elevated levels of oxidative stress, and metabolic disorders in the body, which can lead to chronic diseases such as type 2 diabetes and cardiovascular disease [55,56]. This is closely related to the pathogenesis of frailty.

Significantly, upon stratifying participants by gender, our findings demonstrated that although the association of the plant-based diet index with the development of frailty was statistically significant for both men and women, higher adherence to PDI and hPDI was more protective against developing frailty in men compared to women. Simultaneously, higher adherence to uPDI was also more significantly detrimental to frailty in men. This gender-specific difference may be attributed to biological, psychological, social, and behavioural distinctions between women and men. Women typically bear a higher burden of chronic disease and more severe disability [57], exhibit lower levels of physical activity [58], are more susceptible to mood disorders and stress [59], and often lack social support [60,61], among other factors contributing to a higher risk of frailty in females [62]. This could diminish the impact of the plant-based diet compared to the animal-based diet on frailty risk in females. Additionally, it has been noted that the relevance of diet in the pathogenesis of female frailty is lower than that of males if the body is already in an inflammatory state due to the influence of other factors [58]. Furthermore, due to differences between sex chromosomes, males exhibit higher innate and pro-inflammatory activity, rendering them more susceptible to inflammatory diets than females [63]. Therefore, based on the multidimensional nature of frailty, the progress of frailty can be interfered in multiple areas such as diet, physical activity, mental health and drug optimization. In addition, since the role of diet can play a more important role in the process of male frailty, it can be effectively prevented and delayed by forming a healthy diet pattern of hypoinsulinemia, low inflammation and reducing the risk of diabetes, providing the necessary macronutrients and micronutrients to ensure body function and maintain homeostasis, thereby effectively preventing and delaying frailty [58,64].

The present study boasts several strengths. Unlike other investigations relying on simple indicators, our study comprehensively assesses frailty status using Frailty Indices (FIs) that encompass all major health domains. Furthermore, the study utilizes nationally representative data with an extended follow-up period. However, certain limitations should be acknowledged. Firstly, participants' dietary information was obtained through interviews, introducing potential recall bias. Secondly, the questionnaire, focusing solely on the frequency of food intake and not addressing the amount consumed, precluded the calculation and adjustment of total energy intake. Thirdly, despite extensive adjustment for confounders, the potential for confounding bias persists. Fourth, the classification of indicators used to construct the plant-based diet indices and frailty index is worth exploring in a more rigorous way to highlight different risk groups. Fifth, this study had a long follow-up period, and this study used baseline dietary information from study subjects to calculate the plant-based diet indices for older adults, which may have overlooked possible changes in participants' dietary patterns. Lastly, the study's primary focus on the Chinese elderly population restricts the generalizability of findings to other ethnic and racial populations.

Older people have limited access to ideal dietary patterns, and the burden of health defects attributed to irrational diets can be very high, especially among older men. Therefore, in the future social policy practice, the diet pattern based on healthy plant food or other healthy diet guidance patterns can be promoted in communities or hospitals, and health education can be carried out among the elderly to change the concept of healthy diet for the elderly. Different interventions should be taken for frail elderly people with different dietary habits, and the role of primary health care should be played to enhance the sustainability of healthy poverty reduction from the source.

## 5. Conclusions

In conclusion, the current study establishes an association between high adherence to PDI and hPDI and a reduced risk of frailty in older adults. Conversely, high adherence to uPDI is associated with an increased risk of frailty in older adults. Furthermore, the protective effects of PDI and hPDI against frailty, as well as the detrimental effects of uPDI, exhibit more pronounced trends in men compared to women. The findings underscore the pivotal role of appropriate dietary behaviours in influencing frailty risk among older adults. This implies that judicious control of plant-based food intake and reduction of animal-based food intake can contribute to preventing the onset and managing the progression of frailty, particularly in the male elderly population.

**Supplementary Materials:** The following supporting information can be downloaded at: https://www.mdpi.com/article/10.3390/nu15245120/s1, Table S1. Scoring of plant-based diet indices. Table S2. Scoring of frailty index. Table S3: Baseline characteristics of participants by sex.

**Author Contributions:** Conceptualization, X.Z.; Methodology, H.L.; Software, R.Q. and Y.Y.; Validation, Y.Y. and B.S.; Formal analysis, R.Q.; Writing—original draft, R.Q.; Writing—review and editing, B.S., H.L. and X.Z.; Funding acquisition, X.Z. All authors have read and agreed to the published version of the manuscript.

**Funding:** Xinyu Zhang received a grant from the National Natural Science Foundation of National Natural Science Foundation of China Youth Project (71904142).

**Institutional Review Board Statement:** The CLHLS was approved by the Biomedical Ethics Committee of Peking University, China (IRB00001052–13074), and all participants signed informed consent.

**Informed Consent Statement:** Informed consent was obtained from all subjects involved in the study.

**Data Availability Statement:** Data are contained within the article and Supplementary Materials.

**Acknowledgments:** All the authors involved in this study thank all the staff of the CLHLS research team for their work.

**Conflicts of Interest:** The authors declare no conflict of interest.

## References

1. Clegg, A.; Young, J.; Iliffe, S.; Rikkert, M.O.; Rockwood, K. Frailty in elderly people. *Lancet* **2013**, *381*, 752–762. [CrossRef]
2. O'caoimh, R.; Sezgin, D.; O'donovan, M.R.; Molloy, D.W.; Clegg, A.; Rockwood, K.; Liew, A. Prevalence of frailty in 62 countries across the world: A systematic review and meta-analysis of population-level studies. *Age Ageing* **2021**, *50*, 96–104. [CrossRef]
3. Dent, E.; Martin, F.C.; Bergman, H.; Woo, J.; Romero-Ortuno, R.; Walston, J.D. Management of frailty: Opportunities, challenges, and future directions. *Lancet* **2019**, *394*, 1376–1386. [CrossRef]
4. Greco, E.A.; Pietschmann, P.; Migliaccio, S. Osteoporosis and Sarcopenia Increase Frailty Syndrome in the Elderly. *Front. Endocrinol.* **2019**, *10*, 255. [CrossRef]
5. Fried, L.P.; Ferrucci, L.; Darer, J.; Williamson, J.D.; Anderson, G. Untangling the concepts of disability, frailty, and comorbidity: Implications for improved targeting and care. *J. Gerontol. A Biol. Sci. Med. Sci.* **2004**, *59*, 255–263. [CrossRef]
6. Lu, Z.; Er, Y.; Zhan, Y.; Deng, X.; Jin, Y.; Ye, P.; Duan, L. Association of Frailty Status with Risk of Fall among Middle-Aged and Older Adults in China: A Nationally Representative Cohort Study. *J. Nutr. Health Aging* **2021**, *25*, 985–992. [CrossRef]
7. Kojima, G.; Iliffe, S.; Walters, K. Frailty index as a predictor of mortality: A systematic review and meta-analysis. *Age Ageing* **2018**, *47*, 193–200. [CrossRef]
8. Ward, D.D.; Ranson, J.M.; Wallace, L.M.; Llewellyn, D.J.; Rockwood, K. Frailty, lifestyle, genetics and dementia risk. *J. Neurol. Neurosurg. Psychiatry* **2022**, *93*, 343–350. [CrossRef]
9. Hoogendijk, E.O.; Afilalo, J.; Ensrud, K.E.; Kowal, P.; Onder, G.; Fried, L.P. Frailty: Implications for clinical practice and public health. *Lancet* **2019**, *394*, 1365–1375. [CrossRef]
10. Van Assen, M.; Helmink, J.H.M.; Gobbens, R.J.J. Associations between lifestyle factors and multidimensional frailty: A cross-sectional study among community-dwelling older people. *BMC Geriatr.* **2022**, *22*, 7. [CrossRef]
11. Balomenos, V.; Ntanasi, E.; Anastasiou, C.A.; Charisis, S.; Velonakis, G.; Karavasilis, E.; Tsapanou, A.; Yannakoulia, M.; Kosmidis, A.H.; Dardiotis, E.; et al. Association Between Sleep Disturbances and Frailty: Evidence From a Population-Based Study. *J. Am. Med. Dir. Assoc.* **2021**, *22*, 551–558.e1. [CrossRef] [PubMed]
12. Zhu, A.; Yan, L.; Wu, C.; Ji, J.S. Residential Greenness and Frailty Among Older Adults: A Longitudinal Cohort in China. *J. Am. Med. Dir. Assoc* **2020**, *21*, 759–765.e2. [CrossRef] [PubMed]
13. Larsen, R.T.; Turcotte, L.A.; Westendorp, R.; Langberg, H.; Hirdes, J.P. Frailty Index Status of Canadian Home Care Clients Improves With Exercise Therapy and Declines in the Presence of Polypharmacy. *J. Am. Med. Dir. Assoc.* **2020**, *21*, 766–771.e1. [CrossRef] [PubMed]
14. Gao, T.; Han, S.; Mo, G.; Sun, Q.; Zhang, M.; Liu, H. Long-term tea consumption reduces the risk of frailty in older Chinese people: Result from a 6-year longitudinal study. *Front. Nutr.* **2022**, *9*, 916791. [CrossRef] [PubMed]
15. Kojima, G.; Taniguchi, Y.; Urano, T. Fruit and Vegetable Consumption and Incident Frailty in Older Adults: A Systematic Review and Meta-Analysis. *J. Frailty Aging* **2022**, *11*, 45–50. [CrossRef] [PubMed]
16. Gao, J.; Jia, Y.; Dai, J.; Fu, H.; Wang, Y.; Yan, H.; Zhu, Y.; Nie, X. Association of Fruit and Vegetable Intake and Frailty among Chinese Elders: A Cross-Sectional Study in Three Cities. *J. Nutr. Health Aging* **2019**, *23*, 890–895. [CrossRef] [PubMed]
17. Struijk, E.A.; Fung, T.T.; Sotos-Prieto, M.; Rodriguez-Artalejo, F.; Willett, W.C.; Hu, F.B.; Lopez-Garcia, E. Red meat consumption and risk of frailty in older women. *J. Cachexia Sarcopenia Muscle* **2022**, *13*, 210–219. [CrossRef]
18. Liang, F.; Fu, J.; Turner-McGrievy, G.; Wang, Y.; Qiu, N.; Ding, K.; Zeng, J.; Moore, J.B.; Li, R. Association of Body Mass Index and Plant-Based Diet with Cognitive Impairment among Older Chinese Adults: A Prospective, Nationwide Cohort Study. *Nutrients* **2022**, *14*, 3132. [CrossRef]
19. Chen, B.; Zeng, J.; Qin, M.; Xu, W.; Zhang, Z.; Li, X.; Xu, S. The Association Between Plant-Based Diet Indices and Obesity and Metabolic Diseases in Chinese Adults: Longitudinal Analyses From the China Health and Nutrition Survey. *Front. Nutr.* **2022**, *9*, 881901. [CrossRef]
20. Chen, Z.; Drouin-Chartier, J.P.; Li, Y.; Baden, M.Y.; Manson, J.E.; Willett, W.C.; Voortman, T.; Hu, H.B.; Bhupathiraju, S.N. Changes in Plant-Based Diet Indices and Subsequent Risk of Type 2 Diabetes in Women and Men: Three U.S. Prospective Cohorts. *Diabetes Care* **2021**, *44*, 663–671. [CrossRef]
21. Dominguez, L.J.; Di Bella, G.; Veronese, N.; Barbagallo, M. Impact of Mediterranean Diet on Chronic Non-Communicable Diseases and Longevity. *Nutrients* **2021**, *13*, 2028. [CrossRef] [PubMed]
22. Rai, S.K.; Fung, T.T.; Lu, N.; Keller, S.F.; Curhan, G.C.; Choi, H.K. The Dietary Approaches to Stop Hypertension (DASH) diet, Western diet, and risk of gout in men: Prospective cohort study. *BMJ* **2017**, *357*, j1794. [CrossRef] [PubMed]
23. Kim, J.; Giovannucci, E. Healthful Plant-Based Diet and Incidence of Type 2 Diabetes in Asian Population. *Nutrients* **2022**, *14*, 3078. [CrossRef] [PubMed]
24. Sotos-Prieto, M.; Struijk, E.A.; Fung, T.T.; Rodríguez-Artalejo, F.; Willett, W.C.; Hu, F.B.; Lopez-Garcia, E. Association between the quality of plant-based diets and risk of frailty. *J. Cachexia Sarcopenia Muscle* **2022**, *13*, 2854–2862. [CrossRef]

25. Maroto-Rodriguez, J.; Delgado-Velandia, M.; Ortolá, R.; Carballo-Casla, A.; García-Esquinas, E.; Rodríguez-Artalejo, F.; Sotos-Prieto, M. Plant-based diets and risk of frailty in community-dwelling older adults: The Seniors-ENRICA-1 cohort. *Geroscience* **2023**, *45*, 221–232. [CrossRef]
26. Duan, Y.; Qi, Q.; Gao, T.; Du, J.; Zhang, M.; Liu, H. Plant-Based Diet and Risk of Frailty in Older Chinese Adults. *J. Nutr. Health Aging* **2023**, *27*, 371–377. [CrossRef] [PubMed]
27. Panza, F.; Lozupone, M.; Solfrizzi, V.; Sardone, R.; Dibello, V.; Di Lena, L.; D'Urso, F.; Stallone, R.; Petruzzi, M.; Giannelli, G.; et al. Different Cognitive Frailty Models and Health- and Cognitive-related Outcomes in Older Age: From Epidemiology to Prevention. *J. Alzheimer's Dis.* **2018**, *62*, 993–1012. [CrossRef]
28. Bai, W.; Zhang, J.; Smith, R.D.; Cheung, T.; Su, Z.; Ng, C.H.; Zhang, Q.; Xiang, Y.T. Inter-relationship between cognitive performance and depressive symptoms and their association with quality of life in older adults: A network analysis based on the 2017-2018 wave of Chinese Longitudinal Healthy Longevity Survey (CLHLS). *J. Affect. Disord.* **2023**, *320*, 621–627. [CrossRef]
29. Pei, Z.; Zhang, J.; Qin, W.; Hu, F.; Zhao, Y.; Zhang, X.; Cong, X.; Liu, C.; Xu, L. Association between Dietary Patterns and Depression in Chinese Older Adults: A Longitudinal Study Based on CLHLS. *Nutrients* **2022**, *14*, 5230. [CrossRef]
30. Fu, Y.C.; Pei, M.Y.; Liao, J.J.; Li, N.; Zhang, F.C.; Liu, H.L. Prevalence and correlates of elder neglect in the community-dwelling Chinese population: New evidence from the CLHLS study. *Front. Public Health* **2023**, *11*, 1123835. [CrossRef]
31. Chen, H.; Shen, J.; Xuan, J.; Zhu, A.; Ji, J.S.; Liu, X.; Cao, Y.; Zong, G.; Zeng, Y.; Wang, X.; et al. Plant-based dietary patterns in relation to mortality among older adults in China. *Nat. Aging* **2022**, *2*, 224–230. [CrossRef] [PubMed]
32. Zhu, A.; Chen, H.; Shen, J.; Wang, X.; Li, Z.; Zhao, A.; Shi, X.; Yan, L.; Zeng, Y.; Yuan, C.; et al. Interaction between plant-based dietary pattern and air pollution on cognitive function: A prospective cohort analysis of Chinese older adults. *Lancet Reg. Health West. Pac.* **2022**, *20*, 100372. [CrossRef] [PubMed]
33. Qi, R.; Sheng, B.; Zhou, L.; Chen, Y.; Sun, L.; Zhang, X. Association of Plant-Based Diet Indices and Abdominal Obesity with Mental Disorders among Older Chinese Adults. *Nutrients* **2023**, *15*, 2721. [CrossRef] [PubMed]
34. Chen, Q.; Tang, B.; Zhai, Y.; Chen, Y.; Jin, Z.; Han, H.; Gao, Y.; Wu, C.; Chen, T.; He, J. Dynamic statistical model for predicting the risk of death among older Chinese people, using longitudinal repeated measures of the frailty index: A prospective cohort study. *Age Ageing* **2020**, *49*, 966–973. [CrossRef] [PubMed]
35. Cao, L.; Zhou, Y.; Liu, H.; Shi, M.; Wei, Y.; Xia, Y. Bidirectional Longitudinal Study of Frailty and Depressive Symptoms Among Older Chinese Adults. *Front. Aging Neurosci.* **2022**, *14*, 791971. [CrossRef] [PubMed]
36. Haghighatdoost, F.; Mahdavi, A.; Mohammadifard, N.; Hassannejad, R.; Najafi, F.; Farshidi, H.; Lotfizadeh, M.; Kazemi, T.; Karimi, S.; Roohafza, H.; et al. The relationship between a plant-based diet and mental health: Evidence from a cross-sectional multicentric community trial (LIPOKAP study). *PLoS ONE* **2023**, *18*, e0284446. [CrossRef] [PubMed]
37. Wu, H.; Gu, Y.; Meng, G.; Wu, H.; Zhang, S.; Wang, X.; Zhang, J.; Huang, T.; Niu, K. Quality of plant-based diet and the risk of dementia and depression among middle-aged and older population. *Age Ageing* **2023**, *52*, afad070. [CrossRef]
38. Satija, A.; Bhupathiraju, S.N.; Rimm, E.B.; Spiegelman, D.; Chiuve, S.E.; Borgi, L.; Willett, W.C.; Manson, J.E.; Sun, Q.; Hu, F.B. Plant-Based Dietary Patterns and Incidence of Type 2 Diabetes in US Men and Women: Results from Three Prospective Cohort Studies. *PLoS Med.* **2016**, *13*, e1002039. [CrossRef]
39. Trautwein, E.A.; Mckay, S. The Role of Specific Components of a Plant-Based Diet in Management of Dyslipidemia and the Impact on Cardiovascular Risk. *Nutrients* **2020**, *12*, 2671. [CrossRef]
40. Coelho-Junior, H.J.; Calvani, R.; Picca, A.; Gonçalves, I.O.; Landi, F.; Bernabei, R.; Cesari, M.; Uchida, M.C.; Marzetti, E. Association between Dietary Habits and Physical Function in Brazilian and Italian Older Women. *Nutrients* **2020**, *12*, 1635. [CrossRef]
41. Zhang, J.; Wang, Q.; Hao, W.; Zhu, D. Long-Term Food Variety and Dietary Patterns Are Associated with Frailty among Chinese Older Adults: A Cohort Study Based on CLHLS from 2014 to 2018. *Nutrients* **2022**, *14*, 4279. [CrossRef] [PubMed]
42. Ygnatios, N.T.M.; Lima-Costa, M.F.; Torres, J.L. Food consumption is associated with frailty in edentulous older adults: Evidence from the ELSI-Brazil study. *Cien. Saude Colet.* **2023**, *28*, 1891–1902. [CrossRef] [PubMed]
43. Sandoval-Insausti, H.; Blanco-Rojo, R.; Graciani, A.; López-García, E.; Moreno-Franco, B.; Laclaustra, M.; Donat-Vargas, C.; Ordovás, J.M.; Rodríguez-Artalejo, F.; Guallar-Castillón, P. Ultra-processed Food Consumption and Incident Frailty: A Prospective Cohort Study of Older Adults. *J. Gerontol. A Biol. Sci. Med. Sci.* **2020**, *75*, 1126–1133. [CrossRef] [PubMed]
44. Soysal, P.; Stubbs, B.; Lucato, P.; Luchini, C.; Solmi, M.; Peluso, R.; Sergi, G.; Isik, A.T.; Manzato, E.; Maggi, S.; et al. Inflammation and frailty in the elderly: A systematic review and meta-analysis. *Ageing Res. Rev.* **2016**, *31*, 1–8. [CrossRef] [PubMed]
45. Kim, S.; Jazwinski, S.M. The Gut Microbiota and Healthy Aging: A Mini-Review. *Gerontology* **2018**, *64*, 513–520. [CrossRef] [PubMed]
46. Abbatecola, A.M.; Paolisso, G. Is there a relationship between insulin resistance and frailty syndrome? *Curr. Pharm. Des.* **2008**, *14*, 405–410. [PubMed]
47. Cleasby, M.E.; Jamieson, P.M.; Atherton, P.J. Insulin resistance and sarcopenia: Mechanistic links between common co-morbidities. *J. Endocrinol.* **2016**, *229*, R67–R81. [CrossRef]
48. Soysal, P.; Arik, F.; Smith, L.; Jackson, S.E.; Isik, A.T. Inflammation, Frailty and Cardiovascular Disease. *Adv. Exp. Med. Biol.* **2020**, *1216*, 55–64.
49. Krentz, A.J.; Viljoen, A.; Sinclair, A. Insulin resistance: A risk marker for disease and disability in the older person. *Diabet. Med.* **2013**, *30*, 535–548. [CrossRef]

50. Bao, B.; Prasad, A.S.; Beck, F.W.; Fitzgerald, J.T.; Snell, D.; Bao, G.W.; Singh, T.; Cardozo, L.J. Zinc decreases C-reactive protein, lipid peroxidation, and inflammatory cytokines in elderly subjects: A potential implication of zinc as an atheroprotective agent. *Am. J. Clin. Nutr.* **2010**, *91*, 1634–1641. [CrossRef]
51. Michelon, E.; Blaum, C.; Semba, R.D.; Xue, Q.-L.; Ricks, M.O.; Fried, L.P. Vitamin and carotenoid status in older women: Associations with the frailty syndrome. *J. Gerontol. A Biol. Sci. Med. Sci.* **2006**, *61*, 600–607. [CrossRef] [PubMed]
52. Park, S.-J.; Park, J.; Won, C.W.; Lee, H.-J. The Inverse Association of Sarcopenia and Protein-Source Food and Vegetable Intakes in the Korean Elderly: The Korean Frailty and Aging Cohort Study. *Nutrients* **2022**, *14*, 1375. [CrossRef] [PubMed]
53. Tomata, Y.; Wang, Y.; Hägg, S.; Jylhävä, J. Protein Nutritional Status and Frailty: A Mendelian Randomization Study. *J. Nutr.* **2022**, *152*, 269–275. [CrossRef] [PubMed]
54. Isanejad, M.; Sirola, J.; Rikkonen, T.; Mursu, J.; Kröger, H.; Qazi, S.L.; Tuppurainen, M.; Erkkilä, A.T. Higher protein intake is associated with a lower likelihood of frailty among older women, Kuopio OSTPRE-Fracture Prevention Study. *Eur. J. Nutr.* **2020**, *59*, 1181–1189. [CrossRef] [PubMed]
55. Ley, S.H.; Sun, Q.; Willett, W.C.; Eliassen, A.H.; Wu, K.; Pan, A.; Grodstein, F.; Hu, F.B. Associations between red meat intake and biomarkers of inflammation and glucose metabolism in women. *Am. J. Clin. Nutr.* **2014**, *99*, 352–360. [CrossRef] [PubMed]
56. Würtz, A.M.L.; Jakobsen, M.U.; Bertoia, M.L.; Hou, T.; Schmidt, E.B.; Willett, W.C.; Overvad, K.; Sun, Q.; E Manson, J.; Hu, F.B.; et al. Replacing the consumption of red meat with other major dietary protein sources and risk of type 2 diabetes mellitus: A prospective cohort study. *Am. J. Clin. Nutr.* **2021**, *113*, 612–621. [CrossRef] [PubMed]
57. Gordon, E.H.; Hubbard, R.E. Do sex differences in chronic disease underpin the sex-frailty paradox? *Mech. Ageing Dev.* **2019**, *179*, 44–50. [CrossRef]
58. Reid, N.; Young, A.; Hanjani, L.S.; Hubbard, R.E.; Gordon, E.H. Sex-specific interventions to prevent and manage frailty. *Maturitas* **2022**, *164*, 23–30. [CrossRef]
59. Holsen, L.M.; Huang, G.; Cherkerzian, S.; Aroner, S.; Loucks, E.B.; Buka, S.; Handa, R.J.; Goldstein, J.M. Sex Differences in Hemoglobin A1c Levels Related to the Comorbidity of Obesity and Depression. *J. Women's Health* **2021**, *30*, 1303–1312. [CrossRef]
60. Bedaso, A.; Adams, J.; Peng, W.; Sibbritt, D. The relationship between social support and mental health problems during pregnancy: A systematic review and meta-analysis. *Reprod. Health* **2021**, *18*, 162. [CrossRef]
61. Cho, H.; Lee, K.; Choi, E.; Cho, H.N.; Park, B.; Suh, M.; Rhee, Y.; Choi, K.S. Association between social support and postpartum depression. *Sci. Rep.* **2022**, *12*, 3128. [CrossRef] [PubMed]
62. Geronikola, N.; Zalonis, I.; Ntanasi, E.; Charisis, S.; Kosmidis, M.H.; Anastasiou, C.A.; Dardiotis, E.; Hadjigeorgiou, G.; Megalou, M.; Velonakis, G.; et al. Sex Differences in Frailty Incidence in Greek Community-Dwelling Older People: The HELIAD Study. *J. Frailty Aging* **2022**, *11*, 250–255. [CrossRef] [PubMed]
63. Park, C.; Ko, F.C. The Science of Frailty: Sex Differences. *Clin. Geriatr. Med.* **2021**, *37*, 625–638. [CrossRef] [PubMed]
64. Wang, P.; Song, M.; Eliassen, A.H.; Wang, M.; Fung, T.T.; Clinton, S.K.; Rimm, E.B.; Hu, F.B.; Willett, W.C.; Tabung, F.K.; et al. Optimal dietary patterns for prevention of chronic disease. *Nat. Med.* **2023**, *29*, 719–728. [CrossRef]

nutrients

Article

# A Comprehensive Examination of Vegan Lifestyle in Italy

Annachiara Stenico [1], Diana Zarantonello [2], Fabio Vittadello [3] and Michael Kob [1,4,*]

1 College of Health Care-Professions "Claudiana", 39100 Bolzano, Italy; annachiarastenico@gmail.com
2 Department of Nephrology, S. Chiara Hospital, APSS, 38122 Trento, Italy; diana.zarantonello@apss.tn.it
3 Explora—Research and Statistical Analysis, 350100 Padova, Italy; fabio.vittadello@centroexplora.it
4 Division of Clinical Nutrition, Hospital of Bolzano (SABES-ASDAA), Teaching Hospital of Paracelsus Medical University (PMU), 39100 Bolzano, Italy
* Correspondence: michael.kob@sabes.it; Tel.: +39-0471-438545

**Abstract:** The popularity of veganism and plant-based diets is rapidly increasing worldwide, including in Italy, where more individuals and families are adopting this lifestyle. However, medical and health professionals often lack the necessary knowledge and are skeptical about this diet despite the scientific evidence. It is important for them to provide support and expertise to those following this diet. The survey evaluated various aspects of the lifestyle of Italian vegans living in Italy and abroad, including food frequency, vitamin and mineral supplementation, relationship with medical and health professionals, and perceived difficulties in daily life. The emphasis was on potentially critical aspects for those following this dietary choice. A cross-sectional survey was conducted in Italy between March and April 2022. A questionnaire was distributed through social media platforms such as Instagram, Facebook, and Telegram, and 2180 Italian adults who follow a vegan diet completed it. The survey found that most of the vegan population surveyed were female, showed a greater sensitivity to ethical issues, were aware of the need for vitamin B12 supplementation, and followed healthy-eating guidelines. It is evident that despite the increasing popularity of plant-based diets, many medical and health professionals remain cautious and hesitant to recommend them.

**Keywords:** plant-based diet; vegan diet; healthy habits and eating trends; dietary patterns

## 1. Introduction

A vegan diet is characterized by the complete exclusion of animal products, including meat, fish, dairy, eggs, and honey. In recent years, there has been a significant increase in the popularity of plant-based diets among Western populations. In the UK, 8% of people claimed to follow a plant-based diet in 2021 [1], while in the US and Australia, the figures were 1.5% in 2023 [2] and 2% in 2020 [3], respectively.

The Eurispes survey reports that the percentage of Italians following a vegan diet will increase from 1.4% in 2022 to 2.4% in 2023 [4]. Respondents cited a broader philosophy of life as their main motivation for adopting a vegan or vegetarian diet, followed by health (mental and physical wellbeing), ethics, and respect for animals. In fourth, fifth, and sixth place, respectively, additional reasons for adopting a vegetarian diet were environmental protection, experimentation with new ways of eating, and the belief in sacrificing quantity for quality by eating less but better [5]. This increase may be due to a growing concern for environmental sustainability, increased popularization of animal welfare issues, and heightened sensitivity towards personal health, as demonstrated in other populations [6].

The scientific literature confirms that a plant-based diet, when supplemented with adequate vitamin B12 and attention to critical nutrients such as protein, omega-3, iron, calcium, zinc, iodine, and vitamin D, promotes health and is associated with a lower risk of all-cause mortality. Additionally, it has been shown to be effective in treating, halting, and reversing some major diseases, including type 2 diabetes, cardiovascular disease, and cancer incidence [7–9]. The Academy of Nutrition and Dietetics (AND) states that plant-based diets, whether vegetarian or vegan, can be healthy, nutritionally adequate, and appropriate for individuals at any stage of life, provided they are properly planned and supplemented [10].

From an environmental perspective, a plant-based diet is considered the most effective dietary model to date. This is because emissions of pollutants, as well as land and water use, are closely related to diet [11]. A vegan diet has a favorable impact on many ecological indicators and is compatible with the 'diet for planetary health' recommended by the EAT-Lancet Commission. This diet has the potential to address the environmental crisis, feed the entire world population, and prevent chronic diseases [12].

Despite the evidence and confirmation, some medical professionals still hold the opinion that a vegan diet is nutritionally deficient and may not be suitable for certain patient groups, particularly pregnant and lactating women and children. A study conducted in Italy found that around half of vegan parents reported that their Primary Care Pediatrician (PCP) was unable to provide sufficient guidance on vegan weaning, while almost 80% stated that their PCP was against vegan weaning [13]. Similarly, 36.2% of parents who raise their children on a plant-based diet did not inform their primary care physician (PCP). In 70.8% of cases, the PCP was skeptical or opposed to the child's fully plant-based diet. The most common professionals involved were dietitians, followed by medical dietitians [14].

Misinformation in this area can have serious consequences. Those who choose to follow a vegan diet by relying on their doctor may not receive the necessary knowledge about supplementation, monitoring, and proper planning of their diet. This can compromise their health and discredit the validity of a plant-based diet. To avoid this risk, VegPlate was created in 2017. VegPlate is a vegetarian food guide based on the Mediterranean diet that follows the established Italian Dietary Reference Intakes (DRIs). Its main objective is to help health professionals and individuals following a vegetarian or vegan diet to conveniently organize well-balanced meal plans [15].

Currently, there is a lack of knowledge regarding the health and supplementation behavior of Italian vegans. The study aimed to investigate the habits and behaviors of the Italian vegan population, including their vitamin and mineral supplementation practices, with a special focus on vitamin B12. Additionally, the study examined the frequency of consumption of processed foods and adherence to the Mediterranean food pyramid. The reasons behind the participants' adoption of a vegan diet were also explored, as well as the main difficulties they faced in social settings and interactions with health professionals. The study aimed to assess possible critical issues. For research purposes, it was important to investigate the relationship between the participants' social and dietary choices and their health status.

The study presents a qualitative analysis of lifestyle and perceived difficulties, as well as a quantitative analysis of supplements and staple foods based on the VegPlate recommendations [16].

## 2. Materials and Methods

### 2.1. Study Design and Participants

The study was conducted from 9 March to 6 April 2022 through a questionnaire. The questionnaire consisted of 46 items divided into 11 sections and was created using Google Forms. The total duration of the questionnaire varied between 8 and 12 min depending on individual responses. Each section explores different topics, including biographical and socio-economic information, motivation for choosing a vegan diet, eating habits and behavior, and questions on vitamin and mineral supplementation. The survey also includes questions on perceived difficulties in dealing with health professionals, as well as other general questions such as anthropometric data, personal choices, and types of vegan diets. The language used is clear, concise, and objective, with a formal register and precise word choice. The text adheres to conventional structure and formatting features, including consistent citation and footnote style. The grammar, spelling, and punctuation are correct. No changes in content have been made. The study employed structured and semi-structured questions, with some allowing for an "other" option to capture unexpected responses. For instance, participants were asked about unintentional exceptions, challenges in finding vegan options, and their interactions with nutrition professionals.

This study is a cross-sectional web-based survey that collects data on the dietary habits and lifestyle choices of the vegan population in Italy and abroad. The subjects were recruited primarily through social media channels, including Instagram, WhatsApp, Telegram, and Facebook. The sample was selected based on specific criteria:

- Italian nationality
- Adopting a vegan diet for more than 365 days
- Over 18 years of age

Prior to its use in this study, we pre-tested our survey for face validity with a sample of ten individuals who provided feedback on its comprehensibility, functionality, content, and completion time. Participation in the survey was voluntary and anonymous, and it could be terminated at any time without justification.

### 2.2. Data Assessment

The questionnaire was online for 1 month, from 9 March 2022 to 6 April 2022.

### 2.3. Data Analysis and Statistics

For each variable considered in the study, the absolute and percentage distributions of the subjects were calculated and supplemented where appropriate by indicators of centrality and variability. For each variable considered in the study, the absolute and percentage distributions of the subjects were calculated. For quantitative variables, the main indicators of centrality and variability were calculated.

Non-parametric tests were used to analyze comparisons between clinical variables in different groups. The normality of the distributions of the variables considered was checked prior to analysis. Numerical variables were analyzed using the Mann–Whitney U test and Kruskal–Wallis test, while categorical variables were analyzed using Pearson's X2 test and Fisher's exact test where appropriate. The correlation between ordinal variables was assessed using Spearman's Rho correlation coefficient. Statistical significance was considered for $p$-values less than 0.05 (two-tailed test). IBM SPSS statistical software (version 20.0) was used for all analyses.

## 3. Results

### 3.1. Study Participants

The study included 2180 subjects who reported being vegan for more than one year (365 days). Of these, 69.1% ($n$ = 1783) reported being vegan for between 1 and 5 years, 10.9% ($n$ = 282) for between 5 and 10 years, and 4.5% ($n$ = 115) for 10 years or more.

### 3.2. Sample Characteristics

The baseline characteristics of participants are shown in Table 1.

**Table 1.** Baseline characteristics.

| Total Subjects, % | 100.0% (2180) |
|---|---|
| Females, % | 90.2% |
| Males, % | 8.4% |
| Others [1], % | 1.4% |
| Age, years (median ± SD [2], range) | 28 ± 8.9 |
| Height, cm (median ± SD [2], range) | 165.0 ± 7.6 (145–203) |
| Weight, kg (median ± SD [2], range) | 58.0 ± 10.7 (37–135) |
| Total weight status | $n$ = 2180 |
| BMI [3], $kg/m^2$ (mean ± SD [2], range) | 21.8 ± 3.4 (14.7–45.1) |

**Table 1.** *Cont.*

| Total Subjects, % | 100.0% (2180) |
| --- | --- |
| Underweight, % (BMI [3] < 18.5) | 10.0% |
| Normal weight, % (BMI [3] 18.5–24.9) | 77.0% |
| Overweight, % (BMI [3] 25–29.9) | 10.2% |
| Obesity, % (BMI [3] > 30) | 2.9% |
| Geographical area | |
| North-West Italy, % | 38.8% |
| North-East Italy, % | 27.3% |
| Central Italy, % | 16.0% |
| South Italy, % | 7.9% |
| Italian islands, % | 4.3% |
| Abroad, % | 5.8% |
| Marital status | |
| Engaged, % | 31.6% |
| Single, % | 28.0% |
| Cohabit, % | 21.7% |
| Married, % | 15.0% |
| Divorced, % | 1.5% |
| Widowed, % | 0.1% |
| Polyamorous relationship, % | 0.1% |
| Profession | |
| Full-time employee, % | 32.9% |
| Student, % | 31.9% |
| Freelance worker, % | 13.5% |
| Part-time employee, % | 10.0% |
| Unemployed, % | 4.4% |
| Housewife, % | 2.2% |
| Student worker, % | 1.9% |
| Retired, % | 0.4% |
| Education | |
| High school diploma, % | 42.3% |
| Bachelor, % | 24.2% |
| MA/MSc, % | 27.8% |
| Secondary school diploma, % | 3.8% |
| PhD, % | 1.7% |

[1] Other: not declared, non-binary, agender, transgender. [2] SD (Standard Deviation). [3] BMI (Body Mass Index) based on self-reported indications of body weight and size and calculated kg/m$^2$.

#### 3.2.1. Weight Status

The BMI of females and males differed by only one point, with females having a BMI of 21.7 kg/m$^2$ and males having a BMI of 22.7 kg/m$^2$. The percentage of underweight subjects (BMI < 18.5) was 10.2% for females and 7.1% for males, while the percentage of overweight subjects (BMI > 24.9) was 9.7% for females and 15.2% for males. Most participants in both groups had a normal weight (BMI 18.5–24.9), with 77.4% of females and 75% of males falling into this category. The rate of obesity (BMI > 30) was very low in both populations, with only 2.7% of females and 2.8% of males being classified as obese.

#### 3.2.2. Type of Vegan Diet

Of the participants, 95.6% ($n$ = 2084) reported following a standard vegan diet, while 1.6% ($n$ = 34) followed a high-protein vegan diet. A Whole-Food Plant-Based (WFPB) diet was followed by 0.4% ($n$ = 8), a gluten-free vegan diet by 0.6% ($n$ = 13), a low carbohydrate diet by 0.8% ($n$ = 17), a raw vegan diet by 0.4% ($n$ = 9), and a macrobiotic vegan diet by 0.7% ($n$ = 15). None of the respondents followed strict fruitarian or liquid/juice-based vegan diets.

#### 3.2.3. Medical Conditions

Out of the 1805 subjects, 83.3% reported not having any chronic pathology. The remaining 16.7% reported suffering from various pathologies, including endometriosis (1.0%), asthma (3.7%), dyslipidemia (1.2%), chronic inflammatory bowel disease (1.5%), thyroiditis (3.3%), and other unidentified pathologies (5.1%).

### 3.3. Vegan Choice: MAIN Motivation

The main reasons for choosing a vegan diet are listed in Table 2.

**Table 2.** What is the MAIN reason that made you turn vegan?

| | Percentage (%) |
|---|---|
| **Total** | **100.0% (2180)** |
| Environmental sustainability | 21.2% |
| Health and general wellbeing | 14.5% |
| Health (suffering from a chronic illness) | 1.3% |
| Ethics/animal rights | 61.2% |
| Food preferences | 0.8% |
| Foods scandals | 0.01% |
| Social influence (from friends, relatives, partner, etc.) | 0.4% |
| Social justice/world's hunger | 0.5% |
| Curiosity/current trend | 0.01% |
| Religious and spiritual beliefs | 0.0% |

A significant association ($p = 0.005$) was found between the level of higher education attained and the importance placed on environmental sustainability and health and wellbeing when adopting a vegan diet (Figure 1). However, no significant association was found for the other aspects analyzed, including ethics and animal rights, religious and spiritual beliefs, curiosity, and current trends.

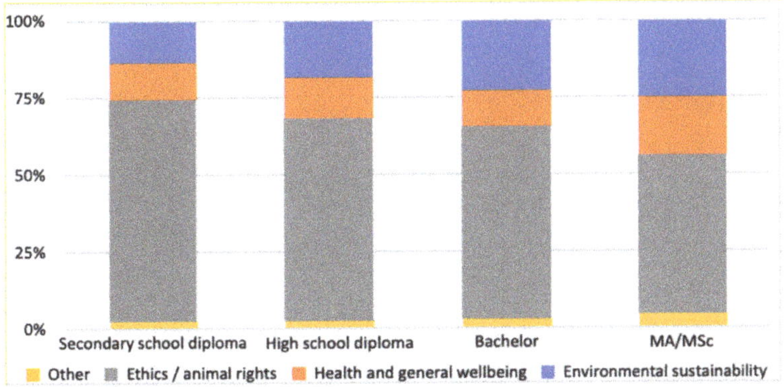


**Figure 1.** Correlation between higher educational qualification and the MAIN reason for the adoption of the vegan diet. Nominal variables were compared using the chi-square test.

A negative significant association ($p = 0.005$) was found between the time of adopting a vegan diet and the importance of switching to such a diet for environmental sustainability reasons (Figure 2). Additionally, a positive significant association ($p = 0.005$) was found between the time of adopting a vegan diet and ethical motivations.

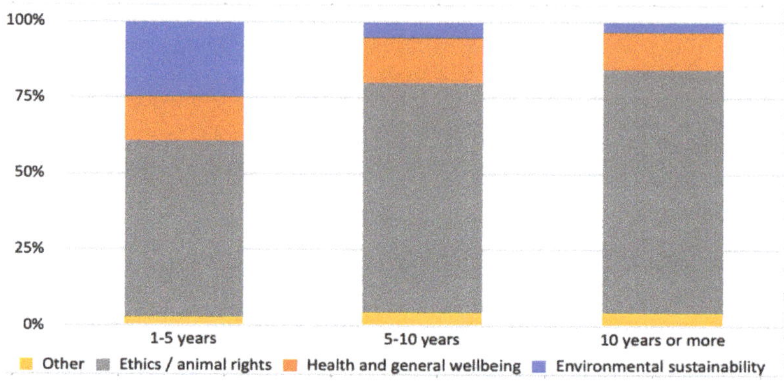


**Figure 2.** Correlation between the time of adoption of the vegan diet and MAIN reason for adopting the vegan diet. Nominal variables were compared using a chi-square test.

### *3.4. Vegan Diet in the Family*

Of the subjects surveyed, 57.4% ($n$ = 1365) claimed to be the only member of their family following a vegan diet. A total of 21.7% ($n$ = 517) reported that their partner also follows this diet. A total of 8.7% ($n$ = 207) declared that other family members are also vegan, 5.9% ($n$ = 140) specified that either their father or mother is vegan, and 5.4% ($n$ = 128) said at least one of their children is vegan. The remaining 0.9% ($n$ = 22) reported that both parents are vegan.

#### 3.4.1. Children

Out of the 2180 participants, 88.6% ($n$ = 1937) reported not having any children between the ages of 0 and 18 years. A total of 6.9% ($n$ = 151) reported having one child, and 4.4% ($n$ = 97) reported having more than one child.

#### 3.4.2. Weaning

Of the 356 children surveyed, 85 (23.9%) were raised with a vegan weaning, 49 (12.8%) with a vegetarian weaning, and 222 (63.3%) with an omnivorous weaning. A total of 37 (14.9%) of the subjects reported that their pediatrician supported vegan weaning, while an equal percentage, 37 (14.9%), reported that their pediatrician was against it. Of the respondents, 14.1% ($n$ = 35) disagreed with the pediatrician but still weaned their child vegan. Meanwhile, 21.1% ($n$ = 60) did not confront their pediatrician, and 32.1% ($n$ = 80) had no intention of vegan weaning. Currently, 33.1% ($n$ = 118) of the children follow an omnivorous diet, 26.7% ($n$ = 95) follow a vegan diet, 14% ($n$ = 50) follow a vegetarian diet, and 26.1% ($n$ = 93) eat vegan at home but consume non-vegan food when outside. Of the children who are not currently following a vegan diet, 45.2% ($n$ = 100) do not consider it a suitable choice at present, while 22.2% ($n$ = 49) cite their partner's opposition as the reason. A total of 17.2% ($n$ = 38) state that their parent does not consider it a suitable choice, and 14.5% ($n$ = 32) report that a vegan menu is not available in the canteen. Only 0.9% ($n$ = 2) of cases cite opposition from the pediatrician as the reason.

#### 3.4.3. Exceptions

In the past year, 48.6% ($n$ = 1060) of the participants reported no intentional deviations from their vegan diet. In 21.5% ($n$ = 468) of cases, there were less than three deviations, while in 12.1% ($n$ = 263) there were between three and five deviations. In 17.8% ($n$ = 389) of cases, there were more than five deviations. Of the exceptions that occurred, 40.4% ($n$ = 668) were due to a lack of other vegan options, 18% ($n$ = 298) were to avoid disappointing others, 17.9% ($n$ = 297) were due to a desire to taste, 14% ($n$ = 231) were for other reasons, and

9.7% ($n$ = 161) were to avoid feeling embarrassed. Overall, 96.1% ($n$ = 2096) of respondents reported difficulty finding vegan options when dining out.

### 3.5. Frequencies

A significant correlation was found between the frequency of food consumption and the time of adoption of the vegan diet for some items (Table 3). Specifically, there was a negative correlation for the consumption of grains ($\rho = -0.140$, $p < 0.001$), legumes ($\rho = -0.110$, $p < 0.001$), soy products ($\rho = -0.068$, $p = 0.002$), and sugary drinks ($\rho = -0.077$, $p < 0.001$). On the other hand, there was a positive correlation for burgers and meat substitutes ($\rho = +0.102$, $p < 0.001$), coconut oil-based vegan cheeses ($\rho = +0.139$, $p < 0.001$), and nut-based vegan cheeses ($\rho = +0.145$ $p < 0.001$).

**Table 3.** Frequency of different foods consumption.

| Food | Frequency % (Total Population $n$ = 2180) | | | | | | |
|---|---|---|---|---|---|---|---|
| | >1/Day | 1/Day | 3–5/Week | 1/Week | 1 Every 2 Weeks | 1/Month | Never |
| Fruit and vegetables | 89.2% | 8.1% | 2.1% | 0.5% | 0.1% | 0.0% | 0.01% |
| Cereals (pasta, rice, bread...) | 75.9% | 19.7% | 3.7% | 0.5% | 0.1% | 0.0% | 0.2% |
| Legumes (beans, lentils...) | 42.9% | 41.0% | 14.5% | 1.0% | 0.2% | 0.2% | 0.1% |
| Soy products (tofu, tempeh...) | 22.3% | 37.8% | 30.0% | 6.6% | 1.7% | 0.8% | 0.7% |
| Seeds and dried fruit | 25.0% | 43.4% | 21.0% | 6.3% | 2.2% | 1.4% | 0.6% |
| Extra virgin olive oil | 74.2% | 20.2% | 3.1% | 1.0% | 0.3% | 0.4% | 0.7% |
| Sugary drinks (Coca-Cola, Sprite...) | 0.6% | 0.6% | 3.1% | 14.6% | 9.9% | 20.3% | 51.0% |
| Other vegetable oils (corn, peanut...) | 3.6% | 9.2% | 21.2% | 27.2% | 12.0% | 15.9% | 10.9% |
| Industrial and packaged products (cookies, chips) | 3.1% | 16.8% | 24.1% | 27.3% | 9.3% | 12.9% | 6.5% |
| Fried foods | 0.0% | 0.3% | 3.4% | 19.2% | 22.6% | 39.0% | 15.4% |
| Meat alternatives (meatballs, burgers...) | 0.5% | 2.7% | 20.4% | 40.9% | 14.3% | 13.1% | 8.3% |
| Coconut oil-based cheese substitutes | 0.2% | 0.5% | 6.1% | 15.0% | 15.3% | 27.0% | 35.9% |
| Nuts-based cheeses | 0.2% | 0.8% | 4.7% | 11.9% | 12.7% | 29.1% | 40.6% |
| Frozen ready meals (pizza, lasagna...) | 0.01% | 0.4% | 2.4% | 12.9% | 10.1% | 23.5% | 50.5% |
| Preserved ready products (hummus, noodles...) | 0.01% | 0.7% | 5.9% | 10.9% | 11.6% | 20.7% | 51.1% |
| High-protein products (bars, protein powder) | 0.5% | 3.2% | 5.2% | 4.6% | 4.5% | 9.3% | 72.7% |
| Meal replacements | 0.2% | 0.1% | 0.4% | 0.7% | 0.7% | 1.7% | 96.2% |

In addition, when comparing the time of adoption of a vegan diet with the importance of factors that determine the choice of frozen foods, preserved convenience foods, high-protein products, and meal replacements, a significant inverse correlation was found for speed ($\rho = -0.52$, $p = 0.014$) and curiosity ($\rho = -0.86$, $p < 0.001$).

No significant differences were found between the frequency of consumption of the analyzed food groups and educational qualifications, except in subjects with higher university qualifications who consumed more fruit and vegetables ($p = 0.001$) and nut-based vegan cheeses ($p = 0.018$) and fewer packaged and industrial products ($p < 0.001$).

### 3.6. *Lifestyle*

#### 3.6.1. Physical Activity, Tobacco and Alcohol

Of the respondents, 75.4% ($n$ = 1643) reported practicing regular physical activity several times a week for 1–2 h, while 24.6% ($n$ = 537) reported doing so sporadically. Non-smokers accounted for 56.7% ($n$ = 1237) of the respondents, while ex-smokers accounted for 20% ($n$ = 435). Occasional smokers and those who smoke less than 20 cigarettes per day accounted for 13.1% ($n$ = 285) and 7.8% ($n$ = 170), respectively. Only 0.3% ($n$ = 7) reported smoking more than 20 cigarettes per day. In terms of alcohol consumption, 16.7% ($n$ = 636) of participants reported never drinking alcohol, 27.6% ($n$ = 602) reported drinking it a maximum of once per month, 37.8% ($n$ = 824) reported drinking it 2 to 4 times per month, 15.9% ($n$ = 347) reported drinking it 2 to 4 times per week, and 2.0% ($n$ = 44) reported drinking it 5 or more times per week. Additionally, 80.7% ($n$ = 1466) of participants reported drinking less than 2 alcoholic units.

#### 3.6.2. Medical Aspects

The results indicate that 49.2% ($n$ = 1073) of the respondents undergo blood exams at least once a year to monitor their vitamin-mineral status. A total of 19.3% ($n$ = 420) do so once every two years, while 21.4% ($n$ = 466) and 10.1% ($n$ = 221) do not undergo regular exams or rarely do so, respectively.

### 3.7. *Relationship with Professionals in Nutrition*

Of the participants, 69% ($n$ = 1547) did not receive professional nutritional advice. Among those who did, 17.2% ($n$ = 385) received advice from a nutritionist, 7% ($n$ =158) from a dietitian, 6.3% ($n$ = 142) from a medical dietitian, and 0.4% ($n$ = 10) from a non-professional figure not belonging to any of the above categories. Of the total participants ($n$ = 1209), 51.3% reported experiencing reticence from their general practitioner, 12.6% from gynecologists ($n$ = 297), 10% from nutritionists ($n$ = 235), 6% from pediatricians ($n$ = 141), 5.3% from dietitians ($n$ = 126), 6.5% from medical dietitians, and 8.3% from other medical professionals.

### 3.8. *Source of Nutritional Knowledge*

Of the respondents, 28.8% ($n$ = 1761) usually source information about the vegan diet from the Internet (Instagram, blogs, groups, etc.), while 23.4% ($n$ = 1426) rely on scientific articles. Additionally, 20.7% ($n$ = 1238) seek advice from nutritional practitioners, 18.8% read books and magazines on the topic, 4.2% ($n$ = 256) obtain information from acquaintances and friends, and 3.6% ($n$ = 221) attend courses and seminars. Only 0.4% ($n$ = 22) report never searching for nutritional information.

## 4. Discussion

This study examines the eating habits and behavior of the Italian vegan population, with particular attention to food frequency consumption, vitamin-mineral supplementation (Table 4), and their relationship with medical professionals. Most of the sample has followed a vegan diet for one year, with less than 5% following it for longer. These data further confirm the increasing interest in plant-based diets in recent years in Italy, as already shown in the Eurispes Italy Report [4].

In this study, most vegans were female (90.2%) and young (median age of 28 years), with a normal weight status. Only a small percentage of the total population was found to be underweight or overweight.

The surveyed population did not show any interest in restrictive and potentially dangerous dietary patterns, such as fruitarian or raw diets. In fact, almost all participants followed a standard vegan diet with no particular dietary restrictions within the plant food groups.

**Table 4.** Vitamin-mineral supplementation.

| Supplement | Regularly % | Occasionally % | By Prescription % | Never % |
|---|---|---|---|---|
| Vitamin B12 | 89.0% | 6.3% | 0.9% | 3.7% |
| Vitamin D | 28.9% | 16.8% | 9.3% | 45.0% |
| Omega 3 (EPA [1]/DHA [2]) | 8.2% | 11.1% | 1.7% | 79.1% |
| Iron | 4.2% | 7.6% | 7.3% | 80.9% |
| Calcium | 1.8% | 4.0% | 1.3% | 92.9% |
| Multivitamin | 6.0% | 18.1% | 2.8% | 73.1% |
| Protein powder/BCAA [3]/EAA [4] | 5.7% | 9.0% | 0.6% | 84.7% |
| Other | 5.6% | 4.4% | 1.8% | 88.1% |

[1] EPA (Eicosapentenoic Acid). [2] DHA (Docosahexaenoic Acid). [3] BCAA (Branched-Chain Amino Acids). [4] EAA (Essential Amino Acids).

Over 80% of the total subjects did not have chronic pathologies. Less than 5% of the subjects had diseases associated with incorrect lifestyles, such as heart disease, type 2 diabetes mellitus, IBD (Inflammatory Bowel Disease), dyslipidemia, and arterial hypertension. Although the low average age of the sample must be taken into consideration, these results could confirm two hypotheses. First, an entirely plant-based diet may have positive effects on individuals' health. Second, as suggested by the literature, those who follow a plant-based diet not only make more careful and conscious food choices but also tend to have a healthier and more active lifestyle in general than the omnivorous population, taking care of their health in all respects, as shown in other studies [10,17]. Further investigation is required to confirm this hypothesis.

Among the studied population, over half of the subjects shifted towards a plant-based diet due to ethical and animal rights concerns, followed by environmental sustainability, and lastly, health and general wellbeing. This is consistent with previous studies conducted in Australia, America, Canada, Great Britain, and Holland [18–21].

The study found a statistically significant positive correlation between higher reported educational qualifications and motivation for veganism related to environmental sustainability and general health and welfare. Conversely, a statistically significant negative correlation was found between higher reported educational qualifications and ethical motivation regarding animal welfare. With a higher level of education, individuals may become more aware of the impact of their diet on animal welfare, environmental sustainability, and personal health.

The study found a statistically significant negative correlation between the time of adoption of a vegan diet and motivations related to environmental sustainability and a statistically significant positive correlation between the time of adoption of a vegan diet and ethical motivations. It is possible that this finding reflects the fact that the younger generation is more aware of the environmental impact of their diet.

Regarding weaning, most children follow an omnivorous diet rather than a vegan or vegetarian one. This is consistent with other research that has shown that pediatricians are generally opposed to vegan weaning, a position that is also supported by the position paper of the Italian Society of Preventive and Social Pediatrics [13,14]. However, it is worth noting that a significant proportion of the subjects had no intention of introducing a vegan diet to their child(ren), indicating that the pediatrician's opposition may not always be a decisive factor.

Although there is ample literature supporting the validity of a vegan diet even during early human development, some professionals remain unconvinced, possibly due to a lack of academic resources on the subject [10]. To eliminate uncertainties regarding plant-based diets in childhood, it is necessary to implement and offer educational and training courses aimed at pediatricians.

Currently, most children who are not vegan do not consider this dietary model suitable for themselves at this stage of their lives. The remaining percentage of non-vegan students is due to opposition from one or both parents or the unavailability of a fully vegan option at school. To address this issue, there is a strong need to incentivize canteens and the government to provide a fully plant-based menu in schools.

According to the survey, a significant challenge faced by those transitioning to a vegan diet is the absence of entirely vegan options during social events. This often leads to intentional deviations from the plant-based diet. Although half of the participants claimed to have never strayed from their vegan diet, the other half admitted to making exceptions to their diet for various reasons, such as the desire to try new foods, avoid disappointing others, or avoid embarrassment. All the motivations mentioned in this study are also reflected in another research [22] and are confirmed by other results of this study. According to most respondents, it is still quite or very difficult to find a vegan option when eating out. For this reason, more than three quarters of the population analyzed in the study almost always eat meals at home. Promoting the integration of plant-based options into the menus of restaurants, canteens, hospitals, bakeries, and fast-food outlets to listen to consumer demands is therefore becoming an increasingly pressing need. This can help not only normalize this dietary pattern but also more easily convey that the vegan choice is not restrictive nor limiting.

However, research suggests that cooking at home more frequently is associated with a higher score on the Healthy-Eating Index 2015 [23]. Additionally, the literature shows that the vegan population adheres more closely to the Mediterranean diet than the vegetarian and omnivorous populations, consuming significantly more fruit, vegetables, pulses, and dried oleaginous fruit [24]. The study's sample confirms that most subjects consume fruit and vegetables at least once a day, while over 80% of respondents consume legumes at least once a day. The consumption of oilseeds and nuts, as well as extra virgin olive oil, also followed similar trends. Regarding all the aforementioned categories, the frequency is in line with the guidelines for cereals and cereal products [25].

As per the same guidelines [25], sugary soft drinks and fried foods, referred to as "indulgent" foods, should be consumed occasionally and limited to special events. This recommendation is followed by almost all subjects. A very similar trend is also evident for frozen and preserved convenience products, coconut oil-based vegan cheeses, and ready meals, again demonstrating a similarity with what is stated in the frequency of consumption indications.

A deviation from the trends described above can be observed in the frequency of consumption of the category "burgers and meat substitutes": one fifth of the respondents consume these products three to five times a week. As these are processed foods, their consumption should be limited as much as possible. However, this figure shows that vegans tend to consume more ultra-processed foods than vegetarians and omnivores [26]. Despite this, it is important to note that a vegan diet is still entirely plant-derived, cholesterol-free, often lower in calories and contains a fair proportion of fiber. Compared to their animal counterparts, plant-based products have demonstrated several health benefits [27,28]. Therefore, it would be inaccurate to categorize the vegan diet as nutritionally poor or unbalanced.

However, despite low consumption, a significant inverse correlation was found between the time of adoption of the vegan diet and the frequency of consuming grains, legumes, soy products, and sugary soft drinks. Conversely, a direct correlation was observed with the consumption of burgers and meat substitutes, coconut oil-based vegan cheeses, and nut-based vegan cheeses. This finding contrasts with previous studies [26]. A possible explanation for this phenomenon may be attributed to the increased purchasing power and knowledge of the aforementioned products over time.

The study found a statistically significant negative correlation between the duration of adopting a vegan diet and the selection of frozen foods, preserved convenience foods, high-protein products, and meal replacements that are associated with quick preparation and curiosity. This statement suggests that individuals who are more familiar with a vegan diet may be less inclined towards novelty and experimentation when it comes to their food choices.

The popularity of these foods among consumers can be attributed to their taste, which is the primary factor influencing their purchase. Many vegans reject the production methods of certain products but still desire the pleasure and enjoyment of eating. This is why the market for plant-based alternatives is rapidly expanding [29].

It is worth noting that respondents with higher educational qualifications consume fruit, vegetables, and fermented nut-based vegan cheeses more frequently, while packaged products are more commonly consumed by those with lower educational qualifications. This may be because individuals with higher educational qualifications are more health-conscious.

Focusing on lifestyle, it is evident from numerous reports in the literature that regular physical activity leads to better general health status, including clinical-metabolic, psychological, and behavioral benefits [30]. Sedentary behavior and unhealthy eating habits, which are often associated [31], play a decisive role in the spread of serious pathological frameworks, defined as "diseases of wellbeing" [32]. Based on these data, it is evident that over three quarters of the sample engage in regular physical activity several times a week for an average duration of 1–2 h, which is in line with WHO recommendations [33]. Additionally, the results indicate positive trends in smoking and alcohol consumption, with most of the sample being non-smokers or ex-smokers, as well as teetotalers or occasional drinkers. Alcohol consumption is widely recognized as a significant risk factor for cancer development, alongside smoking, obesity, physical inactivity, and poor fruit and vegetable consumption [34]. It is also a risk factor for blood diseases. Smoking, on the other hand, is a major risk factor for a range of diseases, including cancer and cardiovascular diseases.

As numerous position papers from various institutions have emphasized, vitamin B12 supplementation is essential for a nutritionally balanced and healthy vegan diet [10]. B12 is crucial for regulating hemoglobin and DNA synthesis, as well as for the proper functioning of the central nervous system. It is worth noting that no plant-based food contains B12. A deficiency in this area may lead to a range of health issues, including depression, memory disorders up to dementia, spinal cord problems up to tetra-paresis, and neuropathies affecting the peripheral nervous system [35].

It is worth noting that almost 90% of the sample is aware of these indications and regularly supplements accordingly. However, it is important to note and monitor the small percentage of the investigated population that claims never to use the supplement. Although this is a very small share, the health risks are significant and cannot be ignored. Therefore, it is crucial to continue informing patients and instructing medical professionals to ensure they have taken this recommendation on board. However, supplementing with iron, omega-3, and multivitamins is not as crucial as vitamin D supplementation. Almost one third of the analyzed sample regularly supplements with vitamin D. The body's vitamin D levels are dependent on sun exposure. In the absence of adequate sun exposure, it must be obtained through fortified plant foods or supplements. This recommendation applies to the general population, not just vegans, as vitamin D intake is not dependent on diet [36].

It is noteworthy that despite less than 70% of the sample seeking support and having direct experience with a nutrition professional for vegan eating, almost three quarters of the total encountered resistance or skepticism from medical professionals, including general practitioners (GPs) who were reported to be the most skeptical among all other nutrition professionals. On one hand, this could indicate a potential lack of expertise and knowledge regarding vegan diets. On the other hand, this higher frequency could be due to medical figures being the most frequently addressed.

The reasons why professionals do not recommend a vegan diet are repeatedly refuted by the literature, as reported above. There is a need to educate health professionals, including nutrition specialists, about the validity of 100% plant-based diets. These diets can be applied to every patient at every stage of life and may have a preventive role in the onset of certain diseases if correctly planned and integrated. This issue could be addressed by implementing academic lessons during university and training courses for all health-related medical professionals, as previously mentioned.

Almost all the participants showed a strong desire to learn about vegan nutrition and actively sought out information from various sources, including nutrition professionals, scientific articles, books, magazines, friends, acquaintances, and online platforms such as Instagram, blogs, and groups. It is important to note that Instagram plays a significant role in disseminating content and facilitating the conscious and effective sharing of messages.

The study presented valuable results that can serve as a benchmark and for monitoring purposes. Additionally, the data can be used as a reference for other studies aimed at collecting information on the same indicators in specific contexts, which can then be compared with national-level data.

*Limitations of the Study*

The study has some limitations. First, the sample only includes Italian participants, so it cannot be considered representative of other nations' populations.

Additionally, there may be biases present in the study, including selection bias, performance bias, and recall bias.

The study may be subject to selection bias as participants were recruited on a voluntary basis through social media platforms such as Instagram, Facebook, and Telegram. The sample is limited to users subscribed to these channels and accounts of those who participated in the study's dissemination. Therefore, any Italian vegans who did not fit into the aforementioned categories were excluded from the survey.

The study may be affected by performance bias since participants were aware that they were taking part in a study analyzing the eating habits of the vegan population in Italy, which could have influenced their responses. Furthermore, conducting the questionnaire online may result in less control over the respondent when compared to an in-person questionnaire.

Under this type of administration, it is not possible to verify the accuracy of the answers provided or the identity of the questionnaire respondent. Recall bias, however, may result from the possible inaccuracy or incompleteness of memories retrieved from study participants, particularly regarding food consumption frequency, vitamin-mineral supplementation, and other past experiences investigated.

## 5. Conclusions

In conclusion, our results indicate an increasing number of people choosing the vegan option, with a greater involvement among females compared to males. The main reasons for choosing a completely plant-based diet are ethics and animal rights.

Eating meals primarily at home is linked to better diet quality. In fact, the surveyed vegan population demonstrated greater attention to their eating habits compared to the general omnivorous population. The consumption of fruit, vegetables, cereals, legumes, oleaginous nuts, and extra virgin olive oil fully complies with the guidelines' recommendations. Additionally, the use of processed and sugary products does not exceed the maximum intake limits indicated. Most of the survey sample also respects proper supplementation of vitamin B12, demonstrating widespread knowledge of the medical and nutritional indications reported by institutions.

Those who adopt a vegan diet, whether out of desire or necessity, often increase their nutritional knowledge and indirectly improve various other aspects of their lifestyle. This increased awareness is likely due to the desire to avoid potential deficiencies. The respondents showed a lower percentage of smokers and drinkers and a higher number of individuals who engage in regular physical activity.

The skepticism encountered by many individuals when approaching medical and health professionals about a plant-based diet is unfounded. Hypothesized deficiencies or the occurrence of physical and nutritional problems derived from the vegan diet are concepts that have been disproven by the literature. It is necessary to overcome these misconceptions.

Based on the findings, it may be beneficial to introduce educational courses and seminars or implement nutrition education classes in medical and health-profession degree programs. These courses should be led by professionals with expertise in plant-based nutrition, such as dietitians and specialized nutritional biologists. The purpose of this is to raise awareness among health professionals about the feasibility and validity of an all-plant-based diet and to provide their patients with up-to-date and scientifically based information. The main objective of the proposed interventions is to inform and educate health professionals about plant-based diets and thus reduce the risk of nutritional deficiencies in patients.

**Author Contributions:** Conception and design, A.S. and M.K.; methodology, A.S. and M.K.; data collection, A.S.; statistical analysis, M.K. and F.V.; data interpretation, A.S., D.Z. and M.K.; writing—original draft: A.S.; writing—review and editing: A.S., M.K., D.Z., and F.V. All authors have read and agreed to the published version of the manuscript.

**Funding:** This research received no external funding.

**Institutional Review Board Statement:** Not applicable.

**Informed Consent Statement:** Informed consent was obtained from all subjects involved in the study.

**Data Availability Statement:** The data presented in this study are available on request from the corresponding author.

**Conflicts of Interest:** The authors declare no conflict of interest.

## References

1. Dietary Choices of Brits (e.g., Vegetarian, Flexitarian, Meat-Eater etc.). *YouGov*, 30 December 2021. Available online: https://www.google.com/url?sa=t&rct=j&q=&esrc=s&source=web&cd=&ved=2ahUKEwiO7ouPg6KDAxUSz2EKHSsSA1sQFnoECBIQAQ&url=https://yougov.co.uk/topics/society/trackers/dietery-choices-of-brits-eg-vegeterian-flexitarian-meat-eater-etc&usg=AOvVaw1v1kB5SVT83_HFy95SDifv&opi=89978449 (accessed on 4 July 2022).
2. Jons, J.M. In U.S., 4% Identify as Vegetarian, 1% as Vegan. *Gallup*, 24 August 2023. Available online: https://news.gallup.com/poll/510038/identify-vegetarian-vegan.aspx (accessed on 8 September 2023).
3. Vegan FAQ. Available online: veganaustralia.org (accessed on 22 September 2022).
4. Rapporto Italia Eurispes Il Dovere di Avere Coraggio. 2023. Available online: https://eurispes.eu/wp-content/uploads/2023/05/sintesi-rapporto-italia-2023.pdf (accessed on 7 July 2023).
5. Rapporto Italia Eurispes Per una nuova Ri-Costruzione. 2021. Available online: https://eurispes.eu/wp-content/uploads/2021/05/eurispes_sintesi-rapporto-italia-2021.pdf (accessed on 7 July 2023).
6. Dedehayir, O.; Riverola, C.; Velasquez, S.; Smidt, M. Diffusion of Vegan Food Innovations: A Dual-Market Perspective. In *Responsible Consumption and Production*; Leal Filho, W., Azul, A.M., Brandli, L., Özuyar, P.G., Wall, T., Eds.; Springer International Publishing: Cham, Switzerland, 2019; pp. 1–9.
7. Chen, Z.; Zuurmond, M.G.; van der Schaft, N.; Nano, J.; Wijnhoven, H.A.H.; Ikram, M.A.; Franco, O.H.; Voortman, T. Plant versus animal based diets and insulin resistance, prediabetes and type 2 diabetes: The Rotterdam Study. *Eur. J. Epidemiol.* **2018**, *33*, 883–893. [CrossRef] [PubMed]
8. Kim, H.; Caulfield, L.E.; Rebholz, C.M. Healthy Plant-Based Diets Are Associated with Lower Risk of All-Cause Mortality in US Adults. *J. Nutr.* **2018**, *148*, 624–631. [CrossRef] [PubMed]
9. Dinu, M.; Abbate, R.; Gensini, G.F.; Casini, A.; Sofi, F. Vegetarian, vegan diets and multiple health outcomes: A systematic review with meta-analysis of observational studies. *Crit. Rev. Food Sci. Nutr.* **2017**, *57*, 3640–3649. [CrossRef] [PubMed]
10. Melina, V.; Craig, W.; Levin, S. Position of the Academy of Nutrition and Dietetics: Vegetarian Diets. *J. Acad. Nutr. Diet.* **2016**, *116*, 1970–1980. [CrossRef] [PubMed]
11. Springmann, M.; Godfray, H.C.J.; Rayner, M.; Scarborough, P. Analysis and valuation of the health and climate change cobenefits of dietary change. *Proc. Natl. Acad. Sci. USA* **2016**, *113*, 4146–4151. [CrossRef] [PubMed]
12. Willett, W.; Rockström, J.; Loken, B.; Springmann, M.; Lang, T.; Vermeulen, S.; Garnett, T.; Tilman, D.; DeClerck, F.; Wood, A.; et al. Food in the Anthropocene: The EAT-Lancet Commission on healthy diets from sustainable food systems. *Lancet* **2019**, *393*, 447–492, Erratum in: *Lancet* **2019**, *393*, 530; Erratum in: *Lancet* **2019**, *393*, 2590; Erratum in: *Lancet* **2020**, *395*, 338; Erratum in: *Lancet* **2020**, *396*, e56. [CrossRef] [PubMed]
13. Baldassarre, M.E.; Panza, R.; Farella, I.; Posa, D.; Capozza, M.; Mauro, A.D.; Laforgia, N. Vegetarian and Vegan Weaning of the Infant: How Common and How Evidence-Based? A Population-Based Survey and Narrative Review. *Int. J. Environ. Res. Public Health* **2020**, *17*, 4835. [CrossRef]

14. Mauro, G.; Caroli, M.; Verga, M.; Scaglioni, S.; Francavilla, R.; Barberi, S.; Bergamini, M.; Bernardo, L.; Berni Canani, R.; Biasucci, G.; et al. Position Paper Sipps-Fimp-Simp. Diete Vegetariane in Gravidanza ed età Evolutiva. *Pediatr. Prev. Soc.* **2017**, *12* (Suppl. S3), 120–193.
15. Bivi, D.; Di Chio, T.; Geri, F.; Morganti, R.; Goggi, S.; Baroni, L.; Mumolo, M.G.; de Bortoli, N.; Peroni, D.G.; Marchi, S.; et al. Raising Children on a Vegan Diet: Parents' Opinion on Problems in Everyday Life. *Nutrients* **2021**, *13*, 1796. [CrossRef]
16. Baroni, L.; Goggi, S.; Battino, M. VegPlate: A Mediterranean-Based Food Guide for Italian Adult, Pregnant, and Lactating Vegetarians. *J. Acad. Nutr. Diet.* **2018**, *118*, 2235–2243. [CrossRef]
17. García-Conesa, M.T.; Philippou, E.; Pafilas, C.; Massaro, M.; Quarta, S.; Andrade, V.; Jorge, R.; Chervenkov, M.; Ivanova, T.; Dimitrova, D.; et al. Exploring the Validity of the 14-Item Mediterranean Diet Adherence Screener (MEDAS): A Cross-National Study in Seven European Countries around the Mediterranean Region. *Nutrients* **2020**, *12*, 2960. [CrossRef] [PubMed]
18. Jabs, J.; Devine, C.M.; Sobal, J. Model of the Process of Adopting Vegetarian Diets: Health Vegetarians and Ethical Vegetarians. *J. Nutr. Educ.* **1998**, *30*, 196–202. [CrossRef]
19. North, M.; Klas, A.; Ling, M.; Kothe, E. A qualitative examination of the motivations behind vegan, vegetarian, and omnivore diets in an Australian population. *Appetite* **2021**, *167*, 105614. [CrossRef] [PubMed]
20. Fox, N.; Ward, K. Health, ethics and environment: A qualitative study of vegetarian motivations. *Appetite* **2008**, *50*, 422–429. [CrossRef] [PubMed]
21. Hopwood, C.J.; Bleidorn, W.; Schwaba, T.; Chen, S. Health, environmental, and animal rights motives for vegetarian eating. *PLoS ONE* **2020**, *15*, e0230609. [CrossRef]
22. Fehér, A.; Gazdecki, M.; Véha, M.; Szakály, M.; Szakály, Z. A Comprehensive Review of the Benefits of and the Barriers to the Switch to a Plant-Based Diet. *Sustainability* **2020**, *12*, 4136. [CrossRef]
23. Wolfson, J.A.; Leung, C.W.; Richardson, C.R. More frequent cooking at home is associated with higher Healthy Eating Index-2015 score. *Public Health Nutr.* **2020**, *23*, 2384–2394. [CrossRef]
24. Avital, K.; Buch, A.; Hollander, I.; Brickner, T.; Goldbourt, U. Adherence to a Mediterranean diet by vegetarians and vegans as compared to omnivores. *Int. J. Food Sci. Nutr.* **2020**, *71*, 378–387. [CrossRef]
25. Centro di ricerca Alimenti e Nutrizione. Linee Guida per una sana Alimentazione—Revisione 2018. 2018. Available online: https://www.crea.gov.it/en/web/alimenti-e-nutrizione/-/linee-guida-per-una-sana-alimentazione-2018 (accessed on 14 September 2022).
26. Gehring, J.; Touvier, M.; Baudry, J.; Julia, C.; Buscail, C.; Srour, B.; Hercberg, S.; Péneau, S.; Kesse-Guyot, E.; Allès, B. Consumption of Ultra-Processed Foods by Pesco-Vegetarians, Vegetarians, and Vegans: Associations with Duration and Age at Diet Initiation. *J. Nutr.* **2021**, *151*, 120–131. [CrossRef]
27. Khandpur, N.; Martinez-Steele, E.; Sun, Q. Plant-Based Meat and Dairy Substitutes as Appropriate Alternatives to Animal-Based Products? *J. Nutr.* **2021**, *151*, 3–4. [CrossRef]
28. Messina, M.; Duncan, A.M.; Glenn, A.J.; Mariotti, F. Perspective: Plant-Based Meat Alternatives Can Help Facilitate and Maintain a Lower Animal to Plant Protein Intake Ratio. *Adv. Nutr.* **2023**, *14*, 392–405. [CrossRef] [PubMed]
29. BIS Research. Fermented Plant-Based Alternatives Market. A Global and Regional Analysis. Focus on Applications, Products, Patent Analysis, and Country Analysis—Analysis and Forecast, 2019–2026. 2021. Available online: https://bisresearch.com/industry-report/fermented-plant-based-alternatives-market.html (accessed on 14 May 2023).
30. Warburton, D.E.; Nicol, C.W.; Bredin, S.S. Health benefits of physical activity: The evidence. *CMAJ* **2006**, *174*, 801–809. [CrossRef] [PubMed]
31. Pearson, N.; Biddle, S.J. Sedentary behavior and dietary intake in children, adolescents, and adults. A systematic review. *Am. J. Prev. Med.* **2011**, *41*, 178–188. [CrossRef] [PubMed]
32. Kohl, H.W., 3rd; Craig, C.L.; Lambert, E.V.; Inoue, S.; Alkandari, J.R.; Leetongin, G.; Kahlmeier, S. Lancet Physical Activity Series Working Group. The pandemic of physical inactivity: Global action for public health. *Lancet* **2012**, *380*, 294–305. [CrossRef]
33. World Health Organization. *Obesity: Preventing and Managing the Global Epidemic*; Report on a WHO Consultation; WHO: Geneva, Switzerland, 2000; Technical Report Series, 894.
34. Danaei, G.; Vander Hoorn, S.; Lopez, A.D.; Murray, C.J.; Ezzati, M. Comparative Risk Assessment collaborating group (Cancers). Causes of cancer in the world: Comparative risk assessment of nine behavioral and environmental risk factors. *Lancet* **2005**, *366*, 1784–1793. [CrossRef]
35. Ankar, A.; Kumar, A. Vitamin B12 Deficiency. 22 October 2022. In *StatPearls [Internet]*; StatPearls Publishing: Treasure Island, FL, USA, 2023.
36. Wacker, M.; Holick, M.F. Sunlight and vitamin D: A global perspective for health. *Derm. Endocrinol.* **2013**, *5*, 51–108. [CrossRef]

nutrients

MDPI

*Article*

# Associations of Dietary Intake with Cardiovascular Risk in Long-Term "Plant-Based Eaters": A Secondary Analysis of a Cross-Sectional Study

**Boštjan Jakše [1,*], Uroš Godnov [2], Zlatko Fras [3,4] and Nataša Fidler Mis [5]**

[1] Independent Researcher, 1000 Ljubljana, Slovenia
[2] Department of Computer Science, Faculty of Mathematics, Natural Sciences and Information Technologies, University of Primorska, 6000 Koper, Slovenia; uros.godnov@gmail.com
[3] Division of Medicine, Centre for Preventive Cardiology, University Medical Centre Ljubljana, 1000 Ljubljana, Slovenia; zlatko.fras@kclj.si
[4] Faculty of Medicine, University of Ljubljana, 1000 Ljubljana, Slovenia
[5] Ministry of Health, 1000 Ljubljana, Slovenia; natasa.fidler-mis@gov.si
* Correspondence: bj7899@student.uni-lj.si

**Abstract:** A plant-based diet rich in whole foods and fiber is beneficial for cardiovascular (CV) health. This impact is often linked to specific food groups and their preparation methods, reflecting the overall dietary pattern. However, research on the long-term effects of a carefully designed plant-based diet on adults transitioning from a typical Western lifestyle is limited. Notably, studies on people managing CV risk factors effectively are scarce. As part of a cross-sectional study, we examined 151 individuals committed to a long-term, well-designed plant-based diet and active lifestyle. We investigated how specific food groups and macronutrient intake are related to various CV health markers. In this secondary analysis, our comprehensive approach encompassed several methods: 3-day weighted dietary records, fasting blood lipid and blood pressure measurements, body composition assessments, and evaluations of lifestyle status. We adjusted our analysis for multiple variables, such as age, sex, current body mass index, smoking status, physical activity, and time (years) following the plant-based diet. Our findings revealed several associations between macronutrient intake (per 50 g) and CV risk markers, although these associations were generally weak. Individuals who consumed more whole grains and fruits had lower levels of total, low-density lipoprotein (LDL-C), and high-density lipoprotein (HDL-C) cholesterol. We also found associations between the intake of legumes and nuts/seeds and reduced HDL-C levels. These findings suggested that these food groups might influence the lipid profile, contributing to CV health in a plant-based diet. A greater intake of spices/herbs was associated with lower uric acid levels, while diets rich in plant-based fast food and pasta (made from white flour) were associated with higher uric acid levels. A greater intake of various macronutrients, such as fiber, carbohydrates (from whole-food sources), proteins, and different types of fats (saturated fatty acids [SFAs], monounsaturated fatty acids [MUFAs], and polyunsaturated fatty acids [PUFAs]), was associated with lower levels of total cholesterol, LDL-C (only for carbohydrates), and HDL-C. We found a unique negative correlation between PUFA intake and LDL-C, suggesting that PUFAs might significantly affect LDL-C levels. In contrast, increased fiber, protein and SFA consumption were associated with increased uric acid levels. These findings support the impact of dietary patterns on CV risk factors, highlighting that even small amounts of unhealthy food groups can significantly influence specific CV risk markers, regardless of the overall diet.

**Keywords:** plant-based diet; whole food; plant based; active lifestyle; food groups; macronutrients; cardiovascular risk factors; LDL cholesterol

## 1. Introduction

Over the past two decades, various dietary patterns have garnered considerable attention. One of these patterns is the exclusive plant-based (vegan) diet, which is characterized by the complete exclusion of all animal products [1]. Once considered a niche dietary choice, plant-based diets, particularly vegetarian diets, have recently surged in popularity due to their reported health benefits [2–6] and contribution to environmental sustainability [7–9].

However, there is some confusion about the definition of a "plant-based diet". This term is used interchangeably with vegan or vegetarian diets in certain studies. However, in other studies, it refers to a diet mainly consisting of plant-based foods. In some cases, it may include animal products in smaller amounts than a typical omnivorous diet recommended by the governmental healthy nutrition guidelines [1,10]. Table 1 describes the basic plant-based dietary patterns.

**Table 1.** Basic plant-based dietary patterns [1,11–15].

| | Plant-Based Diets | Vegan Diet | WFPB Diet | WFPB Lifestyle ‡ |
|---|---|---|---|---|
| Does not include | Large amounts of animal food (the amount is not specified) | Flesh and animal food sources (meat, dairy, eggs, and fish). On average, a WFPB diet typically primarily excludes processed foods. | | |
| Includes | A smaller amount of animal products compared to general dietary recommendations (the amount is not specified) | Plant and nonplant food sources † | Whole-food, plant-based food sources †† | Whole-food, plant-based food sources †† |
| Description | This term usually includes vegetarian and vegan diets and should be used in combination with a comprehensive dietary explanation | It may contain processed foods high in caloric content, free sugars, fats, salt, preservatives, and/or refined flour. It may not necessarily incorporate whole foods. It can also include less appropriate food preparation methods. | This is a whole-food, plant-based diet that can be implemented with a low or high proportion of energy from fat-source foods. | It also includes a lifestyle, usually healthy and active |
| Dietary supplements | Depends on the quality of the planning and how restrictive the diet is regarding the elimination of animal food sources | At least vitamin B12, possibly eicosapentaenoic acid (EPA), docosahexaenoic acid (DHA), and vitamin D (depending on geographical areas with either lower or higher UV indices). Depending on the quality of the diet, there is the potential for deficient iodine and calcium intake †††. | | |

WFPB diet = whole-food, plant-based diet, † Grains, legumes, vegetables, fruits, nuts/seeds, spices/herbs, fungi/mushrooms, some algae, bacteria. †† The consensus regarding the percentage of energy derived from non-whole-food, plant-based diet sources is at the discretion of the authors and the individual's interpretation of the strictness while still being able to classify the dietary pattern as a whole-food, plant-based diet. ††† Other supplements, such as meal replacements (MRs), protein shakes, sports drinks, and other nutritional supplements, are not essential. However, people usually add more or less of them to any kind of diet. ‡ Studied an ongoing whole-food, plant-based lifestyle program.

Cardiovascular diseases (CVDs) are the leading cause of global public health challenges responsible for a substantial burden of mortality and disability globally [16], as well as in Slovenia [17]. The interplay between diet and CV health is well established, making dietary interventions a crucial component of preventative and therapeutic strategies [18–22]. Several dietary patterns, such as plant-based diets, the Mediterranean diet, and the Nordic dietary pattern, have been found to be effective in reducing the risk of CVDs [2,23–28]. The common characteristics of these nutritional patterns are the consumption of whole-food groups, reduced or eliminated animal food intake, and increased consumption of plant-based foods. In contrast, Western dietary habits are characterized by excessive energy intake and the overconsumption of added and/or free sugars, added fats, saturated fatty acids (SFAs), dietary cholesterol, and salt, while at the same time lacking sufficient whole foods (e.g., whole grains, legumes, fruits, vegetables, and nuts). This nutritional imbalance contributes to the increasing incidence of obesity, type 2 diabetes, hypertension, hyperlipidemia, and coronary artery disease [29–31]. The abundance of fiber, antioxidants, and phytochemicals in plant-based and healthy plant-based diets may contribute to decreased blood pressure, improved lipid profiles, and reduced risk of CVDs [32–35].

By exploring how different food groups affect CV health, we found that some groups played a pivotal role. Understanding which food groups play a crucial role in CV health is critical in the formulation of effective dietary strategies for the prevention and management of CVDs. Whole grains, legumes, fruits, vegetables, and nuts/seeds consistently show protective effects against CVDs. These foods are packed with fiber, which can help to reduce cholesterol levels, lower blood pressure, and improve blood sugar control [19,36–43]. It is essential to understand that not all plant-based diets are the same. Just as omnivorous diets differ significantly in terms of nutritional sufficiency and health benefits, plant-based diets also fall along a broad spectrum, from very healthy to less nutritious, and consequently, having more or less favorable health benefits [14,44]. An unhealthy plant-based diet might include many highly processed foods, sweetened drinks, and plant-based versions of unhealthy junk foods, resulting in a less healthy dietary pattern [45,46]. Therefore, specific food groups within the plant-based diet, as well as meal preparation methods, require careful consideration. For example, ultra-processed plant-based foods, such as plant-based fast food and sweets, tend to contain high levels of sodium, added sugars, and unhealthy fats. Consuming these foods regularly, and in excessive amounts, can lead to weight gain, insulin resistance, and high blood pressure, increasing the risk of CVDs [47–50].

In nutrition science, contradictions regarding the associations between various food groups or macronutrients and CVD are common. These disparities can be attributed to several factors, such as differences in study design; sample size; inclusion criteria; methods used to assess dietary intake (which can impact the accuracy of reporting); the duration participants adhere to the diet; quantity, quality, and diversity of the diet; and the influence of lifestyle factors, such as physical activity (PA), smoking, alcohol consumption, and age. Therefore, these factors can impact how diet relates to various CV risk factors. Our previous study compared the nutritional, cardiovascular, and lifestyle status of health-conscious adults following plant-based and omnivorous diets. We observed significant differences in dietary intake (e.g., fiber and SFA intake) and CV risk factor status (e.g., LDL-C levels), although the dietary intake and LDL-C levels in both groups were within the recommended ranges. Using multivariate linear regression analysis, we estimated that the combined effects of fiber, SFA intake, and age accounted for 47% of the variability in LDL-C levels [51].

The present study aimed to investigate the relationships between dietary intake (i.e., specific food groups and macronutrients) and several CV health markers in individuals who adhered to a long-term, well-designed plant-based diet and practiced an active lifestyle. This secondary analysis can provide important contextual insight into which food groups have a distinctive effect on CV risk factors, even when consumed in small amounts. We hypothesize that the consumption of a well-designed plant-based diet is generally associated with favorable CV health profiles. A well-designed plant-based diet is characterized by the consumption of a variety of plant-based food groups daily and weekly. The meals are prepared using healthy cooking methods, such as boiling, steaming, or baking on parchment paper. Therefore, the definition of "well-designed" (also called "healthy") must meet core dietary principles, such as adequacy, diversity, balance, and moderation, ultimately aiming to satiate and provide health benefits [11,14,15,52–55].

## 2. Materials and Methods

### 2.1. Study Design and Eligibility

A study was conducted on healthy adults who followed the WFPB lifestyle program. This study utilized various methods, including 3-day weighted dietary records, fasting blood lipids and blood pressure measurements, body composition assessments using a medically approved and calibrated electrical bioimpedance monitor, and evaluations of lifestyle using standardized questionnaires for physical activity (Long International Physical Activity Questionnaire (L-IPAQ), sleep (Pittsburgh Sleep Quality Index (PSQI), and stress (30-question Perceived Stress Questionnaire (PSQ)) [56–58]. The methods used are briefly described in Section 2.3, while detailed information about the methodology and the enrolment process can be found in previous publications [59–61]. This cross-sectional study was conducted in Slovenia, a European Union member, from June to August 2019.

All participants were provided a complete explanation of this study, and written informed consent was obtained from all participants.

The study protocol received approval from the Slovenian Ethical Committee on the Field of Sport (approval document No. 05:2019; the application was submitted on 16 May 2019, and was approved on 27 May 2019) and the National Medical Ethics Committee of Slovenia (approval document 0120-380/2019/17; the application was submitted on 7 July 2019, and was approved on 20 August 2019). The trial was registered with ClinicalTrials.gov under the number NCT03976479, with registration on 6 June 2019 (this study was submitted on 1 May 2019, and passed the quality control review by the National Library of Medicine on 4 June 2019).

### 2.2. Subjects

Our final data analysis included 151 adults, consisting of 109 females and 42 males. Study participants adhered to a plant-based diet, specifically the WFPB lifestyle program, for a duration ranging from 0.5 to 10 years (average of four years) [59–61]. Before adopting the WFPB lifestyle, these participants followed a Western diet/lifestyle. The primary motive for transitioning to the WFPB lifestyle was to achieve health benefits and manage body mass effectively [61]. The program was designed for primary prevention. Therefore, none of the participants were simultaneously using medications for lipids, blood pressure, or blood sugar control [59].

### 2.3. Participant Characteristics, Nutritional Status, CV Risk Factor, and Lifestyle Status Assessment

Our study assessed participant characteristics, including sociodemographic, economic, and lifestyle status, using the questionnaire developed by the National Institute of Public Health of the Republic of Slovenia [62] and standardized electronic questionnaires [56–58,61]. To determine body composition, we employed an 8-electrode bioelectrical impedance body composition monitor (Tanita 780 S MA, Tanita Corporation, Tokyo, Japan) that has been medically approved, calibrated, and validated across several demographic conditions [61,63–65]. We utilized the abovementioned body composition analyzer for body mass assessment, while body height was measured using a body height gauge (Kern MPE 250K100HM, Kern and Sohn, Balingen, Germany). The characteristics of mean age, sex, current BMI, smoking status, PA status, and years on a WFPB lifestyle were adjusted for in our analysis when examining our primary objectives.

Nutritional status, which encompasses dietary intake and body composition, was evaluated using 3-day weighted dietary records and the dietary software Open Platform for Clinical Nutrition (OPEN) [66,67], a web-based application developed by the Jozef Stefan Institute [68] and supported by the European Food Information Resource Network (EuroFIR); the European Federation of the Association of Dietitians (EFAD); the European Society for Paediatric Gastroenterology, Hepatology, and Nutrition (ESPGHAN); and the American Dietetic Association (AND) [66]. The participants were given detailed instructions on recording their food intake for three consecutive days. The participants were asked to weigh all consumed foods and beverages using our calibrated electronic kitchen scales and to record the type, amount, and flavor of plant-based meal replacements (PB MRs) and dietary supplements. Semiquantitative recording of standard household measures or a picture booklet was allowed when exact weighing was impossible [69]. We used a recipe simulator to estimate the energy and nutrient contents of commercial or home-prepared foods, which involved the use of labeled ingredients and nutrient contents. Participants were asked to specify the form in which they weighed the foods (raw or cooked) and the form in which they consumed them (e.g., raw, cooked in water, baked in the oven). We used appropriate conversion factors [70] when entering the dietary data into the OPEN. Finally, nutritional intake from dietary supplements plus PB MRs was calculated by Res-Pons, a company that professionally manages a database with all dietary supplements and medicinal products available in the Slovenian market [71]. For this study, the average intake of calories and nutrients is presented as the sum of intakes from food, dietary supplements, and PB MRs.

As part of this study, 10–15 mL of blood was taken from participants after a 10–12 h fast. Lipid levels and other biochemical parameters were assessed using conventional laboratory procedures at national medical biochemical facilities employing uniform analytical methodologies. Total cholesterol (total C), HDL-C, and triglyceride plasma levels were directly measured, while LDL-C levels were determined using the Friedewald formula. Blood pressure was assessed using the oscillometric method while participants were in the supine position after five minutes of rest. Two measurements taken three minutes apart were averaged and recorded. The results were reviewed by a specialist in medical chemistry who headed the protein–lipid laboratory at the University Medical Centre in Ljubljana [59].

### 2.4. Outcomes

In this secondary analysis, we aimed to assess the correlation between the intake of various plant-based food groups (per 50 g) and macronutrients (per 10 g) and selected CV risk factors among 151 individuals following a WFPB diet.

Various food groups were considered to assess their correlation with CV risk factors. These food groups included vegetables (processed and unprocessed separately), fruits (processed and unprocessed separately), whole grains (and products), legumes, potatoes, nuts/seeds, PB MRs, bread and bakery products, spices/herbs, pasta (made from white flour), fast food (ready-to-eat meals, processed vegetables, sugary foods, sugary drinks, vegetable-based fats, and sweeteners), sweet products, alcoholic drinks, vegetable fats, and sweeteners (all of which showed statistical significance) [59,60]. However, only food groups that showed a characteristic correlation are highlighted in the correlation table for food groups, macronutrients, and CV risk factors.

The macronutrients that were included in the correlation assessment with CV risk factors were carbohydrates, fiber, proteins, total fats, SFAs, MUFAs, and PUFAs. Furthermore, to better understand dietary habits, we have presented the energy content and nutritional composition of the two most frequently consumed foods from each of the nine food groups. Finally, we evaluated the correlation of different food groups and macronutrients with CV factors, including total cholesterol, LDL-C, HDL-C, non-HDL-C, triglycerides, systolic and diastolic blood pressure, and uric acid.

## 3. Statistical Analysis

Statistical analysis was performed using R 4.1.1. with the tidyverse [72], ggstatsplot [73], and arsenal [74] packages. The data were normalized and examined for approximate normality, and we carried out linear regression with multivariable adjustments (including age, sex, current BMI, smoking status, PA, and years on a plant-based diet). The significance threshold was set at $p < 0.05$, and no missing data were present. We did not perform a sensitivity analysis. The data are presented as the means (standard deviations).

## 4. Results

On average, the study participants showed a high consumption of vegetables (455 g/d), legumes (166 g/d), (nonfried) potatoes (140 g/d), nuts/seeds (52 g/d), and spices/herbs (32 g/d). On average, they preferred cooking, stewing, and roasting on a baking sheet as their usual food preparation methods. Vegetable oil consumption was infrequent and mostly restricted to salad preparation. Additionally, the average daily intake of vegetable oils was only one gram. The participants mostly used cooking, stewing, and roasting potatoes on a baking sheet as food preparation methods [59]. The average sodium intake was 2043 g/day, with the primary source being iodized salt. The participants' average daily vitamin C intake was 337 mg/day, potassium intake was 4933 g/day, magnesium intake was 895 mg/day, and calcium intake was 1081 mg/day. The average intake of plant-based food groups is presented in Table 2.

**Table 2.** Average intake of plant-based food groups.

| Food Groups | Vegetables | Fruit | Whole Grains | Legumes | Potatoes | Nuts/ Seed | PB MRs | Spices/ Herbs | Pasta | PB Fast Foods |
|---|---|---|---|---|---|---|---|---|---|---|
| g/d | 455 ± 190 | 363 ± 187 | 178 ± 114 | 166 ± 115 | 140 ± 123 | 52 ± 46 | 43 ± 72 | 32 ± 40 | 17 ± 35 | 6 ± 34 |

Vegetables: cruciferous, leafy green, and colored vegetables; fruits: unprocessed, berries included; grains: whole grains; legumes: beans, lentils, and soy; nuts/seed: walnuts, sesame, and flaxseed; spices/herbs: fresh and dried; pasta: from white flour; PB MRs = plant-based meal replacements; PB fast foods = plant-based fast foods: ready-to-eat meals, processed vegetables, sugary products, sugary drinks and alcoholic beverages, vegetable-based fats, and sweeteners.

The dietary pattern used (Table 3) resulted in a high intake of fiber (approximately 70 g per day) and a low intake of SFAs (approximately 7.5 g per day or 3% of energy intake). Previous publications contain comprehensive and detailed information about food groups and dietary intake categorized by sex. The results are standardized to 2000 kcal/d [59,60].

**Table 3.** Average energy and macronutrient intake.

| Energy Intake, Macronutrients | Energy | Fiber | Carbohydrates | Protein | Total Fat | SFA | MUFA | PUFA |
|---|---|---|---|---|---|---|---|---|
| kcal/d, g/d, mg/d | 2057 ± 689 | 70 ± 21 | 295 ± 101 | 78 ± 25 | 47 ± 23 | 7.5 ± 3.6 | 13 ± 8 | 20 ± 11 |
| % E | | 7 ± 1 | 57 ± 5 | 15 ± 2 | 20 ± 5 | 3 ± 1 | 6 ± 2 | 9 ± 3 |

Kcal/d = kilocalories per day, g/d = grams per day, mg/d = milligrams per day, % E = percent per daily energy intake, SFAs = saturated fatty acids, MUFAs = monounsaturated fatty acids, PUFAs = polyunsaturated fatty acids.

On average, the study participants displayed a standard blood lipid profile and blood pressure levels (Table 4) and had a normal BMI, with the majority being nonsmokers or former smokers (Table 5) and showing low stress levels (PSQ score, 0.29) and good sleep quality (PSQI score, 2.7). Additionally, during the study, they engaged, on average, in a relatively high amount of PA, according to the recommendations (metabolic equivalent (MET), 5541 MET minutes/week on average vs. the recommended 3000 MET minutes/week from a combination of walking-equivalent, moderate-intensity PA or vigorous-intensity PA). Furthermore, the participants performed resistance training 2.7 times/week, with each session lasting for at least 30 min [61].

**Table 4.** Cardiovascular risk factor status.

| CV Risk Factors | Total C | LDL-C | HDL-C | Non-HDL-C | Triglycerides | Systolic BP | Diastolic BP | Uric Acid |
|---|---|---|---|---|---|---|---|---|
| mmol/L, mmHg, µmol/L | 3.7 ± 0.8 | 2.0 ± 0.7 | 1.4 ± 0.4 | 2.6 ± 0.5 | 0.9 ± 0.4 | 115 ± 11 | 71 ± 9 | 273 ± 68 |

CV = cardiovascular, total C = total cholesterol, LDL-C = low density lipoprotein cholesterol, HDL-C = high-density lipoprotein cholesterol, BP = blood pressure.

**Table 5.** Adjusted variables.

| Adjusted Variables | Mean Age (Years) | Sex n (F/M) | Current BMI (kg/m$^2$) | Smoking % (Never) | PA (Total METs) | WFPB Lifestyle (Mean Years) |
|---|---|---|---|---|---|---|
| | 39 ± 13 | 109/42 | 23.9 ± 3.8 | 78 | 5541 ± 4677 | 4.1 ± 2.5 |

BMI = body mass index; PA = physical activity; WFPB = whole-food, plant-based.

Table 6 outlines the nutritional content of selected nutrients in the two most commonly consumed foods (per 50 g) across each food group to highlight the nutritional diversity and quality of these foods.

**Table 6.** The energy content and nutritional composition of selected nutrients (per 50 g) for the most commonly consumed foods within each of the nine food groups [66].

| | **Vegetables** | | **Fruits** | | **Whole Grains** | | **Legumes** | | **Potatoes** | **Nuts/Seeds** | | **PB MR** | **Spices/Herbs** | | **Pasta** |
|---|---|---|---|---|---|---|---|---|---|---|---|---|---|---|---|
| Food group (per 50 g) | Broccoli/tomato | | Berries/apples | | Oatmeal/bread [wg] | | Beans/tofu | | White potatoes | Walnuts/flaxseeds | | PB MR | Onions/parsley | | Pasta |
| Energy (Kcal) | 14 | 10 | 32 | 30 | 197 | 120 | 165 | 81 | 36 | 360 | 245 | 199 | 27 | 46 | 163 |
| Macronutrients | | | | | | | | | | | | | | | |
| Carbohydrates (g) | 1.3 | 2.0 | 7.3 | 7.2 | 35 | 23 | 28 | 0.8 | 7.4 | 5.5 | 14 | 16 | 5.7 | 3.7 | 33 |
| Dietary fiber (g) | 1.5 | 0.2 | 1.2 | 1.0 | 6.8 | 1.0 | 15 | 0.2 | 1.0 | 3.1 | 19 | 9 | 0.9 | 2.1 | 1.5 |
| Total fat (g) | 0.1 | 0 | 0.2 | 0.1 | 3.8 | 0.8 | 0.5 | 5.1 | 0.1 | 35 | 15 | 4.8 | 0 | 0.2 | 0.8 |
| SFA (g) | 0 | 0 | 0 | 0.1 | 0.6 | 0.4 | 0 | 0.7 | 0.01 | 3.4 | 1.5 | 0.9 | 0.1 | 0 | 0.1 |
| MUFA (g) | 0 | 0 | 0 | 0 | 1.4 | 0.4 | 0 | 0 | 0 | 5.8 | 2.8 | 1.0 | 0.1 | 0 | 0.1 |
| PUFA (g) | 0 | 0.1 | 0.1 | 0.1 | 1.3 | 0.7 | 0 | 0 | 0 | 21 | 10 | 2.8 | 0 | 0.1 | 0.3 |
| LA (g) | 0 | 0 | 0 | 0 | 1.1 | 0.4 | 0 | 0.2 | 0 | 17 | 2.9 | 0 | 0 | 0.1 | 0.3 |
| ALA (g) | 0 | 0 | 0 | 0 | 0 | 0.1 | 0 | 0.1 | 0 | 4.5 | 11 | 0 | 0 | 0 | 0 |
| Protein | 1.9 | 0.4 | 0.4 | 0.1 | 5.8 | 4.8 | 12 | 8 | 1.4 | 7 | 12 | 17 | 0.8 | 7.2 | 5.8 |
| Micronutrients | | | | | | | | | | | | | | | |
| *Vitamins* | | | | | | | | | | | | | | | |
| B9 (folate) (μg) | 57 | 11 | 3.0 | 3.8 | 44 | 15 | 0 | 0 | 11 | 38 | 43 | 125 | 5.5 | 74 | 21 |
| C (ascorbic acid) (mg) | 24 | 12 | 5 | 2 | 0 | 0 | 0 | 0 | 10 | 1.3 | 0.3 | 60 | 9.8 | 19 | 0 |
| Retinol equ. [re] (mg) | 0.1 | 0.1 | 0 | 0 | 0 | 0 | 0 | 0 | 0.4 | 0 | 0 | 0.6 | 0 | 0.9 | 0 |
| E (α-tocopherol) (mg) | 0.3 | 0.4 | 0.3 | 0.3 | 0.7 | 0.4 | 0 | 0 | 0 | 0.9 | 0.2 | 0.9 | 0 | 1.8 | 0.1 |
| *Minerals* | | | | | | | | | | | | | | | |
| Calcium (mg) | 29 | 4.8 | 3.0 | 12 | 19 | 21 | 94 | 90 | 12 | 43 | 99 | 230 | 13 | 89 | 10 |
| Magnesium (mg) | 9.0 | 5.5 | 3.0 | 18 | 65 | 30 | 70 | 30 | 55 | 64 | 196 | 215 | 4.8 | 22 | 26 |
| Phosphorus (mg) | 31 | 12 | 6.0 | 5.5 | 151 | 75 | 298 | 0 | 25 | 204 | 331 | 0 | 21 | 43 | 94 |
| Potassium (mg) | 128 | 104 | 38 | 60 | 168 | 765 | 765 | 0 | 208 | 272 | 362 | 785 | 89 | 658 | 111 |
| Sodium (mg) | 11 | 1.7 | 0.5 | 0.6 | 3.4 | 0 | 12 | 1 | 1 | 1.2 | 30 | 0 | 1.3 | 86 | 1 |
| *Trace elements* | | | | | | | | | | | | | | | |
| Iron (mg) | 0.4 | 0.3 | 0.1 | 0.3 | 1.4 | 1.9 | 4.7 | 0 | 0.9 | 1.2 | 4.1 | 11 | 0.5 | 1.8 | 0.6 |
| Iodine (μg) | 7.5 | 0.6 | 0.5 | 0.4 | 2.3 | 3.0 | 0 | 0 | 1.2 | 1.5 | 5.0 | 115 | 0.9 | 1.7 | 0 |
| Zinc (mg) | 0.2 | 0.1 | 0.1 | 0.1 | 1.2 | 0.7 | 1.3 | 0 | 0.7 | 1.3 | 2.8 | 6 | 0.1 | 0.4 | 0.7 |
| Selenium (mg) | 0.4 | 1.0 | 0.1 | 0.7 | 4.8 | 1.2 | 1.6 | 0 | 0 | 2.7 | 13 | 39 | 0 | 0.5 | 32 |

[re] Retinol equivalents = vitamin A + α-carotene (1 mg retinol equivalent = 12 mg α-carotene) + β-carotene (1 mg retinol equivalent = 6 mg β-carotene) + γ-carotene (1 mg retinol equivalent = 12 mg γ-carotene) [75]. [wg] = whole-grain bread, PB MR = plant-based meal replacement [76].

Notably, all the significant associations we observed exhibited weak or very weak coefficients, with values ranging from $0.16 < r < 0.32$. All adjusted variables are presented in Table 6. Notably, linear regression was adjusted for sex, current BMI, smoking status, PA, and years on a plant-based diet. Nevertheless, regarding the intake of food groups (all per 50 g), we found that whole grain and fruit intake were negatively associated with total C, LDL-C, and HDL-C levels. Moreover, legume and nut/seed intake were only negatively associated with HDL-C. Interestingly, spice/herb intake was negatively associated with uric acid, but plant-based fast food and pasta (made from white flour) intake were positively associated with uric acid. The plant-based fast food group comprises a variety of foods and drinks, including ready-to-eat meals, processed vegetables, sugary products, vegetable-based fats, sweeteners, sugary drinks, and alcoholic beverages. Interestingly, none of these food groups significantly impacted triglyceride levels.

Regarding the intake of macronutrients (all per 10 g), all micronutrients, including fiber, were negatively associated with total C and HDL-C, with no significant association with LDL-C, except for carbohydrates and PUFAs. Furthermore, the intake of all macronutrients, except for total fat intake, showed a positive association with uric acid levels, with SFAs having the most significant impact, followed by carbohydrates. No macronutrient intake had a significant effect on triglycerides. Statistically significant correlations between food groups, macronutrients, and CV risk factors are presented in Table 7.

**Table 7.** Correlations between food groups and macronutrients and CV risk factors.

| | **Total C (mmol/L)** | | **LDL-C (mmol/L)** | | **HDL-C (mmol/L)** | | **Systolic BP (mmHg)** | | **Diastolic BP (mmHg)** | | **Uric Acid (μmol/L)** | |
|---|---|---|---|---|---|---|---|---|---|---|---|---|
| Food groups (per 50 g) | ↑↓ | *p*-value | ↑↓ | *p*-value | ↑↓ | *p*-value | ↑↓ | *p*-value | ↑↓ | *p*-value | ↑↓ | *p*-value |
| Whole grains | −0.10 | 0.001 | −0.05 | 0.032 | −0.03 | 0.017 | | | | | | |
| Fruits | −0.22 | 0.024 | −0.23 | 0.003 | −0.02 | 0.004 | | | | | | |
| Legumes | | | | | −0.03 | 0.033 | | | | | | |
| Nuts/seeds | | | | | −0.10 | 0.003 | | | | | | |
| Spices/herbs | | | | | | | | | | | −3.6 | 0.013 |
| PB MR | | | | | | | | | 1.0 | 0.044 | | |
| PB fast food | | | | | | | | | | | 3.9 | 0.017 |
| Pasta | | | | | | | | | | | 3.9 | 0.023 |
| Macronutrient (per 10 g) | ↑↓ | *p*-value | ↑↓ | *p*-value | ↑↓ | *p*-value | ↑↓ | *p*-value | ↑↓ | *p*-value | ↑↓ | *p*-value |
| Fiber | −0.12 | 0.001 | | | −0.06 | 0.001 | | | | | 7.9 | 0.006 |
| Carbohydrates | −0.03 | 0.001 | −0.01 | 0.021 | −0.01 | 0.001 | | | | | 18 | 0.003 |
| Protein | −0.09 | 0.001 | | | −0.04 | 0.004 | | | | | 5.1 | 0.038 |
| Total fat | −0.10 | 0.001 | | | −0.05 | 0.001 | | | | | | |
| SFAs | −0.68 | 0.001 | | | −0.31 | 0.001 | | | | | 38 | 0.019 |
| MUFAs | −0.26 | 0.001 | | | −0.12 | 0.001 | | | | | | |
| PUFAs | −0.25 | 0.002 | −0.10 | 0.037 | −0.12 | 0.002 | | | | | | |

↑↓ = the direction of association (an arrow pointing up means a positive association, while an arrow pointing down means a negative association). LDL-C = low-density lipoprotein cholesterol; HDL-C = high-density lipoprotein cholesterol; PB MR = plant-based meal replacement; PB fast food = plant-based fast food; SFAs = saturated fatty acids; MUFAs = monounsaturated fatty acids; PUFAs = polyunsaturated fatty acids. The data were adjusted for age, sex, current BMI, smoking status, PA, and years on a plant-based diet.

## 5. Discussion

### *5.1. Main Findings*

The present study provides a comprehensive understanding of the impact of various food groups and macronutrients on selected CV risk factors in individuals following a long-term WFPB lifestyle. We expected that individuals who follow the WFPB lifestyle program would have blood lipid, blood pressure, and BMI profiles that meet the recommendations in evidence-based guidelines. In addition, as part of this secondary associative evaluation analysis, we predicted that high dietary fiber intake and low SFA consumption would contribute to favorable CV risk factor outcomes.

Regarding our first hypothesis, this study partially confirmed that a well-designed plant-based diet rich in dietary fiber and low in SFAs is associated with favorable markers of

CV health. Furthermore, these findings underscore that even small quantities of unhealthy food groups can negatively affect specific CV risk markers, regardless of the overall dietary pattern. The phrase "small quantities" is often used to describe the general intake of foods in a typical Western diet but does not have a clear definition. However, the results of a recent secondary analysis of a randomized clinical trial with 244 participants who were randomly assigned to either a well-designed WFPB diet or a control group for 16 weeks suggested that minimizing the consumption of animal foods and animal products, sweets, and vegetable oils could be an effective strategy for weight loss in overweight adults. However, it is difficult to precisely determine the amount of these foods that can have clinically relevant adverse health effects, as published data are limited. The researchers analyzed both groups together, which made it impossible to determine the impact that "small quantities" of these food groups had on both studied groups. It is a poorly defined term compared to the typical Western diet, which is estimated to consist of small quantities of these foods [77,78]. However, the clinical significance of these minor effects found in our study is likely negligible within the context of an overall well-designed nutritional plan.

Interestingly, we did not find some of the expected associations between specific food groups, macronutrients, and CVD risk factors. For example, anticipated links between legumes, nuts/seeds, fiber, SFAs, and LDL-C levels have not been confirmed. This might be attributed to the relatively homogenous nature of the study sample, which limits the diversity of the results. Notably, our study population has much smaller variation than studies on individuals following a typical Western diet/lifestyle, where the relationships between healthy and unhealthy versions of the plant-based diet (indexes), as well as varied omnivorous diets, can be investigated, as well as the impacts of the different ratios of plant and animal food sources on various aspects of health [47–50]. Furthermore, this may be due to the overall nutritional sufficiency (on average, very high fiber intake and very low SFA intake) associated with a well-designed plant-based diet and the effective control of associated CV risk factors. Nevertheless, these findings emphasize that the overall healthfulness of an individual's dietary pattern can significantly influence how individual food groups impact CV risk factors, providing valuable knowledge in this area.

### 5.2. Food Groups Associated with CV Risk Factors

The relationships between plant-based food groups and macronutrients and various CV risk factors are complex and multifaceted, mainly because they accumulate the effects of what we eat, what we do not eat, and how we live [79,80]. Nonetheless, while we found some significant associations, it is essential to emphasize that the observed relationships were generally weak. Specifically, we observed that a greater intake of whole grains and fruits was associated with lower total C, LDL-C, and HDL-C levels, indicating a potential protective effect against adverse blood lipid profiles; these findings are consistent with the findings of meta-analyses of these two food groups. Researchers have consistently identified their role in preventing CVDs [41,42,81,82].

In addition, legumes and nuts/seeds showed some unexpected negative associations, albeit only with HDL-C. While HDL-C has traditionally been regarded as an antiatherosclerotic biomarker, levels lower than the recommended levels of HDL-C represent a risk factor for CVDs [83,84]. However, recent studies have proposed a more complex mechanism—i.e., U-shaped—association between HDL-C and CV risk [83,85,86]. Based on findings from a pooled analysis of 37 prospective cohort studies, it is essential to pay attention not only to individuals with low HDL-C levels but also to those with relatively high HDL-C levels since both subpopulations have an increased risk of mortality [83]. Nevertheless, our participants had relatively high HDL-C levels (i.e., mean 1.4 mmol/L), and the recommended non-HDL-C level (2.6 mmol/L) still falls within the optimal range, which is associated with the lowest mortality risk [83,86,87]. This finding can also be attributed to a physically active lifestyle (5541 MET minutes/week) [61] and weight loss (an average of 7.1 kg) compared to the pre-WFPB lifestyle period. Individuals with a normal BMI lost 2.5 kg on average, overweight individuals lost 7.2 kg, and obese individuals lost 16.1 kg [88].

Regardless, the effect sizes of these dietary factors on CV risk factors were relatively modest. This is particularly notable given that the average daily intake of legumes (including soy foods) was 166 g (corresponding to 1162 g/week), and nuts/seeds were consumed at an average of 52 g (the main sources of nuts and seeds were walnuts, hazelnuts, flax, and sesame seeds) [59]. The relationship between CV risk factors and food group intake was assessed for every 50 g of these foods consumed. Additional legume intakes based on already very high levels (i.e., 1162 g/week) are supposedly above the threshold for additional clinical benefits compared to the scenario of moving from a legume intake being too low towards the recommended intake. Beans, lentils, chickpeas, and soybeans (tofu) were the most commonly consumed subgroups in the legume group [59]. In support of these findings, a recent systematic review and dose–response meta-analysis attempted to identify the optimal legume intake level for reducing CVD risk. The study estimated that 400 g per week provides the optimal CV benefit, beyond which the benefits appear to level off [19]. In addition, a review of 26 randomized controlled trials revealed that consuming pulses can significantly lower LDL-C levels compared to consuming controlled diets. The review estimated that a median intake of 130 g/day (i.e., 910 g/week) of pulses could lead to a 5% reduction in LDL-C, and a 5–10% reduction is expected from heart-healthy diets alone. It is worth noting that the authors highlighted that most trials included in the review were conducted on a foundation of heart-healthy diets. These diets consist of more than 20–25 g/day of fiber (2.8–3.5 times less than in our study) and less than 10% of the energy from saturated fat (up to 3.3 times more than in our study) [89]. Therefore, the cumulative intake of legumes needs to be considered in terms of its overall effect on HDL-C and LDL-C levels and other aspects of health.

Interestingly, we found that spice/herb intake was negatively associated with uric acid levels, potentially affecting CV health. The participants recorded their intake of all locally grown spices, herbs, bulbs, celery, rosemary, and turmeric [60]. Conversely, the intake of pasta (made from white flour) and plant-based fast food (usually a source of added oils/fat and free/added sugar) was positively associated with increased uric acid levels, suggesting that these food choices could contribute to increased CV risk through mechanisms related to uric acid metabolism [90,91]. While the observed effect size was statistically significant, it is essential to note that the effect size was relatively small. Furthermore, our study participants had limited consumption of these two food groups on average, with an average daily intake of only 17 g of white flour pasta and 6 g of PB fast food.

Importantly, our study participants had relatively high average potato consumption, averaging 140 g daily. However, despite this, we did not observe the typical adverse association with uric acid levels found in a meta-analysis of population-based cohorts [92]. The likely reason for this discrepancy lies in the method of preparation. In the group following the WFPB lifestyle program, the recommended methods of potato preparation were healthy and included cooking, steaming, or baking on baking paper—without frying or adding extra fat (i.e., vegetable oils or butter).

Our study did not reveal a significant relationship between food groups and systolic blood pressure. This could be attributed not only to the plant-based diet per se but also to its well-designed nature (predominantly from whole-food sources) and the influence of lifestyle factors, such as BMI, PA, nonsmoking status, or smoking cessation [93–95]. We considered factors, such as appropriate sodium and high potassium intake (averaging 2043 mg/day and 4933 g/day, respectively) and regular consumption of herbal teas [59], which likely played a role in these findings, in addition to a high intake of many micronutrients, which are also associated with controlled blood pressure (for example, vitamin C (in too low intake), magnesium, and calcium) [96]. Several studies conducted on the general population have shown that dietary supplements containing vitamin C, magnesium, and calcium favorably impact blood pressure control [97]. In our previous publication, we presented the results of a detailed assessment of nutrient intake separately from foods, dietary supplements, and PB MRs. Specifically, we standardized the estimated dietary intake to 2000 kcal/day; therefore, individuals' average vitamin C intake from food, dietary supplements, and PB MRs was 197 mg/day and 152 mg/day, respectively. Similarly, magnesium intake was 616 mg/day and 272 mg/day, and calcium intake was 690 mg/day and 408 mg/day, respectively [60]. Hence, the well-controlled blood pressure in our study participants (115/71 mmHg) may be partly due to the WFPB lifestyle, especially dietary intake (whole foods consumed and highly processed food omitted), as well as PA, sleeping, nonsmoking, and stress management.

The final relationship we observed between food groups and CV risk factors was a positive association between PB MR and diastolic blood pressure. However, the association was weak, and the effect size was relatively small (i.e., 1 mmHg) based on an intake of 50 g per day. Our study participants consumed approximately 43 g of this specific food group per day.

Notably, recently, the researchers performed a secondary analysis on a clinical trial involving overweight adults randomly assigned to either a vegan or omnivorous diet. The study used plant-based diet indices and 3-day dietary records. Vegetable oils were inversely associated with body mass loss within the study sample [77]. However, further studies need to clarify how and at what quantity of intake potentially unhealthy (ultra-processed/refined) plant-based food groups (e.g., fruit juice, sugar-sweetened beverages, sweets, refined grains, or French fries) impact body mass (change) and CV risk factors within the vegan group, as well as their clinical relevance.

### 5.3. Macronutrients Associated with CV Risk Factors

Our observations revealed that a greater intake of fiber, which is a crucial component of plant-based diets and is derived from whole-food grains, legumes, fruits, vegetables, and nuts/seeds, with an average intake of 70 g per day, was associated with lower levels of total C and HDL-C. However, only the intake of PUFAs was significantly associated with lower LDL-C levels. A systematic review with a meta-analysis of 38 studies indicated a positive association between total C intake and total blood cholesterol levels. Notably, the most significant reduction in risk for various relevant outcomes was observed when daily dietary fiber intake was within 25 to 29 g [98]. However, our study revealed a notably high average fiber intake. This could explain why we did not find a typical beneficial association between fiber intake (per 10 g) and LDL-C levels. In a recent study, we examined 80 health-conscious adults who consumed either a plant-based or nonplant-based diet. We examined the relationship between the intake of fiber (75 g/day vs. 34 g/day) or SFAs (3% of energy intake vs. 9% of energy intake) and LDL-C levels (1.7 mmol/L vs. 2.8 mmol/L). This information was briefly mentioned in the introduction. Through multivariate linear regression adjusted for age, sex, and smoking status, the analysis revealed that fiber and SFA intake alone accounted for 43% of the variation in LDL-C levels, and age contributed an additional 4%. Notably, each 10 g increase in total fiber intake was associated with a 0.12 mmol/L reduction in LDL-C levels [51]. Furthermore, our study revealed a noteworthy relationship between PUFAs and lower LDL-C levels. The beneficial effect of PUFAs on LDL-C is well known [99,100]. However, it should be emphasized that PUFAs also include eicosapentaenoic acid/docosahexaenoic acid (average intake of 565 g per day) based on a greater intake of nuts/seeds, including flaxseed [59], which also has a beneficial effect [101]. Notably, a relatively weak positive correlation was detected between carbohydrate intake and LDL-C levels. This is probably because our participants consumed the majority of carbohydrates from whole-food sources. Additionally, the typical source of PUFAs (which also showed beneficial effects on LDL-C) was nuts and seeds (52 g, including walnuts and flaxseeds) and legumes (66 g, including soy), which also represent a typical source of carbohydrates. Therefore, this combination had a favorable effect on the negative correlation between the intake of carbohydrates and LDL-C.

Consistent with the expected associations between specific food groups and HDL-C levels, we also observed negative associations between all macronutrients and HDL-C levels (discussed above in the food groups section). We revealed an intriguing but weak negative correlation between SFA consumption and LDL-C levels. However, two key factors likely influenced the observed correlation. The study participants had a notably low average SFA intake—just 7.5 g/day or 3% of their total energy intake. Additionally, the subjects exhibited relatively low LDL-C levels, averaging 2.0 mmol/L. A prospective urban–rural epidemiology (*PURE*) observational study revealed a significant association between a higher intake of saturated fat and a reduced risk of stroke, which could explain our results. Although this contradicts the general belief that SFA increases LDL-C levels, the PURE study included subjects from different countries with varying socioeconomic backgrounds. For instance, the study included approximately 80,000 Asian and 50,000 non-Asian participants. In predominantly Asian individuals, SFAs constitute only 2.3–3.9% of the total energy consumed and are associated with general malnutrition [102]. In a recent study, researchers evaluated the dietary intake of a well-designed theoretical WFPB diet. The results of their research on participants consuming a 2000 kcal diet per day hardly achieved 3% of their energy from SFAs [53], which further explains the associations observed in our study and the PURE study. In addition, in our previous study mentioned above [51], we found strong correlations between lower/higher intakes of SFAs, fiber intake, and LDL-C levels. We explored the differences in LDL-C between individuals on a plant-based diet (consuming only 3% of their energy from SFAs) and individuals on an omnivorous diet (consuming approximately 9% of their energy from SFAs) via multivariate regression analysis [51].

Furthermore, regarding macronutrient intake, we observed positive associations with uric acid levels for all macronutrients except for total fat, MUFAs, and PUFAs. Notably, SFAs had the most pronounced negative impact on uric acid levels, followed by carbohydrates. Caution is crucial when interpreting the potential effects of the amount of SFAs consumed on uric acid levels. This is because, out of the sample size of 151 individuals, 72% were women. Women generally exhibit lower uric acid values than men and have different reference ranges. Therefore, it is essential to consider this when analyzing the results. As a result, the data provided in our case can only be utilized to estimate the effect of SFAs, and it is important again to emphasize their very low intake in our participants (3% of energy). However, further research is needed to determine the potential clinical relevance of these findings.

Our findings highlight the vital importance of maintaining a healthy diet to decrease cardiovascular (CV) risk factors. In a recent umbrella review of nine published meta-analyses, which included both observational and randomized controlled studies, researchers explored the impact of plant-based diets (vegetarian and vegan) on cardiovascular health. The study's findings revealed a clear association between healthier dietary choices and a lower risk of cerebrovascular disease, CVD incidence, ischemic heart disease mortality, and ischemic stroke [103].

### 5.4. Strengths and Limitations

The strengths of our study are that it provides a comprehensive and detailed analysis of participants' dietary intake, particularly their adherence to a well-designed plant-based diet, including the consumption of specific food groups and macronutrients. In addition, it includes a thorough assessment of participants' CV health profiles, BMI, and lifestyle status. Such an approach allows a more holistic understanding of their health status. Furthermore, the participants represented a relatively homogeneous group in terms of diet and lifestyle, reducing the confounding variables and increasing the internal validity of our findings. For analyses, we adjusted for critical confounding variables, such as sex, BMI, smoking status, PA, and years on a plant-based diet, strengthening the credibility of the results.

However, this study's cross-sectional design limits its ability to establish causation, as it can only show simultaneous associations between different variables measured. Furthermore, the limited sample size could constrain the generalization of the findings obtained to larger populations on a plant-based diet. It is worth noting that some of the data, such as dietary intake and PA, might be susceptible to recall and social desirability bias, as participants enrolled in this study were part of the WFPB lifestyle program. However, dietary intake was evaluated using a 3-day weighted dietary record in the most extensive sample of adults on a long-term WFPB lifestyle. The web-based software tool OPEN, designed for assessing the nutritional intake of recipes, was developed by the Jozef Stefan Institute, a renowned research institution. Additionally, there is a risk of inaccurate reporting due to under- or overreporting [104] and accuracy issues when entering menus into the system. In addition, this study focused on cholesterol and blood pressure as CV risk factors. Including a broader range of CV risk factors (e.g., LDL-C particles, fasting glucose, hemoglobin A1C, predicted insulin sensitivity index, oral glucose insulin sensitivity) and other health outcomes would provide a more comprehensive view of the impact of a diet practiced by the study participants.

## 6. Conclusions

Our study provides comprehensive insight into individuals who adhere to a WFPB lifestyle, namely, high vegetable, fruit, legume, potato, nut/seed, or spice/herb consumption and PA, while avoiding smoking (with the majority being nonsmokers or former smokers) and alcohol consumption. This results in a substantial fiber intake, low SFA consumption, and an active lifestyle. These dietary and lifestyle choices corresponded with favorable CV health profiles, encompassing, on average, normal lipid levels, blood pressure, and BMI. Additionally, the study participants engaged in a relatively high amount of PA compared to the general sedentary or physically nonactive population but within the recommended guidelines.

However, while we identified some significant associations between various food groups and CV risk/health factors, these were relatively weak with small effect sizes. These findings, adjusted for important confounders, suggest that CV health outcomes are influenced by a combination of dietary and lifestyle factors, underscoring the complexity of these interactions. Furthermore, they highlighted the need for careful dietary planning to optimize CV well being. Regardless of food group or macronutrient intake, our results emphasize that the composition and quality of a plant-based diet play vital roles in CV health, underscoring the multifaceted nature of these diet–health relationships.

**Author Contributions:** Conceptualization; B.J. and N.F.M.; writing—original draft preparation; B.J., N.F.M. and Z.F.; writing—review and editing; B.J., U.G., Z.F. and N.F.M.; statistical analyses and interpretation of the data; U.G., B.J. and Z.F.; supervision; N.F.M. and U.G. All authors have read and agreed to the published version of the manuscript.

**Funding:** This work was partly financially supported by the Slovenian Research Agency (Research Program P3-0395: Nutrition and Public Health) and partly financed by Barbara Jakše, the sole proprietor. Z.F. received funding from the Slovenian Research Agency [P3-0308: Atherosclerosis and throm-bosis, J3-4525: Synchronized cardiorespiratory coronary rehabilitation, and J3-4526: Chimeric au-tologous vaccine against PCSK9], N.F.M. received funding from the Slovenian Research Agency [P3-0395: Nutrition and Public Health]. B.J. received no research funding.

**Institutional Review Board Statement:** The study protocol received approval from the Slovenian Ethical Committee on the Field of Sport (approval document No. 05:2019) and the National Medical Ethics Committee of Slovenia (approval document 0120-380/2019/17). The trial was registered with ClinicalTrials.gov under the number NCT03976479, with registration on 6 June 2019.

**Informed Consent Statement:** Written informed consent was obtained from all participants.

**Data Availability Statement:** The data used to support the findings of this study are included within the article.

**Conflicts of Interest:** N.F.M., U.G. and Z.F. declare that they have no conflicts of interest and have collaborated as independent researchers. B.J. received royalty compensation from Herbalife Nutrition, which did not have any role in the design; interpretation; course (e.g., collection; analysis; and interpretation of the data); or results of the study; or the writing of this manuscript.

## References


1. Storz, M.A. What makes a plant-based diet? a review of current concepts and proposal for a standardized plant-based dietary intervention checklist. *Eur. J. Clin. Nutr.* **2022**, *76*, 789–800. [CrossRef] [PubMed]
2. Selinger, E.; Neuenschwander, M.; Koller, A.; Gojda, J.; Kühn, T.; Schwingshackl, L.; Barbaresko, J.; Schlesinger, S. Evidence of a vegan diet for health benefits and risks—An umbrella review of meta-analyses of observational and clinical studies. *Crit. Rev. Food Sci. Nutr.* **2022**, *63*, 9926–9936. [CrossRef] [PubMed]
3. Dinu, M.; Abbate, R.; Gensini, G.F.; Casini, A.; Sofi, F. Vegetarian, vegan diets and multiple health outcomes: A systematic review with meta-analysis of observational studies. *Crit. Rev. Food Sci. Nutr.* **2017**, *57*, 3640–3649. [CrossRef] [PubMed]
4. Kelly, J.; Karlsen, M.; Steinke, G. Type 2 Diabetes Remission and Lifestyle Medicine: A Position Statement From the American College of Lifestyle Medicine. *Am. J. Lifestyle Med.* **2020**, *14*, 406–419. [CrossRef] [PubMed]
5. Tran, E.; Dale, H.F.; Jensen, C.; Lied, G.A. Effects of Plant-Based Diets on Weight Status: A Systematic Review. *Diabetes, Metab. Syndr. Obes. Targets Ther.* **2020**, *13*, 3433–3448. [CrossRef]
6. Oussalah, A.; Levy, J.; Berthezène, C.; Alpers, D.H.; Guéant, J.L. Health outcomes associated with vegetarian diets: An umbrella review of systematic reviews and meta-analyses. *Clin. Nutr.* **2020**, *39*, 3283–3307. [CrossRef] [PubMed]
7. Chai, B.C.; van der Voort, J.R.; Grofelnik, K.; Eliasdottir, H.G.; Klöss, I.; Perez-Cueto, F.J.A. Which Diet Has the Least Environmental Impact on Our Planet? A Systematic Review of Vegan, Vegetarian and Omnivorous Diets. *Sustainability* **2019**, *11*, 4110. [CrossRef]
8. Gibbs, J.; Cappuccio, F.P. Plant-Based Dietary Patterns for Human and Planetary Health. *Nutrients* **2022**, *14*, 1614. [CrossRef]
9. O'Malley, K.; Willits-Smith, A.; Rose, D. Popular diets as selected by adults in the United States show wide variation in carbon footprints and diet quality. *Am. J. Clin. Nutr.* **2023**, *17*, 701–708. [CrossRef]
10. Key, T.J.; Papier, K.; Tong, T.Y.N. Plant-based diets and long-term health: Findings from the EPIC-Oxford study. *Proc. Nutr. Soc.* **2022**, *81*, 190–198. [CrossRef]
11. Jakše, B. Placing a Well-Designed Vegan Diet for Slovenes. *Nutrients* **2021**, *13*, 4545. [CrossRef]
12. Campbell, T.C.; Campbell, T.M. *The China Study: The Most Comprehensive Study of Nutrition ever Conducted and the Startling Implications for Diet, Weight Loss and Long-Term Health*; BenBella Books: Dallas, TX, USA, 2005; ISBN 1932100660.
13. Solway, J.; McBride, M.; Haq, F.; Abdul, W.; Miller, R. Diet and Dermatology: The Role of a Whole-food, Plant-based Diet in Preventing and Reversing Skin Aging—A Review. *J. Clin. Aesthet. Dermatol.* **2020**, *13*, 38–43.
14. Neufingerl, N.; Eilander, A. Nutrient Intake and Status in Adults Consuming Plant-Based Diets Compared to Meat-Eaters: A Systematic Review. *Nutrients* **2021**, *14*, 29. [CrossRef]
15. Jakše, B.; Fras, Z.; Fidler Mis, N. Vegan Diets for Children: A Narrative Review of Position Papers Published by Relevant Associations. *Nutrients* **2023**, *15*, 4715. [CrossRef] [PubMed]
16. Roth, G.A.; Johnson, C.; Abajobir, A.; Abd-Allah, F.; Abera, S.F.; Abyu, G.; Ahmed, M.; Aksut, B.; Alam, T.; Alam, K.; et al. Global, Regional, and National Burden of Cardiovascular Diseases for 10 Causes, 1990 to 2015. *J. Am. Coll. Cardiol.* **2017**, *70*, 1–25. [CrossRef] [PubMed]
17. Fras, Z.; Jakše, B.; Kreft, S.; Malek, Ž.; Kamin, T.; Tavčar, N.; Fidler Mis, N. The Activities of the Slovenian Strategic Council for Nutrition 2023/24 to Improve the Health of the Slovenian Population and the Sustainability of Food: A Narrative Review. *Nutrients* **2023**, *15*, 4390. [CrossRef] [PubMed]
18. Chareonrungrueangchai, K.; Wongkawinwoot, K.; Anothaisintawee, T.; Reutrakul, S. Dietary factors and risks of cardiovascular diseases: An umbrella review. *Nutrients* **2020**, *12*, 1088. [CrossRef]
19. Mendes, V.; Niforou, A.; Kasdagli, M.I.; Ververis, E.; Naska, A. Intake of legumes and cardiovascular disease: A systematic review and dose–response meta-analysis. *Nutr. Metab. Cardiovasc. Dis.* **2023**, *33*, 22–37. [CrossRef]
20. Esselstyn, C.B.; Ellis, S.G.; Edendorp, S.V.M.; Ph, M.; Crowe, T.D. A Strategy to Arrest and Reverse Coronary Artery Disease: A 5-Year Longitudinal Study of a Single Physician's Practice. *J. Fam. Pract.* **1995**, *41*, 560–568.
21. Choi, Y.; Larson, N.; Steffen, L.M.; Schreiner, P.J.; Gallaher, D.D.; Duprez, D.A.; Shikany, J.M.; Rana, J.S.; Jacobs, D.R. Plant-centered diet and risk of incident cardiovascular disease during young to middle adulthood. *J. Am. Heart Assoc.* **2021**, *10*, 20718. [CrossRef]
22. Ornish, D.; Scherwitz, L.W.; Billings, J.H.; Brown, S.E.; Gould, K.L.; Merritt, T.A.; Sparler, S.; Armstrong, W.T.; Ports, T.A.; Kirkeeide, R.L.; et al. Intensive lifestyle changes for reversal of coronary heart disease. *JAMA* **1998**, *280*, 2001–2007. [CrossRef] [PubMed]
23. Barnard, N.D.; Alwarith, J.; Rembert, E.; Brandon, L.; Nguyen, M.; Goergen, A.; Horne, T.; do Nascimento, G.F.; Lakkadi, K.; Tura, A.; et al. A Mediterranean Diet and Low-Fat Vegan Diet to Improve Body Weight and Cardiometabolic Risk Factors: A Randomized, Cross-over Trial. *J. Am. Coll. Nutr.* **2021**, *41*, 127–139. [CrossRef] [PubMed]
24. Grosso, G.; Marventano, S.; Yang, J.; Micek, A.; Pajak, A.; Scalfi, L.; Galvano, F.; Kales, S.N. A comprehensive meta-analysis on evidence of Mediterranean diet and cardiovascular disease: Are individual components equal? *Crit. Rev. Food Sci. Nutr.* **2017**, *57*, 3218–3232. [CrossRef] [PubMed]
25. Chiavaroli, L.; Nishi, S.K.; Khan, T.A.; Braunstein, C.R.; Glenn, A.J.; Mejia, S.B.; Rahelić, D.; Kahleová, H.; Salas-Salvadó, J.; Jenkins, D.J.A.; et al. Portfolio Dietary Pattern and Cardiovascular Disease: A Systematic Review and Meta-analysis of Controlled Trials. *Prog. Cardiovasc. Dis.* **2018**, *61*, 43–53. [CrossRef]
26. Chew, H.S.J.; Heng, F.K.X.; Tien, S.A.; Thian, J.Y.; Chou, H.S.; Loong, S.S.E.; Ang, W.H.D.; Chew, N.W.S.; Lo, K.H.K. Effects of Plant-Based Diets on Anthropometric and Cardiometabolic Markers in Adults: An Umbrella Review. *Nutrients* **2023**, *15*, 2331. [CrossRef]

27. Koch, C.A.; Kjeldsen, E.W.; Frikke-Schmidt, R. Vegetarian or vegan diets and blood lipids: A meta-analysis of randomized trials. *Eur. Heart J.* **2023**, *44*, 2609–2622. [CrossRef]
28. Tomé-Carneiro, J.; Visioli, F. Plant-Based Diets Reduce Blood Pressure: A Systematic Review of Recent Evidence. *Curr. Hypertens. Rep.* **2023**, *25*, 127–150. [CrossRef]
29. Esselstyn, C.B.; Gendy, G.; Doyle, J.; Golubic, M.; Roizen, M.F. A way to reverse CAD? *J. Fam. Pract.* **2014**, *63*, 356–364.
30. Ley, S.H.; Hamdy, O.; Mohan, V.; Hu, F.B. Prevention and management of type 2 diabetes: Dietary components and nutritional strategies. *Lancet* **2014**, *383*, 1999–2007. [CrossRef]
31. Freeman, A.M.; Morris, P.B.; Barnard, N.; Esselstyn, C.B.; Ros, E.; Agatston, A.; Devries, S.; O'Keefe, J.; Miller, M.; Ornish, D.; et al. Trending Cardiovascular Nutrition Controversies. *J. Am. Coll. Cardiol.* **2017**, *69*, 1172–1187. [CrossRef]
32. Kahleova, H.; Levin, S.; Barnard, N.D. Vegetarian Dietary Patterns and Cardiovascular Disease. *Prog. Cardiovasc. Dis.* **2018**, *61*, 54–61. [CrossRef]
33. Yokoyama, Y.; Nishimura, K.; Barnard, N.D.; Takegami, M.; Watanabe, M.; Sekikawa, A.; Okamura, T.; Miyamoto, Y. Vegetarian Diets and Blood Pressure. *JAMA Intern. Med.* **2014**, *174*, 577. [CrossRef]
34. Koutentakis, M.; Surma, S.; Rogula, S.; Filipiak, K.J.; Gąsecka, A. The Effect of a Vegan Diet on the Cardiovascular System. *J. Cardiovasc. Dev. Dis.* **2023**, *10*, 94. [CrossRef]
35. Thomas, M.S.; Calle, M.; Fernandez, M.L. Healthy plant-based diets improve dyslipidemias, insulin resistance, and inflammation in metabolic syndrome. A narrative review. *Adv. Nutr.* **2023**, *14*, 44–54. [CrossRef]
36. Balakrishna, R.; Bjørnerud, T.; Bemanian, M.; Aune, D.; Fadnes, L.T. Consumption of Nuts and Seeds and Health Outcomes Including Cardiovascular Disease, Diabetes and Metabolic Disease, Cancer, and Mortality: An Umbrella Review. *Adv. Nutr.* **2022**, *13*, 2136–2148. [CrossRef]
37. Madsen, H.; Sen, A.; Aune, D. Fruit and vegetable consumption and the risk of hypertension: A systematic review and meta-analysis of prospective studies. *Eur. J. Nutr. 2023* **2023**, *62*, 1941–1955. [CrossRef]
38. Halvorsen, R.E.; Elvestad, M.; Molin, M.; Aune, D. Fruit and vegetable consumption and the risk of type 2 diabetes: A systematic review and dose-response meta-analysis of prospective studies. *BMJ Nutr. Prev. Heal.* **2021**, *4*, 519–531. [CrossRef] [PubMed]
39. Xi, H.; Zhou, W.; Sohaib, M.; Niu, Y.; Zhu, R.; Guo, Y.; Wang, S.; Mao, J.; Wang, X.; Guo, L. Flaxseed supplementation significantly reduces hemoglobin A1c in patients with type 2 diabetes mellitus: A systematic review and meta-analysis. *Nutr. Res.* **2023**, *110*, 23–32. [CrossRef] [PubMed]
40. Li, L.; Li, H.; Gao, Y.; Vafaei, S.; Zhang, X.; Yang, M. Effect of flaxseed supplementation on blood pressure: A systematic review, and dose–response meta-analysis of randomized clinical trials. *Food Funct.* **2023**, *14*, 675–690. [CrossRef] [PubMed]
41. Tieri, M.; Ghelfi, F.; Vitale, M.; Vetrani, C.; Marventano, S.; Lafranconi, A.; Godos, J.; Titta, L.; Gambera, A.; Alonzo, E.; et al. Whole grain consumption and human health: An umbrella review of observational studies. *Int. J. Food Sci. Nutr.* **2020**, *71*, 668–677. [CrossRef] [PubMed]
42. McRae, M.P. Health Benefits of Dietary Whole Grains: An Umbrella Review of Meta-analyses. *J. Chiropr. Med.* **2017**, *16*, 10–18. [CrossRef]
43. Mirrafiei, A.; Jayedi, A.; Shab-Bidar, S. Total and different dietary fiber subtypes and the risk of all-cause, cardiovascular, and cancer mortality: A dose–response meta-analysis of prospective cohort studies. *Food Funct.* **2023**, *14*, 10667–10680. [CrossRef]
44. Wang, Y.; Liu, B.; Han, H.; Hu, Y.; Zhu, L.; Rimm, E.B.; Hu, F.B.; Sun, Q. Associations between plant-based dietary patterns and risks of type 2 diabetes, cardiovascular disease, cancer, and mortality—A systematic review and meta-analysis. *Nutr. J.* **2023**, *22*, 46. [CrossRef]
45. Gallagher, C.T.; Hanley, P.; Lane, K.E. Pattern analysis of vegan eating reveals healthy and unhealthy patterns within the vegan diet. *Public. Health Nutr.* **2021**, *25*, 1310–1320. [CrossRef]
46. Haider, S.; Sima, A.; Kühn, T.; Wakolbinger, M. The Association between Vegan Dietary Patterns and Physical Activity-A Cross-Sectional Online Survey. *Nutrients* **2023**, *15*, 1847. [CrossRef]
47. Satija, A.; Bhupathiraju, S.N.; Spiegelman, D.; Chiuve, S.E.; Manson, J.A.E.; Willett, W.; Rexrode, K.M.; Rimm, E.B.; Hu, F.B. Healthful and Unhealthful Plant-Based Diets and the Risk of Coronary Heart Disease in U.S. Adults. *J. Am. Coll. Cardiol.* **2017**, *70*, 411–422. [CrossRef] [PubMed]
48. Satija, A.; Malik, V.; Rimm, E.B.; Sacks, F.; Willett, W.; Hu, F.B. Changes in intake of plant-based diets and weight change: Results from 3 prospective cohort studies. *Am. J. Clin. Nutr.* **2019**, *110*, 574–582. [CrossRef] [PubMed]
49. Satija, A.; Bhupathiraju, S.N.; Rimm, E.B.; Spiegelman, D.; Chiuve, S.E.; Borgi, L.; Willett, W.C.; Manson, J.E.; Sun, Q.; Hu, F.B. Plant-Based Dietary Patterns and Incidence of Type 2 Diabetes in US Men and Women: Results from Three Prospective Cohort Studies. *PLOS Med.* **2016**, *13*, e1002039. [CrossRef] [PubMed]
50. Huang, Y.; Li, X.; Zhang, T.; Zeng, X.; Li, M.; Li, H.; Yang, H.; Zhang, C.; Zhou, Z.; Zhu, Y.; et al. Associations of healthful and unhealthful plant-based diets with plasma markers of cardiometabolic risk. *Eur. J. Nutr.* **2023**, *62*, 2567–2579. [CrossRef] [PubMed]
51. Jakše, B.; Jakše, B.; Godnov, U.; Pinter, S. Nutritional, Cardiovascular Health and Lifestyle Status of 'Health Conscious' Adult Vegans and Non-Vegans from Slovenia: A Cross-Sectional Self-Reported Survey. *Int. J. Environ. Res. Public. Health* **2021**, *18*, 5968. [CrossRef] [PubMed]
52. Hever, J. Plant-Based Diets: A Physician's Guide. *Perm. J.* **2016**, *20*, 15–082. [CrossRef] [PubMed]

53. Karlsen, M.; Rogers, G.; Miki, A.; Lichtenstein, A.; Folta, S.; Economos, C.; Jacques, P.; Livingston, K.; McKeown, N.; Karlsen, M.C.; et al. Theoretical Food and Nutrient Composition of Whole-Food Plant-Based and Vegan Diets Compared to Current Dietary Recommendations. *Nutrients* **2019**, *11*, 625. [CrossRef] [PubMed]
54. Barnard, N.D.; Cohen, J.; Jenkins, D.J.A.; Turner-McGrievy, G.; Gloede, L.; Green, A.; Ferdowsian, H. A low-fat vegan diet and a conventional diabetes diet in the treatment of type 2 diabetes: A randomized, controlled, 74-wk clinical trial. *Am. J. Clin. Nutr.* **2009**, *89*, 1588S–1596S. [CrossRef] [PubMed]
55. World Health Organization; Food and Agriculture Organization of the United Nations. Defining Healthy Diets: The FAO-WHO Approach. Available online: https://www.who.int/news-room/events/detail/2023/07/13/default-calendar/launch-event-for-who-healthy-diet-guidelines-and-fao-who-concept-of-healthy-diets?fbclid=IwAR3HDr1O3Zl3R6mHbL2BfQe8P4FhU-EqUSzcF60Wta5US1dg1BfhoN7nCkc (accessed on 26 February 2024).
56. Hagströmer, M.; Oja, P.; Sjöström, M. The International Physical Activity Questionnaire (IPAQ): A study of concurrent and construct validity. *Public. Health Nutr.* **2006**, *9*, 755–762. [CrossRef]
57. Buysse, D.J.; Reynolds, C.F.; Monk, T.H.; Berman, S.R.; Kupfer, D.J. The Pittsburgh Sleep Quality Index: A new instrument for psychiatric practice and research. *Psychiatry Res.* **1989**, *28*, 193–213. [CrossRef]
58. Levenstein, S.; Prantera, C.; Varvo, V.; Scribano, M.L.; Berto, E.; Luzi, C.; Andreoli, A. Development of the Perceived Stress Questionnaire: A new tool for psychosomatic research. *J. Psychosom. Res.* **1993**, *37*, 19–32. [CrossRef]
59. Jakše, B.; Jakše, B.; Pinter, S.; Jug, B.; Godnov, U.; Pajek, J.; Fidler Mis, N. Dietary Intakes and Cardiovascular Health of Healthy Adults in Short-, Medium-, and Long-Term Whole-Food Plant-Based Lifestyle Program. *Nutrients* **2019**, *12*, 55. [CrossRef]
60. Jakše, B.; Jakše, B.; Pinter, S.; Pajek, J.; Godnov, U.; Fidler Mis, N. Nutrient and Food Intake of Participants in a Whole-Food Plant-Based Lifestyle Program. *J. Am. Coll. Nutr.* **2020**, *40*, 333–348. [CrossRef]
61. Jakše, B.; Jakše, B.; Pinter, S.; Pajek, J.; Fidler Mis, N. Characteristics of Slovenian Adults in Community-Based Whole-Food Plant-Based Lifestyle Program. *J. Nutr. Metab.* **2020**, *2020*, 6950530. [CrossRef]
62. National Institute of Public Health of Slovenia & Partners. EU Menu Slovenija. Potek Ankete Mladostnik/Odrali LOT 2. Available online: https://www.nijz.si/sites/www.nijz.si/files/uploaded/p-5_priloga_k_specifikaciji_2_a.pdf (accessed on 10 August 2019).
63. Verney, J.; Schwartz, C.; Amiche, S.; Pereira, B.; Thivel, D. Comparisons of a Multi-Frequency Bioelectrical Impedance Analysis to the Dual-Energy X-Ray Absorptiometry Scan in Healthy Young Adults Depending on their Physical Activity Level. *J. Hum. Kinet.* **2015**, *47*, 73–80. [CrossRef]
64. Miller, R.M.; Chambers, T.L.; Burns, S.P. Validating InBody[R] 570 multi-frequency bioelectrical impedance analyzer versus DXA for body fat percentage analysis. *J. Exerc. Physiol. Online* **2016**, *19*, 71–79. [CrossRef]
65. Ballesteros-Pomar, M.D.; González-Arnáiz, E.; Pintor-de-la Maza, B.; Barajas-Galindo, D.; Ariadel-Cobo, D.; González-Roza, L.; Cano-Rodríguez, I. Bioelectrical impedance analysis as an alternative to dual-energy x-ray absorptiometry in the assessment of fat mass and appendicular lean mass in patients with obesity. *Nutrition* **2022**, *93*, 111442. [CrossRef] [PubMed]
66. Institut Jožef Stefan. Computer Systems Department Computer Web-Based Software: The Open Platform for Clinical Nutrition (OPEN). Available online: http://opkp.si/en_GB/cms/introduction (accessed on 7 February 2024).
67. Korošec, M.; Golob, T.; Bertoncelj, J.; Stibilj, V.; Seljak, B.K. The Slovenian food composition database. *Food Chem.* **2013**, *140*, 495–499. [CrossRef] [PubMed]
68. JSI—Institut "Jozef Stefan". Available online: https://www.ijs.si/ijsw/JSI (accessed on 2 July 2019).
69. NIJZ. Picture Material for Determining Food Intake. Available online: https://www.nijz.si/sl/publikacije/slikovno-gradivo-za-dolocanje-vnosa-zivil (accessed on 28 July 2019).
70. Bognár, A. Tables on Weight Yield of Food and Retention Factors of Food Constituents for the Calculation of Nutrient Composition of Cooked Foods (Dishes). Available online: https://www.fao.org/uploads/media/bognar_bfe-r-02-03.pdf (accessed on 28 July 2019).
71. Res-Pons Pretehtajte Prehranska Dopolnila. Available online: https://pretehtajte.si/ (accessed on 28 July 2019).
72. Wickham, H.; Averick, M.; Bryan, J.; Chang, W.; D', L.; Mcgowan, A.; François, R.; Grolemund, G.; Hayes, A.; Henry, L.; et al. Welcome to the Tidyverse. *J. Open Source Softw.* **2019**, *4*, 1686. [CrossRef]
73. Patil, I. Visualizations with statistical details: The "ggstatsplot" approach. *J. Open Source Softw.* **2021**, *6*, 3167. [CrossRef]
74. Heinzen, E.; Sinnwell, J.; Atkinson, E.; Gunderson, T.; Dougherty, G.; Votruba, P.; Lennon, R.; Lundt, E.; Broderick, B.; McCullough, M. *An Arsenal of "R" Functions for Large-Scale Statistical Summaries [R Package Arsenal Version 3.6.3]*; Comprehensive R Archive Network (CRAN). 2021. Available online: https://cran.r-project.org/web/packages/arsenal/arsenal.pdf (accessed on 26 September 2022).
75. German Nutrition Society, Austrian Nutrition Society, Swiss Society of Nutrition Research, the S.A. for N. Ergaenzlieferung D-A-CH Referenzwerte für die Nährstoffzufuhr (Reference Values for Nutrient Intake), 4th ed. 2018, pp. 1–56. Available online: https://www.dge-medienservice.de/d-a-ch-referenzwerte-fur-die-nahrstoffzufuhr.html (accessed on 21 October 2019).
76. Herbalife Nutrition. Formula 1 Smooth Chocolate 550 g Label. Available online: https://assets.herbalifenutrition.com/content/dam/regional/emea/sl_si/consumable_content/product-catalog-assets/pdfs/2020/10-Oct/LPR4468SI-00_OP1_HiR.pdf (accessed on 20 February 2024).
77. Kahleova, H.; Brennan, H.; Znayenko-Miller, T.; Holubkov, R.; Barnard, N.D. Does diet quality matter? A secondary analysis of a randomized clinical trial. *Eur. J. Clin. Nutr.* **2023**. [CrossRef]

78. Kahleova, H.; Znayenko-Miller, T.; Uribarri, J.; Holubkov, R.; Barnard, N.D. Dietary advanced glycation products and their associations with insulin sensitivity and body weight: A 16-week randomized clinical trial. *Obes. Sci. Pract.* **2023**, *9*, 235–242. [CrossRef]
79. Marrone, G.; Guerriero, C.; Palazzetti, D.; Lido, P.; Marolla, A.; Di Daniele, F.; Noce, A. Vegan Diet Health Benefits in Metabolic Syndrome. *Nutrients* **2021**, *13*, 817. [CrossRef]
80. Kotseva, K.; De Backer, G.; De Bacquer, D.; Rydén, L.; Hoes, A.; Grobbee, D.; Maggioni, A.; Marques-Vidal, P.; Jennings, C.; Abreu, A.; et al. Lifestyle and impact on cardiovascular risk factor control in coronary patients across 27 countries: Results from the European Society of Cardiology ESC-EORP EUROASPIRE V registry. *Eur. J. Prev. Cardiol.* **2019**, *26*, 824–835. [CrossRef] [PubMed]
81. Sun, L.; Liang, X.; Wang, Y.; Zhu, S.; Ou, Q.; Xu, H.; Li, F.; Tan, X.; Lai, Z.; Pu, L.; et al. Fruit consumption and multiple health outcomes: An umbrella review. *Trends Food Sci. Technol.* **2021**, *118*, 505–518. [CrossRef]
82. Wallace, T.C.; Bailey, R.L.; Blumberg, J.B.; Burton-Freeman, B.; Chen, C.Y.O.; Crowe-White, K.M.; Drewnowski, A.; Hooshmand, S.; Johnson, E.; Lewis, R.; et al. Fruits, vegetables, and health: A comprehensive narrative, umbrella review of the science and recommendations for enhanced public policy to improve intake. *Crit. Rev. Food Sci. Nutr.* **2020**, *60*, 2174–2211. [CrossRef] [PubMed]
83. Zhong, G.C.; Huang, S.Q.; Peng, Y.; Wan, L.; Wu, Y.Q.L.; Hu, T.Y.; Hu, J.J.; Hao, F.B. HDL-C is associated with mortality from all causes, cardiovascular disease and cancer in a J-shaped dose-response fashion: A pooled analysis of 37 prospective cohort studies. *Eur. J. Prev. Cardiol.* **2020**, *27*, 1187–1203. [CrossRef] [PubMed]
84. Lippman, D.; Stump, M.; Veazey, E.; Guimarães, S.T.; Rosenfeld, R.; Kelly, J.H.; Ornish, D.; Katz, D.L. Foundations of Lifestyle Medicine and its Evolution. *Mayo Clin. Proc. Innov. Qual. Outcomes* **2024**, *8*, 97–111. [CrossRef] [PubMed]
85. Mach, F.; Baigent, C.; Catapano, A.L.; Koskinas, K.C.; Casula, M.; Badimon, L.; Chapman, M.J.; De Backer, G.G.; Delgado, V.; Ference, B.A.; et al. 2019 ESC/EAS Guidelines for the management of dyslipidaemias: Lipid modification to reduce cardiovascular risk. *Eur. Heart J.* **2019**, *41*, 111–188. [CrossRef] [PubMed]
86. Madsen, C.M.; Varbo, A.; Nordestgaard, B.G. Extreme high high-density lipoprotein cholesterol is paradoxically associated with high mortality in men and women: Two prospective cohort studies. *Eur. Heart J.* **2017**, *38*, 2478–2486. [CrossRef]
87. Zeng, R.X.; Xu, J.P.; Kong, Y.J.; Tan, J.W.; Guo, L.H.; Zhang, M.Z. U-Shaped Relationship of Non-HDL Cholesterol With All-Cause and Cardiovascular Mortality in Men Without Statin Therapy. *Front. Cardiovasc. Med.* **2022**, *9*, 903481. [CrossRef] [PubMed]
88. Jakše, B.; Jakše, B.; Pinter, S.; Pajek, J.; Fidler Mis, N. Whole-Food Plant-Based Lifestyle Program and Decreased Obesity. *Am. J. Lifestyle Med.* **2022**, *16*, 260–270. [CrossRef]
89. Ha, V.; Sievenpiper, J.L.; de Souza, R.J.; Jayalath, V.H.; Mirrahimi, A.; Agarwal, A.; Chiavaroli, L.; Mejia, S.B.; Sacks, F.M.; Di Buono, M.; et al. Effect of dietary pulse intake on established therapeutic review and meta-analysis of randomized controlled trials. *Can. Med. Assoc. J.* **2014**, *186*, 252–262. [CrossRef]
90. Jakše, B.; Jakše, B.; Pajek, M.; Pajek, J. Uric Acid and Plant-Based Nutrition. *Nutrients* **2019**, *11*, 1736. [CrossRef]
91. Choi, J.W.J.; Ford, E.S.; Gao, X.; Choi, H.K. Sugar-sweetened soft drinks, diet soft drinks, and serum uric acid level: The Third National Health and Nutrition Examination Survey. *Arthritis Rheum.* **2008**, *59*, 109–116. [CrossRef]
92. Major, T.J.; Topless, R.K.; Dalbeth, N.; Merriman, T.R. Evaluation of the diet wide contribution to serum urate levels: Meta-analysis of population based cohorts. *BMJ* **2018**, *363*, k3951. [CrossRef]
93. Tsai, S.Y.; Huang, W.H.; Chan, H.L.; Hwang, L.C. The role of smoking cessation programs in lowering blood pressure: A retrospective cohort study. *Tob. Induc. Dis.* **2021**, *19*, 82. [CrossRef]
94. Veronese, N.; Li, Y.; Manson, J.E.; Willett, W.C.; Fontana, L.; Hu, F.B. Combined associations of body weight and lifestyle factors with all cause and cause specific mortality in men and women: Prospective cohort study. *BMJ* **2016**, *355*, i5855. [CrossRef] [PubMed]
95. Pescatello, L.S.; Buchner, D.M.; Jakicic, J.M.; Powell, K.E.; Kraus, W.E.; Bloodgood, B.; Campbell, W.W.; Dietz, S.; Dipietro, L.; George, S.M.; et al. Physical Activity to Prevent and Treat Hypertension: A Systematic Review. *Med. Sci. Sports Exerc.* **2019**, *51*, 1314–1323. [CrossRef] [PubMed]
96. Chiu, H.F.; Venkatakrishnan, K.; Golovinskaia, O.; Wang, C.K. Impact of Micronutrients on Hypertension: Evidence from Clinical Trials with a Special Focus on Meta-Analysis. *Nutrients* **2021**, *13*, 588. [CrossRef] [PubMed]
97. Behers, B.J.; Melchor, J.; Behers, B.M.; Meng, Z.; Swanson, P.J.; Paterson, H.I.; Mendez Araque, S.J.; Davis, J.L.; Gerhold, C.J.; Shah, R.S.; et al. Vitamins and Minerals for Blood Pressure Reduction in the General, Normotensive Population: A Systematic Review and Meta-Analysis of Six Supplements. *Nutrients* **2023**, *15*, 4223. [CrossRef] [PubMed]
98. Reynolds, A.; Mann, J.; Cummings, J.; Winter, N.; Mete, E.; Te Morenga, L. Carbohydrate quality and human health: A series of systematic reviews and meta-analyses. *Lancet* **2019**, *393*, 434–445. [CrossRef] [PubMed]
99. Wang, Y.; Fang, Y.; Witting, P.K.; Charchar, F.J.; Sobey, C.G.; Drummond, G.R.; Golledge, J. Dietary fatty acids and mortality risk from heart disease in US adults: An analysis based on NHANES. *Sci. Rep.* **2023**, *13*, 1614. [CrossRef]
100. Sacks, F.M.; Lichtenstein, A.H.; Wu, J.H.Y.; Appel, L.J.; Creager, M.A.; Kris-Etherton, P.M.; Miller, M.; Rimm, E.B.; Rudel, L.L.; Robinson, J.G.; et al. Dietary Fats and Cardiovascular Disease: A Presidential Advisory From the American Heart Association. *Circulation* **2017**, *136*, e1–e23. [CrossRef]
101. Hadi, A.; Askarpour, M.; Ziaei, R.; Venkatakrishnan, K.; Ghaedi, E.; Ghavami, A. Impact of flaxseed supplementation on plasma lipoprotein(a) concentrations: A systematic review and meta-analysis of randomized controlled trials. *Phyther. Res.* **2020**, *34*, 1599–1608. [CrossRef]

102. Dehghan, M.; Mente, A.; Zhang, X.; Swaminathan, S.; Li, W.; Mohan, V.; Iqbal, R.; Kumar, R.; Wentzel-Viljoen, E.; Rosengren, A.; et al. Associations of fats and carbohydrate intake with cardiovascular disease and mortality in 18 countries from five continents (PURE): A prospective cohort study. *Lancet* **2017**, *390*, 2050–2062. [CrossRef] [PubMed]
103. Ocagli, H.; Berti, G.; Rango, D.; Norbiato, F.; Chiaruttini, M.V.; Lorenzoni, G.; Gregori, D. Association of Vegetarian and Vegan Diets with Cardiovascular Health: An Umbrella Review of Meta-Analysis of Observational Studies and Randomized Trials. *Nutrients* **2023**, *15*, 4103. [CrossRef] [PubMed]
104. Castro-Quezada, I.; Ruano-Rodríguez, C.; Ribas-Barba, L.; Serra-Majem, L. Misreporting in nutritional surveys: Methodological implications. *Nutr. Hosp.* **2015**, *31* (Suppl. S3), 119–127. [PubMed]

MDPI AG
Grosspeteranlage 5
4052 Basel
Switzerland
Tel.: +41 61 683 77 34

*Nutrients* Editorial Office
E-mail: nutrients@mdpi.com
www.mdpi.com/journal/nutrients